Type 2 Diabetes in 2024 - From Early Suspicion to Effective Management

Edited by Rudolf Chlup

Published in London, United Kingdom

Type 2 Diabetes in 2024 - From Early Suspicion to Effective Management
http://dx.doi.org/10.5772/intechopen.1000405
Edited by Rudolf Chlup

Contributors
Adina Mitrea, Alejandra Hernández Suárez, Altaf Makwana, Andrea Martínez Echauri, Angélica Araújo Cortines Laxe Renó, Arantza Maya Gómez, Ashutosh Kakkad, Charles Billington, Dana Weberová, Diana Clenciu, Dov Gal, Eugen Mota, Fernando Grover-Páez, Hana Meluzinova, Hana Zálešáková, Heta Shukla, Ionela Mihaela Vladu, Iulia Huluţă, Jana Zapletalová, Jiřina Gottwaldová, Jonathan Waataja, Lada Hanáčková, Leonardo da Cruz Renó, Leslie Bahn Kawa, Loudry Amsal Elfa Gustanar, Maria Magdalena Rosu, Maria Mota, Martin Nezval, Michal Trefil, Mick John Kumwenda, Milena Bretšnajdrová, Mohammed Zaid Aljulifi, Nanang Miftah Fajari, Nicolae Gică, Noemi Nováková, Pankaj Kumar Jha, Pavel Weber, Přemysl Falt, Richard Kaňa, Rudolf Chlup, Sayeed Ikramuddin, Taoreed Adegoke Azeez, Uwe Gudat, Viktória Molnárová, Zdenka Polzerová

First published in London, United Kingdom, 2024 by IntechOpen
IntechOpen is the global imprint of INTECHOPEN LIMITED, registered in England and Wales, registration number: 11086078, 167-169 Great Portland Street, London, W1W 5PF, United Kingdom

British Library Cataloguing-in-Publication Data
A catalogue record for this book is available from the British Library

Additional hard and PDF copies can be obtained from orders@intechopen.com

Type 2 Diabetes in 2024 - From Early Suspicion to Effective Management
Edited by Rudolf Chlup
p. cm.
Print ISBN 978-0-85466-002-5
Online ISBN 978-0-85466-001-8
eBook (PDF) ISBN 978-0-85466-003-2

For EU product safety concerns:
IN TECH d.o.o., Prolaz Marije Krucifikse Kozulić 3, 51000 Rijeka, Croatia,
info@intechopen.com or visit our website at intechopen.com.

Meet the editor

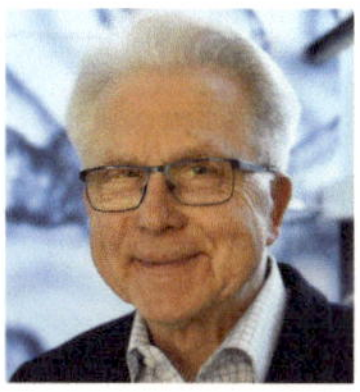

Rudolf Chlup graduated from Palacký University Olomouc, Czechia, and attended postgraduate courses in Prague, Karlsburg, Edinburgh, London, Bucharest, Moscow, Sophia, Düsseldorf, and San Francisco. He is a consultant for internal medicine and diabetology at the Teaching Hospital Olomouc, Czechia. He became Dr. Med Habil at the University of Greifswald, Germany in 1993. He has been a Professor of Medicine at Palacký University Olomouc since 2020. His research interests include diabetes management comprising diet, exercise, education, medication, and technology. He is a member of the Czech, German, European, and American Diabetes Associations and the executive committee of the Diabetes Education Study Group of the European Association for the Study of Diabetes (DESG/EASD). In 2015, Dr. Chlup received the Rudolf Korec Award from the Slovakian Diabetes Association.

Contents

Preface

This book provides a short overview of the pathophysiology, early diagnosis, and professional management of type 2 diabetes (T2D). The purpose of this edition is to support healthcare professionals in transferring recent knowledge to routine diabetes practice.

The book includes fifteen chapters organized into four sections.

The first section includes four chapters that address the development of T2D from early signs and key markers to advanced stages.

The second section includes five chapters that examine hyperlipidemia, multiorgan damage, cardiovascular complications, and risk factors for diabetes such as pregnancy and old age.

The third section describes various methods of diabetes management, including complementary and alternative medicines as well as newer pharmacotherapy options and neuromodulation of nervus vagus.

The final section demonstrates the effectiveness of routine pathophysiology-based management of T2D using selected case reports as well as analyzing a cohort of 200 people in a single-center study.

Written by specialists in diabetes from around the world, including Africa, America, Asia, and Europe, chapters include figures and tables to illustrate important concepts and ideas.

With its comprehensive coverage of the state of the art in T2D, this volume is a useful resource for family physicians, diabetologists, educators, nurses, students, and other interested readers.

I would like to thank the staff at IntechOpen, especially Author Service Manager Ms. Helena Recic and Publishing Process Manager Ms. Zrinka Tomicic, for their continuous assistance throughout the publication process.

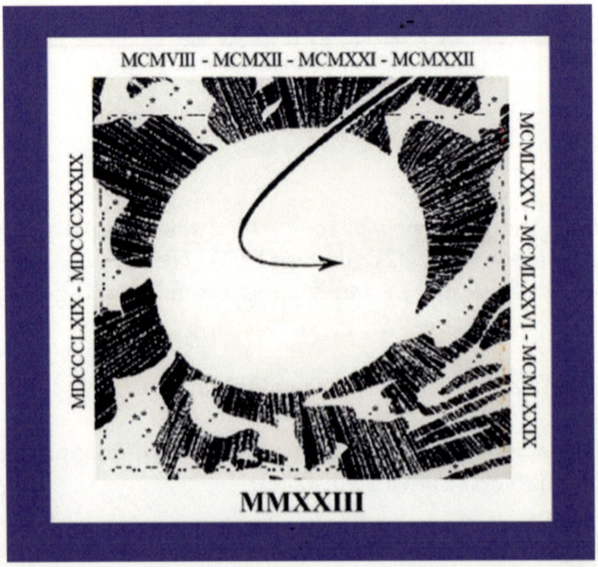

Mission: from recent history to dawning future (years of milestones in diabetes management). Roman numerals at figure margins serve as reminders of important dates related to pancreas function [1, 2], insulin implementation to human medicine [3], technology for insulin substitution and supplementation [4–8], therapeutic exercise [9], risk of atherosclerosis [10], trials on experimental diabetes in the rat [11], and implementation of incretins to type 2 management [12], all of which created a base for the topics presented in this book [13].

Rudolf Chlup
2nd Department of Medicine, Gastroenterology and Geriatrics,
Teaching Hospital Olomouc,
Olomouc, Czech Republic

Department of Diabetes Moravskýu Beroun
Institute of Specialized Treatments Paseka
Paseka, Czech Republic

Department of Physiology,
Faculty of Medicine and Dentistry,
Palacký University Olomouc, Olomouc, Czech Republic

References

[1] Langerhans P. Beiträge zur mikroscopischen Anatomie der Bauchspeicheldrüse. (Contributions to microscopic anatomy of Pancreas. German.) Wilhelms-Friedrich Wilhelm Universität zu Berlin, printed by G. Lange; 1869

[2] Mering J, Minkowski O. Diabetes mellitus nach Pankreas extirpation. (Diabetes mellitus following the pancreatectomy. German.). Zbl Klin Med. 1889;**10**:393-394

[3] Banting FG, Best CH. Pancreatic extracts. Journal of Laboratory and Clinical Medicine. May 1922;7(8):3-11

[4] Pickup JC, Keen H, Parsons JS, et al. Continuous subcutaneous insulin infusion: an approach to achieving normoglycaemia. British Medical Journal. 1978;**282**:347-350

[5] Paton JS, Wilson M, Ireland JT, Reith SB. Convenient pocket insulin syringe. The Lancet. 1981;**317**(8213):189-190

[6] Janů K, Chlup R, Chleboun J. Ruční mechanický dávkovač kapaliny Úřad pro patenty a objevy v Praze: Číslo žádosti PV 6160, podaná dne 24. 8. 1983, číslo patentu 237521, datum udělení patentu 24. 4. 1985. (Manual mechanical device for fluid dosing. Patent and Inventions Office Prague: Application number PV 6160 submitted on 24. 8. 1983, Patent number 237521, was granted by the patent office on 24. 4. 1985. Czech.)

[7] Rex J, Vogeley OA. Dispenser. U.S.patent number 4,592,745 [Application Number 06/584,876], submitted on 1984-02-29, was granted by the patent office on 1986-06-03

[8] Berger M, Jörgens V, Mühlhauser I. Rationale for the use of insulin therapy alone as the pharmacological treatment of type 2 diabetes. Diabetes Care 1999;**22**(Suppl 3):C71-C75

[9] Koivisto VA, Shervin RS. Exercise in diabetes. Therapeutic implications. Postgraduate Medicine 1979;**66**:87

[10] Stout RW. Diabetes and atherosclerosis – the role of insulin. Diabetologie 1979;**16**:14110

[11] Korec R. Experimental and spontaneous diabetes mellitus in the rat and mouse. Edition Center of University PJ Šafárik, Košice, ČSFR, Košice. 1991. pp. 1-246

[12] Bruns W, Fiedler H, Altman B, Lundershausen R, Menzel R, Worms F, et al. Insulintherapie bei Typ 2 Diabetes Pathophysiologisch begründete Therapie mit Insulin unter besonderer Berücksichtigung der Insulinresistenz und des Inkretineffektes. (Insulin treatment in T2D Pathophysiology-based insulin treatment with particular consideration of insulin resistance and incretins. German.) 2. Auflage; UNIMED Verlag, AG, Bremen, 2010

[13] Type 2 Diabetes in 2024 – From Early Suspicion to Effective Management. London, UK: IntechOpen; 2024

Section 1

Paradigms of Prediabetes and Diabetes

Chapter 1

Present State and Perspectives of Type 2 Diabetes Management

Taoreed Adegoke Azeez

Abstract

Diabetes mellitus is a common metabolic disorder characterised by chronic hyperglycaemia that results from a defect in insulin secretion, action, or both. There are different types of diabetes mellitus, but type 2 diabetes mellitus is the most common type globally. Type 2 diabetes mellitus results from a complex interaction between predisposing genes and unhealthy lifestyle choices. The risk factors for type 2 diabetes include obesity, prediabetes, sedentary lifestyle, unhealthy diets, and hypertension. Poorly controlled diabetes causes microvascular and macrovascular complications. The goals of management are to prevent these complications and optimise quality of life. Fasting plasma glucose, 2-hours post glucose load, random plasma glucose or HbA1c above a certain threshold diagnoses diabetes in the presence or classic symptoms otherwise, the tests are repeated on a second occasion. HbA1c is convenient and reliable but, it is affected by conditions affecting the turnover of red cells. Management of type 2 diabetes is individualised with focus on diabetes education, lifestyle changes, pharmacological therapy, management of co-morbidities, and monitoring of treatment. Various factors determine the drugs used, but metformin remains the cornerstone. Other cardiovascular risk factors must be adequately controlled.

Keywords: type 2 diabetes mellitus, diagnosis, management, glycated haemoglobin, pharmacotherapy, diabetes education

1. Introduction

Diabetes mellitus (DM) is a heterogeneous group of metabolic disorders characterised by chronic hyperglycaemia, which results from insufficient insulin secretion or impaired action of insulin or both [1]. B-cells depletion as well as insulin resistance are the key mechanisms driving the hyperglycaemia seen in diabetes. Underlying the myriad of complications of diabetes mellitus is chronic hyperglycaemia. Chronic hyperglycaemia is primarily responsible for the microvascular and macrovascular complications of diabetes [2]. DM is closely linked with gradual and sustained damage to different organs, especially the nerves, kidneys, eyes, heart and blood vessels. Diabetes raises the risk of cardiovascular disease by 2 to 4 folds. The aetiopathogenesis of DM depends on the type.

According to the latest World Health Organisation (WHO) classification of diabetes mellitus, there are six basic types, namely, type I DM, type 2 DM, hybrid forms of diabetes, other specific types, hyperglycaemia first detected during pregnancy, and unclassified diabetes [3]. The most common type of DM (90–95%) is T2D (T2D) [4]. In T2D, insulin resistance accompanied by inadequate compensatory insulin secretion from the β-cells is the central theme in its pathogenesis. Insulin resistance is defined as the deficient responsiveness of cells to insulin. Essentially, insulin resistance results from an interplay of genetic predisposition and unhealthy lifestyle choices. Genome wide association studies (GWAS) have isolated some genetic variants implicated in β-cell dysfunction and insulin resistance [5]. Some of the reported genes include *PPARG, GCK, TCF7L2, WFS1* and *IGF2BP2* [6].

The treatment of a disorder is often dependent on the pathophysiology. The current thinking in the pathophysiology of T2D, which also influences the therapeutic approach, is termed the ominous octet [7]. The ominous octets represent eight fundamental defects in the body homeostasis that contributes to the development of T2D. These defects are β-cells dysfunction, enhanced hepatic glucose production, reduced insulin-mediated uptake of glucose in the muscles, and increased release of free fatty acids from adipose tissue. Others include reduced incretin secretion, hyperglucagonemia, and impaired appetite regulation in the brain. So, there are pharmacological agents which target one or more of these pathways in controlling plasma glucose concentration.

Obesity, especially the central type, has been repeatedly fingered as the central phenomenon in the development of insulin resistance seen in T2D. Basically, insulin resistance is surmounted by enhanced secretion of insulin, but this counterbalancing response attenuates over time and T2D ensues. When insulin fails to exert its expected effects on the cells, the metabolism of carbohydrates, proteins and fats is greatly impaired [8]. The risk factors for T2D include obesity, western diets, sedentary lifestyle, hypertension, dyslipidaemia, gestational diabetes, prediabetes and polycystic ovarian syndrome [9]. In T2D, typically, insulin is not required for survival, although there are rare exceptions, especially in the late stage of the disease.

B-cell dysfunction, characterised initially by the impaired first phase of insulin secretion and later the second phase, is a crucial factor in the pathogenesis of T2D [10]. The defective first phase of insulin secretion is depicted by crippled intake of glucose into B-cell. The second phase problem is a result of the paradoxical suppression of insulin secretion by hyperglycaemia, a phenomenon termed glucotoxicity. B-cell dysfunction, in the presence of insulin resistance, progresses to type 2 diabetes. Insulin resistance could be peripheral or hepatic (in which hepatic glucose production is unchecked). Inappropriate glucagon secretion, enhanced gluconeogenesis and alteration of incretin dynamics have also been implicated in the pathogenesis of T2D.

1.1 The burden of type 2 diabetes

There are ongoing global concerns about the unrelenting burden of T2D. Diabetes is a pandemic. According to the International Diabetes Federation (IDF), 10.5% of the adult population (20–79) years are living with diabetes, of which about 98% is T2D [11]. In terms of absolute numbers, China, India, Pakistan, USA, Indonesia, and Brazil have the highest tally of individuals living with diabetes in the world. This global estimate of diabetes prevalence is projected to increase significantly in the coming years. Interestingly, about 50% of individuals living with type 2 diabetes are undiagnosed [12]. Africa has the largest prevalence of undiagnosed diabetes globally [13]. Diabetes is more common in urban areas when compared with rural areas. Similarly, type 2 diabetes is mainly a disease of middle and old age, but the prevalence among the young is rising significantly. The recent upsurge of T2D among young adults, adolescents and children is principally accounted for by the parallel rise in obesity, sedentary lifestyle and widespread adoption of unhealthy Western diets [14]. It is also slightly more common among males compared with females, partly due to a higher frequency of central obesity among men.

The economic impact of the high prevalence of T2D is further worsened by the fact the majority of the persons affected live in low and middle-income countries where healthcare funding is mainly out-of-pocket and largely suboptimal [15]. Apart from economic distress, there are also undesirable psychological and social consequences of being diagnosed with T2D. It is equally noteworthy that a significant proportion of individuals with type 2 diabetes fail to achieve their treatment goals. Since type 2 diabetes is underdiagnosed and sub-optimally managed, it is imperative to intensify efforts in harnessing resources, empowering the clinicians and educating the population to minimise the immense impact of the disease on the general population. Early diagnosis and prompt treatment have been found to have a noteworthy impact long term. The bulk of the overall cost of care in diabetes is spent on managing the complications.

Over a variable period, poorly controlled diabetes may cause neuropathy, nephropathy or retinopathy. DM is the most common cause of peripheral neuropathy. Among adults (20–74 years), DM is the most prominent aetiological factor leading to blindness [16]. Globally, DM is equally the principal cause of end-stage kidney disease. Foot ulcerations, limb amputation, erectile dysfunction, non-alcoholic steatohepatitis, peripheral arterial disease, stroke and coronary artery disease are other potential complications of DM [17, 18]. Cognitive decline is common in type 2 diabetes when compared with individuals of similar age groups but without diabetes. Atrophy of the hippocampus, limbic system and frontal lobe have been documented in type 2 diabetes, and this could be responsible for the observed cognitive dysfunction [19]. Cardiovascular disease is the principal cause of mortality in individuals living with type 2 diabetes. Moreover, DM is commonly associated with other co-morbidities such as hypertension, dyslipidaemia, hyperuricaemia and hypovitaminosis D.

1.2 Objectives

1. To discuss how type 2 diabetes mellitus is diagnosed

2. To examine the principles of managing type 2 diabetes mellitus

2. Diagnosis

The diagnosis would involve taking a comprehensive history, performing a targeted physical examination, and ordering some specific investigations. T2D remains undiagnosed for a long period because the degree of hyperglycaemia in the early stages is not severe enough to produce the classic symptoms. However, a dynamic test such as the oral glucose tolerance test may be helpful for early detection. So, it is important to emphasise that a significant proportion of individuals with diabetes are diagnosed without having any of the classic symptom. Interestingly, diagnosed or not, the microangiopathy and macroangiopathy associated with T2D tend to start at this stage.

2.1 History taking

The classic symptoms of diabetes are polyuria, polydipsia, weight loss and fatigue. Other symptoms include recurrent infections, especially vaginal candidiasis/balanitis, polyphagia, poorly healing wounds, paraesthesia in the feet or hands, and visual blurriness. Sometimes, the first presentation comes in the form of a hyperglycaemic emergency- hyperglycaemic hyperosmolar state (HHS) or diabetic ketoacidosis (DKA).

Family history of diabetes should be asked. Immunisation history is equally important. Prior diagnoses of hypertension, dyslipidaemia need to be sought. It is important to know if the person smokes and how much of alcohol he/she takes.

2.2 Physical examination

Anthropometric metrics such as the body mass index, waist circumference, and hip-to-waist ratio are determined to assess adiposity. A preliminary fundoscopy is done, while the individual is later sent for a comprehensive eye examination with the ophthalmologist to document the presence and the grade of diabetic retinopathy or any other diabetic eye disease such as cataract or glaucoma. Cardiovascular examination entails checking for evidence of peripheral artery disease, measuring the blood pressure and examining the praecordium. The presence of neuropathy is noted by conducting a full neurological examination, 10-g monofilament test and possibly biothesiometry. The signs of autonomic neuropathy should be carefully looked out for as well. A detailed examination of the feet for dystrophic nails, fissures, ulcers, corns, calluses and small muscle integrity needs to be performed. Biomechanical assessment of the feet should also be done before a person is sent for a specialist podiatry review. A yearly foot examination is of crucial importance in the management of diabetes.

2.3 Screening for type 2 diabetes

The American Diabetes Association (ADA) and the American Association of Clinical Endocrinologists (AACE) recommend screening for diabetes in individuals who are 45 years and above, irrespective of the presence or absence of the risk factors [20, 21]. The interval between screenings is three years, if the prior result is normal. This is to minimise the chances of false negative results. Screening for T2D should be done earlier if a person is overweight, with an additional risk factor for type 2 diabetes. These risk factors include having a family history of diabetes, a sedentary lifestyle, high-risk ethnic groups like Africans or Asians, prior diagnosis of prediabetes, gestational diabetes, and delivery of macrosomic babies. About one-third of individuals with prediabetes will eventually develop type 2 diabetes. Other relevant risk factors are hypertension, dyslipidaemia, prior diagnosis of polycystic ovarian syndrome, insulin resistance-related conditions such as acanthosis nigricans, and the presence of cardiovascular disease.

2.4 Laboratory parameters for diagnosis

To diagnose diabetes, the parameters of interest include glycated haemoglobin (HbA1c), fasting plasma glucose, random plasma glucose or 2-hour post-glucose load (during an oral glucose tolerance test). In persons with the classic symptoms of diabetes (polyuria, polydipsia, weight loss and fatigue), glycated haemoglobin of ≥48 mmol/mol (6.5%) and/or fasting plasma glucose (FPG) of ≥7.0 mmol/L and/or 2 hours post-glucose load (2HPGL) of ≥11.1 mmol/L and/or random plasma glucose (RPG) ≥ 11.1 mmol/L is sufficient to diagnose diabetes. So, HbA1c can be used to diagnose diabetes or identify individuals who are predisposed to developing diabetes later in life.

However, if a person is asymptomatic, a repeat sample has to be analysed later before establishing the diagnosis of diabetes mellitus. It is imperative to repeat the same test for the sake of consistency and avoidance of ambiguity. There are differences in the pre-analytic and analytic variability of the various diagnostic tests. For example, a repeat 2HPGL is most likely to be discordant, while HbA1c has the least variability. If another test is done and the results are discordant (one is above the diagnostic cut-off while the other is not), the test with the higher value is repeated. If the repeat is still above the diagnostic threshold, the individual has diabetes. If the discrepancy persists, the test may be repeated after 3–6 months.

The threshold values for diagnosis are based on the cut-off point at which individuals begin to develop retinopathy, from the findings of previous studies. The values below the diagnostic cut-off were associated with a low prevalence of retinopathy. At the diagnostic cut-off, there was a sharp linear spike in the occurrence of retinopathy. It must be stated that there are no perfect correlations among glycated haemoglobin, fasting plasma glucose or 2-hour post-glucose load, but all three can be used for the diagnosis of diabetes. HbA1c diagnoses one-half of individuals with FPG $\geq$ 7.0 mmol/L and one-third of people with 2HPGL $\geq$ 200 mg/dl [22]. Overall, the decision on which diagnostic test to be used is dependent on the accessibility and feasibility of the respective test.

2.4.1 Glycated haemoglobin (HbA1c)

Glycated haemoglobin represents the average blood glucose concentration in the preceding two to three months. Using the ADA criteria, HbA1c of 39–46 mmol/mol (5.7–6.4%) is used to diagnose prediabetes, while HbA1c of $\geq$48 mmol/mol (6.5%) is diagnostic of diabetes mellitus [23]. HbA1c is equally useful in monitoring glycaemic patterns and profiles in persons living with type 2 diabetes. It correlates well with diabetic microangiopathy (retinopathy, neuropathy and nephropathy) but less well with macroangiopathy (stroke, myocardial infarction and peripheral arterial disease).

The advantage of HbA1c as a diagnostic test includes the fact that it is not affected by recent meals, making it very convenient. It does not require fasting or ingestion of glucose. Also, the turnaround time is short, and the result is not significantly affected by the presence of an acute illness. However, the universally acceptable assaying method must be compliant with the National Glycohaemoglobin Standardisation Program (NGSP), as used in the Diabetes Control and Complications Trial (DCCT). This vital criterion makes HbA1c less readily available in many centres, especially in developing nations. Historically, it was a lack of standardisation that precluded HbA1c from being used as a diagnostic tool for diabetes. Lack of uniformity made generalisability problematic to attain. However, since 2010, ADA has recommended HbA1c as a diagnostic test for diabetes, as long as the assay is compliant with the NGSP standard. Based on this, point-of-care HbA1c assays (which are non-compliant with the NGSP protocol) are not approved for the diagnosis of diabetes. Also, any condition, physiological or pathological, that significantly affects the haematocrit or red cell turnover (such as haemoglobinopathies, other haemolytic anaemias, iron deficiency anaemia, pregnancy, blood loss, and haemodialysis) can give false readings.

2.4.2 Fasting plasma glucose (FPG)

The person is requested to fast overnight for 8–12 hours, following which plasma glucose concentration is obtained. Using the ADA guidelines, FPG of 5.6–6.9 mmol/L is consistent with prediabetes, while FPG $\geq$ 7.0 mmol/L diagnoses diabetes mellitus.

The advantages of FPG include convenience, consistency, and a tight relationship with diabetic microangiopathy (retinopathy, nephropathy, and neuropathy).

2.4.3 2-hour post-glucose load (2HPGL)

This is obtained as a part of the oral glucose tolerance test (OGTT). Following the ingestion of 75 mg of glucose in 300 ml of water, plasma glucose concentration is obtained after 2 hours. This is called the 2-hour post-glucose load. 2-HPGL of 7.8–11.0 mmol/L suggests prediabetes, whereas a value ≥11.1 mmol/L is consistent with diabetes. It is widely validated, but it is more expensive than the FPG test and requires the presence of the person at the laboratory for at least 2 hours, making it cumbersome and time-consuming. The person needs to be instructed to take meals of adequate carbohydrates (at least 150 g/day) for about five days before administering an OGTT. If the person can safely stop steroids several days prior to the test, it is better discontinued.

2.4.4 Random plasma glucose (RPG)

In a person with the classic symptoms, random plasma glucose ≥11.1 mmol/L is sufficient to diagnose diabetes. Similarly, any person presenting with features of hyperglycaemic emergency (HHS or DKA), an RPG ≥ 11.1 mmo/L diagnoses diabetes.

3. Management of type 2 diabetes mellitus

The goals of the management of type 2 diabetes are to minimise the risk of developing microvascular and macrovascular complications, as well as optimising the metabolic profile of the person. Therefore, the approach must go beyond glucocentricity (focusing on controlling the glucose only) but must involve modifying the cardiovascular risk factors in general. The management of type 2 diabetes must be individualised.

The management approach can be divided into four domains:

- Health education and counselling
- Lifestyle management
- Pharmacotherapy
- Miscellaneous

3.1 Health education and counselling

The person needs to see a specialist diabetes educator. Diabetes education has gone beyond handing people a pamphlet of instructions. Health education is an active process that must be undertaken by physicians, diabetes nurses, dieticians, other healthcare professionals, and specialist diabetes educators. Studies have shown that diabetes education has a significant impact on optimising glycaemic control and the general well-being of the people [24]. Similarly, diabetes education has been closely correlated with the prevention of diabetes complications. Diabetes education is a lifelong exercise and not a set of visits to the health educators. However, at the very least, persons living with diabetes must visit the diabetes educators at diagnosis, when glycaemic targets are not attained, when complications arise and when new changes are made to the management plan.

The ultimate aim of patient education is self-management of diabetes mellitus. Education empowers the people and equips them with problem-solving tactics and the necessary strategies to manage themselves. Diabetes self-management education (DSME) improves adherence to medications, dietary therapy and exercise regime. DSME has also been linked to improved quality of life among individuals living with type 2 diabetes mellitus. Persons living with diabetes need to be empowered to make informed decisions as regards their management. Comprehensive education is given on how to perform and interpret self-monitoring of blood glucose (SMBG). They must be able to act based on these interpretations also. Persons living with diabetes must be counselled to stop smoking.

The symptoms, causes and correction options for hypoglycaemia need to be discussed with the people affected. The various devices used in the management of diabetes, such as glucometers, flash glucose monitors, continuous glucose monitors, pens and insulin pumps, are also taught during education sessions. Persons living with diabetes who have been thoroughly educated are better capacitated to handle acute stress. "Education to protect tomorrow" was the theme of the 2022 World Diabetes Day, and this underlies the critical role education plays in the management of diabetes.

3.2 Lifestyle management

The lifestyle approach is the bedrock of managing type 2 diabetes or any other form of diabetes. Lifestyle therapies can be subdivided into dietary approach and physical activity. A major objective of lifestyle management is weight loss. The pillars of lifestyle management include healthy eating, exercise, smoking cessation, adequate sleep, stress reduction, and moderation of alcohol intake.

3.2.1 Dietary therapy

People living with diabetes are advised to visit a professional dietician to get comprehensive nutritional advice. This has been found to aid healthy food choices, maintain healthy weight, and improve quality of life. Based on the dietary needs of each person, the dietician assists in drawing a dietary plan for the people. The constituents, timing and quantity of the food eaten play a central role in reaching glycaemic targets. There is nothing called "diabetic diets", and people living with diabetes can eat healthy diets prescribed to other members of the population who have not been diagnosed with DM.

Generally, diets rich in complex carbohydrates, fibres and unsaturated fats are better suited for optimal glycaemic control, while refined sugars and saturated fats are avoided. Complex carbohydrates should constitute about 50–55% of the total caloric intake. The people are advised to select less processed or packaged food and eat small, frequent meals spread throughout the day. Proteins are derived from legumes, lean meat, fish and poultry. Vegetables, fruits and whole grains are highly recommended. Ultimately, dietary therapy, especially in the presence of obesity, is targeted at weight reduction [25].

3.2.2 Physical activity

Increased physical activity must be inculcated as a habit. Exercise reduces insulin resistance through decreased visceral fat mass, enhanced muscular skeleton insulin sensitivity, mopping up of free fatty acids, and augmented blood flow to insulin-sensitive tissues. Exercise helps not only in intensifying glucose disposition but in controlling other cardiovascular risk factors. It lowers blood pressure and plasma triglycerides levels while it raises high-density lipoprotein cholesterol (HDL-C).

WHO recommends at least 150 minutes of moderate-intensity aerobic physical activity per week [26]. The exercise is spread throughout the week. Alternatively, 75–150 minutes of vigorous-intensity physical activity could be adopted if reasonably feasible. The physical activities should be a combination of aerobic and muscle-strengthening activities. Twice-weekly muscle-strengthening physical activities have been found to have an additional advantage over aerobic exercises [27]. Sedentary activities must be minimised, and when possible, replaced with light-intensity physical activities. Habitual physical activities not only help in optimising glycaemic control, but it also helps in enhancing muscular strength (thereby preventing falls) and enhancing cardiorespiratory fitness (which has been associated with prolonged life expectancy). It also helps in promoting weight loss, boosting mental health and minimising the risk of developing a cardiovascular event (acute myocardial infarction and stroke). WHO recommends policies such as walking and cycling in place of motorised transport. Workplaces are also encouraged to provide opportunities that would encourage the physical activities of the personnel.

3.3 Pharmacotherapy

There are various classes of antidiabetic drugs available for individuals with type 2 diabetes [28]. These classes include biguanides (e.g. metformin), sulphonylureas (e.g., glyburide and glipizide), meglitinides (e.g., repaglinide and nateglinide), peroxisome proliferator-activated receptor-gamma (PPAR-γ) agonists, otherwise known as thiazolidinediones (e.g., pioglitazone), and alpha-glucosidase inhibitors (e.g., acarbose and voglibose) [29]. Other classes comprise dipeptidyl peptidase 4 (DPP-4)- inhibitors (e.g., alogliptin and saxagliptin), glucagon-like peptide-1 (GLP-1) receptor agonists (e.g., semaglutide and liraglutide), and sodium-glucose co-transporter-2 (SGLT-2) inhibitors (e,g., dapaglifozin and empaglifozin). Amylin analogues (e,g., pramlintide), and insulins (basal, pre-mixed, or basal-bolus) are sometimes used in the management of type 2 diabetes. Recently, dual incretin receptor agonists (e.g., tirzepatide) have been approved for the treatment of type 2 diabetes. A new class of anti-diabetic drugs (triagonists) acting on GLP-1 receptor, GIP receptor and glucagon receptor [30]. Retatrutide is an example of this class of drugs [31]. Since the treatment of type 2 diabetes mellitus is individualised, several factors are considered before choosing specific medications for the persons. These factors include efficacy, co-morbidities, risk of hypoglycaemia, cardiovascular safety, weight gain, potential side effects, and cost [28]. The patient's desires, values and aspirations must also be taken into account.

In most clinical practice guidelines, such as ADA and AACE, metformin remains the drug of choice for the management of type 2 diabetes, except contraindications are precluding its usage [32]. However, recent paradigm shift entails primary assessment of the cardiovascular risk of the person living with diabetes, and if high, the drugs that have been proven in clinical trials to be cardiovascular-friendly, such as SGLT-2 inhibitors and GLP-1 agonists, may be considered first.

3.3.1 Biguanides

Metformin is widely available and highly efficacious. Phenformin, a first-generation biguanide, has been withdrawn from the market on account of severe toxicity. Metformin's mechanism of action is to decrease hepatic insulin resistance and to a lower extent, the peripheral insulin resistance. Biguanides do not augment insulin release and their chances of hypoglycaemia, independently, are much lower. Metformin is currently the only approved and commercially available member of the class. Metformin does not bring about weight gain, and it mildly lowers total cholesterol as well as triglycerides. In fact, it causes minimal weight loss in about 30% of the people using it. Metformin causes lactic acidosis. Individuals with renal failure, liver failure, or heart failure are more likely to have lactic acidosis. So, it is avoided (or used with extreme caution) in individuals with these organ failures.

3.3.2 Sulphonylureas

Sulphonylureas are insulin secretagogues which means that these drugs act by increasing insulin secretion from B-cells. They bind to specific receptors on the B-cell, which closes potassium ATP channels, ultimately leading to the opening of calcium channels and influx of calcium into the cells. The raised concentration of calcium in the cells is responsible for insulin secretion. This implies that a residual B-cell mass is required for the efficacy of sulphonylureas. Prominent side effects include hypoglycaemia and weight gain. There are inconsistent data on the deleterious cardiovascular effect of sulphonylureas.

3.3.3 Meglitinides

These are also insulin secretagogues. Though dissimilar to sulphonylureas molecularly, they bind to sulphonylureas receptors and elicit a similar effect of augmented insulin secretion. Compared with sulphonylureas, the onset of action of meglitinides is more rapid, and the duration of action is shorter. This implies a lower propensity to hypoglycaemia and weight gain. Additionally, the efficacy of meglitinides is proportionate to that of sulphonylureas.

3.3.4 Thiazolidinediones

Thiazolidinediones are insulin sensitizers, which means that they can lower insulin resistance. They can do this by binding agonistically with peroxisome proliferator-activated receptor gamma (PPARγ), a transcription factor for nuclear hormone receptors. Unlike metformin, thiazolidinediones decrease peripheral insulin resistance and to a lower extent hepatic insulin resistance. Thiazolidinediones facilitate free fatty acid uptake by adipose tissue, thereby mobilising excess fat from the liver and the muscle, which makes them useful for individuals with steatotic liver disease. They promote water retention and weight gain and are better avoided in heart failure, renal failure and liver failure. They have a lower risk of hypoglycaemia and predispose to osteoporosis. There are published data linking rosiglitazone with bladder cancer.

3.3.5 α-glucosidase inhibitors

This class of drugs prevents postprandial hyperglycaemia by binding to an enzyme called α-glucosidase on the brush border of small intestines, thereby inhibiting the absorption of complex polysaccharides. Their side effects include flatulence, diarrhoea, and abdominal pain. These side effects often make them less desirable and promote non-adherence. They are to be avoided in individuals with certain gastrointestinal disorders such as inflammatory bowel disease, gastroparesis and intestinal obstruction.

3.3.6 DPP-4 inhibitors

DPP-4 inhibitors are a class of drugs that block an enzyme called dipeptidyl peptidase-4. The enzyme is responsible for the clearance of endogenous incretins, namely glucagon-like peptide 1 (GLP-1) and glucose-dependent insulinotropic polypeptide (GIP). Incretins augment insulin secretion in a glucose-dependent fashion, but their half-lives are very short, as they are rapidly cleared by DPP-4. So, DPP-4 inhibitors indirectly assist in raising insulin secretion in a glucose-dependent manner. The drugs do not cause weight gain and have a lower risk of hypoglycaemia. Linagliptin, a member of the class, does not need dose adjustment when there is renal failure, but the others do. There are reports that DPP-4 inhibitors can rarely cause pancreatitis. Other documented side effects include upper respiratory tract infection and headache.

3.3.7 GLP-1 receptor agonists

Glucagon-like peptide 1 (GLP-1) is an incretin produced in the L-cells of the small intestine. It amplifies insulin secretion from β-cells in the presence of glucose. Furthermore, incretins suppress appetite, gastric emptying and glucagon secretion. Endogenous incretins are rapidly degraded by DPP-4, but GLP-1 receptor agonists are not metabolised by DPP-4, yet they do elicit the same effect as the endogenous incretins. While most of the GLP-1 agonists are injectables, there is a formulation of semaglutide (Rybelsus) that is given orally. The GLP-1 receptor agonists have gastrointestinal side effects, such as nausea, diarrhoea and vomiting. They promote weight loss and prevent cardiovascular disease, as found in various cardiovascular outcome trials. (CVOT).

3.3.8 SGLT-2 inhibitors

Sodium-glucose cotransporter-2 (SGLT-2) is a membrane-bound transporter protein which reabsorbs glucose in the proximal convoluted tubules of nephrons. About 97% of filtered glucose is reabsorbed by SGLT-2. The reabsorption is in conjunction with sodium reabsorption at the proximal convoluted tubules. In T2D, SGLT-2 is abnormally upregulated, thereby intensifying glucose reabsorption in the kidneys. SGLT-2 inhibitors prevent glucose reabsorption, consequently causing glucosuria, natriuresis and moderate diuresis. SGLT-2 inhibitors have also been approved for the treatment of heart failure and renal failure. The drugs promote weight loss and prevent cardiovascular disease. Their side effects include genitourinary infection and increased propensity to euglycaemic diabetic ketoacidosis.

3.3.9 Insulins

Improvement in medical technology has seen the evolution of injectable insulin from animal insulin to human insulins (produced from recombinant DNA technology), and now, we have insulin analogues (produced from genetic modifications of human insulins). Inhaled insulins are available, although rarely used, and oral insulin is still being developed experimentally. Insulins, just like endogenous insulins, act by stimulating cellular glucose uptake and inhibiting proteolysis, lipolysis and gluconeogenesis. Various insulins used in clinical practice have different pharmacokinetics. Typically, people requiring insulin are started on basal insulins like neutral protamine Hagedorn (NPH) insulin, glargine, detemir or degludec. If basal insulins are not sufficient, prandial insulins (such as soluble insulin, insulin aspart, insulin lispro, and insulin glulisine) may be added. There are also human and analogue premixed insulins. The side effects of insulin are hypoglycaemia, weight gain and local skin reactions.

3.3.10 Amylin analogues

B-cells co-secrete amylin and insulin. Amylin prevents postprandial excursion of blood glucose. Just as it is applicable to insulin, in type 2 diabetes, there may be eventual β-cell failure with resultant insulinopenia and amylinopenia. In terms of mechanisms of action, amylin analogues reduce appetite, suppress gastric emptying, inhibit glucagon secretion and reduce hepatic glucose production. Pramlintide is an amylin mimetic that can be used as an adjunct in the management of type 2 diabetes mellitus. Pramlintide causes weight loss. The reported side effects are gastrointestinal, such as nausea and vomiting.

3.4 Treatment of co-morbidities

Other co-morbidities such as hypertension, obesity and dyslipidaemia must be treated to targets. Cardiovascular disease tends to kill people with diabetes; therefore, it is not enough to control the glucose but to treat all the cardiovascular risk factors holistically. Angiotensin-converting enzyme (ACE) inhibitors or angiotensin receptor blockers (ARB) are preferred in managing hypertension in individuals living with type 2 diabetes. In managing dyslipidaemia, statins (e.g., atorvastatin, rosuvastatin) remain the drugs of choice. However, in individuals who cannot tolerate statins or who are not achieving their targets despite the maximum tolerable doses of statins, ezetimibe or proprotein convertase subtilisin/kexin type 9 (PCSK9) inhibitors can be used.

3.5 Miscellaneous

The management of type 2 diabetes requires a multidisciplinary approach. A person with type 2 diabetes may be referred to a podiatrist, cardiologist, nephrologist, ophthalmologist or vascular surgeon. A yearly fundal examination is recommended for individuals with type 2 diabetes, starting from the time of diagnosis. Urinary albumin: creatinine ratio should be monitored yearly or twice yearly. Foot examinations must be done at each clinic visit, and a yearly schedule with the podiatrist for a comprehensive foot examination is equally essential.

3.6 Targets of treatment

Targets of treatments are individualised. Glycated haemoglobin (HbA1c) is a validated test for monitoring people with T2D undergoing treatment. The target HbA1c is <7.0% (and sometimes <6.5%, provided that safety and affordability have been carefully considered). HbA1c target is <8% in those with low life expectancy or established cardiovascular disease. The target blood pressure, according to the ADA guidelines, is <140/90 mmHg [33]. In people with established atherosclerotic cardiovascular disease, the low-density lipoprotein cholesterol (LDL-C) target is <70 mg/dl. In others who do not have atherosclerotic cardiovascular disease, the LDL-C target is <100 mg/dl. About 60% of persons with type 2 diabetes do not meet their glycaemic, blood pressure and lipid targets [34, 35]. This emphasises that physicians and other health professionals must intensify their efforts in treating the individuals to target. The target for weight loss is 5–7%, and this has been found to contribute immensely to cardiovascular risk control.

3.7 Monitoring of treatment

Monitoring of treatment is individualised. HbA1c is done every three months. In persons with stable and optimal glycaemic profiles, HbA1c interval can be extended to six months. People on intensive insulin therapy need to monitor the fasting, preprandial, occasional postprandial and bedtime glucose values. Glucose checks are encouraged anytime the patient feels unwell. Glucose checks are also vital before (and after) exercise, driving and operations of machines. Suspicion of hypoglycaemia warrants immediate blood glucose check. Using ADA guidelines, the target FPG is 4.4–7.2 mmol/L and 2-hour postprandial value of <10 mmol/L [21]. Glucose checks can be done with glucometers, flash glucose monitors and continuous glucose monitors. Blood pressure is checked at every hospital visit. Fasting lipid profile is checked at least annually.

List of abbreviations

2HPGL	2 hours post-glucose load
AACE	American Association of Clinical Endocrinologists
ACE	Angiotensin-converting enzyme
ADA	American Diabetes Association
ARB	Angiotensin receptor blockers
ATP	Adenosine triphosphate
CVOT	Cardiovascular outcome trials
DCCT	Diabetes Control and Complications Trial
DKA	Diabetic ketoacidosis
DM	diabetes mellitus
DPP-4	Dipeptidyl peptidase 4
DSME	Diabetes self-management education
FPG	Fasting plasma glucose
GIP	Glucose-dependent insulinotropic polypeptide
GLP-1	Glucagon-like peptide-1
GWAS	Genome-wide association studies
HbA1c	Glycated haemoglobin
HDL-C	High-density lipoprotein cholesterol
HHS	Hyperglycaemic hyperosmolar state
IDF	International Diabetes Federation
LDL-C	Low-density lipoprotein cholesterol
NGSP	National Glycohaemoglobin Standardisation Program
NPH	Neutral Protamine Hagedorn
OGTT	Oral glucose tolerance test
PCSK9	Proprotein convertase subtilidin/kexin type 9

PPAR-γ	Peroxisome proliferator-activated receptor-gamma
RPG	Random plasma glucose
SGLT-2	Sodium-glucose co-transporter-2
SMBG	Self-monitoring of blood glucose
T2D	Type 2 diabetes mellitus
WHO	World Health Organisation

Author details

Taoreed Adegoke Azeez
Department of Medicine, Reddington Multi-Specialist Hospital, Lagos, Nigeria

*Address all correspondence to: adegokegalaxy@yahoo.com

References

[1] Karalliedde J, Gnudi L. Diabetes mellitus, a complex and heterogeneous disease, and the role of insulin resistance as a determinant of diabetic kidney disease. Nephrology Dialysis Transplantation. 2016;**31**(2):206-213. DOI: 10.1093/ndt/gfu405

[2] An J et al. Prevalence and incidence of microvascular and macrovascular complications over 15 years among patients with incident type 2 diabetes. BMJ Open Diabetes Research and Care. 2021;**9**(1):e001847. DOI: 10.1136/bmjdrc-2020-001847

[3] WHO. Classification of diabetes mellitus. Classification of diabetes mellitus. 2019. Available from: https://www.who.int/publications-detail-redirect/classification-of-diabetes-mellitus [Accessed: July 04, 2023]

[4] Olokoba AB, Obateru OA, Olokoba LB. Type 2 diabetes mellitus: A review of current trends. Oman Medical Journal. 2012;**27**(4):269-273. DOI: 10.5001/omj.2012.68

[5] Grotz AK, Gloyn AL, Thomsen SK. Prioritising causal genes at type 2 diabetes risk loci. Current Diabetes Reports. 2017;**17**(9):76. DOI: 10.1007/s11892-017-0907-y

[6] Prasad RB, Groop L. Genetics of type 2 diabetes—Pitfalls and possibilities. Genes. 2015;**6**(1):1. DOI: 10.3390/genes6010087

[7] DeFronzo RA. From the triumvirate to the ominous octet: A new paradigm for the treatment of type 2 diabetes mellitus. Diabetes. 2009;**58**(4):773-795. DOI: 10.2337/db09-9028

[8] Petersen MC, Shulman GI. Mechanisms of insulin action and insulin resistance. Physiological Reviews. 2018;**98**(4):2133-2223. DOI: 10.1152/physrev.00063.2017

[9] Galicia-Garcia U et al. Pathophysiology of type 2 diabetes mellitus. International Journal of Molecular Sciences. 2020;**21**(17):17. DOI: 10.3390/ijms21176275

[10] Saisho Y. β-Cell dysfunction: Its critical role in prevention and management of type 2 diabetes. World Journal of Diabetes. 2015;**6**(1):109-124. DOI: 10.4239/wjd.v6.i1.109

[11] IDF. 'Facts & figures'. International Diabetes Federation – Facts and Figures. Available from: https://idf.org/about-diabetes/facts-figures/ [Accessed: July 04, 2023]

[12] Uloko AE et al. Prevalence and risk factors for diabetes mellitus in Nigeria: A systematic review and Meta-analysis. Diabetes Theraphy. 2018;**9**(3):1307-1316. DOI: 10.1007/s13300-018-0441-1

[13] Kibirige D, Lumu W, Jones AG, Smeeth L, Hattersley AT, Nyirenda MJ. Understanding the manifestation of diabetes in sub Saharan Africa to inform therapeutic approaches and preventive strategies: A narrative review. Clinical Diabetes and Endocrinology. 2019;**5**(1):2. DOI: 10.1186/s40842-019-0077-8

[14] Kharroubi AT, Darwish HM. Diabetes mellitus: The epidemic of the century. World Journal of Diabetes. 2015;**6**(6):850-867. DOI: 10.4239/wjd.v6.i6.850

[15] Seuring T, Archangelidi O, Suhrcke M. The economic costs of type 2 diabetes: A global systematic review. PharmacoEconomics.

2015;**33**(8):811-831. DOI: 10.1007/s40273-015-0268-9

[16] Kropp M et al. Diabetic retinopathy as the leading cause of blindness and early predictor of cascading complications—Risks and mitigation. The EPMA Journal. 2023;**14**(1):21-42. DOI: 10.1007/s13167-023-00314-8

[17] Azeez TA. Erectile dysfunction among Nigerian men with diabetes: A systematic review. PRM. 2020;**4**(2):1-8

[18] Azeez TA, Durotoluwa IM, Makanjuola AI. Diabetes mellitus as a risk factor for stroke among Nigerians: A systematic review and meta-analysis. International Journal of Cardiology and Cardiovascular Risk Prevention. 2023;**18**:200189. DOI: 10.1016/j.ijcrp.2023.200189

[19] Li M et al. Changes in the structure, perfusion, and function of the hippocampus in type 2 diabetes mellitus. Frontiers in Neuroscience. 2023;**16**:1070911. Available from: https://www.frontiersin.org/articles/10.3389/fnins.2022.1070911 [Accessed: July 24, 2023] [Online]

[20] Blonde L et al. American Association of Clinical Endocrinology Clinical Practice Guideline: Developing a diabetes mellitus comprehensive care plan—2022 update. Endocrine Practice. 2022;**28**(10):923-1049. DOI: 10.1016/j.eprac.2022.08.002

[21] American Diabetes Association Professional Practice Committee. 6 Glycemic targets: Standards of medical Care in Diabetes—2022'. Diabetes Care. 2021;**45**(Supplement_1):S83-S96. DOI: 10.2337/dc22-S006

[22] Karnchanasorn R et al. Comparison of the current diagnostic criterion of HbA1c with fasting and 2-hour plasma glucose concentration. Journal Diabetes Research. 2016;**2016**:6195494. DOI: 10.1155/2016/6195494

[23] Li G et al. Evaluation of ADA HbA1c criteria in the diagnosis of pre-diabetes and diabetes in a population of Chinese adolescents and young adults at high risk for diabetes: A cross-sectional study. BMJ Open. 2018;**8**(8):e020665. DOI: 10.1136/bmjopen-2017-020665

[24] Celik S et al. Assessment the effect of diabetes education on self-care behaviors and glycemic control in the Turkey nursing diabetes education evaluating project (TURNUDEP): A multi-center study. BMC Nursing. 2022;**21**(1):215. DOI: 10.1186/s12912-022-01001-1

[25] Evert AB et al. Nutrition therapy for adults with diabetes or prediabetes: A consensus report. Diabetes Care. 2019;**42**(5):731-754. DOI: 10.2337/dci19-0014

[26] Harrington D, Henson J. Physical activity and exercise in the management of type 2 diabetes: Where to start? Practical Diabetes. 2021;**38**(5):35-40b. DOI: 10.1002/pdi.2361

[27] Momma H, Kawakami R, Honda T, Sawada SS. Muscle-strengthening activities are associated with lower risk and mortality in major non-communicable diseases: A systematic review and meta-analysis of cohort studies. British Journal of Sports Medicine. 2022;**56**(13):755-763. DOI: 10.1136/bjsports-2021-105061

[28] Chaudhury A et al. Clinical review of antidiabetic drugs: Implications for type 2 diabetes mellitus management. Frontier in Endocrinology (Lausanne). 2017;**8**:6. DOI: 10.3389/fendo.2017.00006

[29] DeMarsilis A et al. Pharmacotherapy of type 2 diabetes: An update and future

directions. Metabolism - Clinical and Experimental. Dec 2022;**137**:155332. DOI: 10.1016/j.metabol.2022.155332

[30] Bossart M et al. Effects on weight loss and glycemic control with SAR441255, a potent unimolecular peptide GLP-1/GIP/GCG receptor triagonist. Cell Metabolism. 2022;**34**(1):59-74.e10. DOI: 10.1016/j.cmet.2021.12.005

[31] Jastreboff AM et al. Triple–hormone-receptor agonist retatrutide for obesity — A phase 2 trial. New England Journal of Medicine. Jun 2023. DOI: 10.1056/NEJMoa2301972 [Online ahead of print]

[32] Yu J, Lee S-H, Kim MK. Recent updates to clinical practice guidelines for diabetes mellitus. Endocrinology Metabolism (Seoul). 2022;**37**(1):26-37. DOI: 10.3803/EnM.2022.105

[33] Kim H-J, Kim K. Blood pressure target in type 2 diabetes mellitus. Diabetes and Metabolism Journal. 2022;**46**(5):667-674. DOI: 10.4093/dmj.2022.0215

[34] Blonde L, Aschner P, Bailey C, Ji L, Leiter LA, Matthaei S. Gaps and barriers in the control of blood glucose in people with type 2 diabetes. Diabetes & Vascular Disease Research. 2017;**14**(3):172-183. DOI: 10.1177/1479164116679775

[35] Alkandari A, Vaucher J, Marques-Vidal P. Trends in glycemic, blood pressure, and lipid control in adults with diabetes in Switzerland: The CoLaus|PsyCoLaus Study. BMJ Open Diabetes Research and Care. 2023;**11**(3):e003377. DOI: 10.1136/bmjdrc-2023-003377

Chapter 2

Screening and Testing for Prediabetes and Type 2 Diabetes in Asymptomatic Adults

Loudry Amsal Elfa Gustanar and Nanang Miftah Fajari

Abstract

Screening for prediabetes and type 2 diabetes risk through an informal assessment of risk factors or with an assessment tool, such as the ADA (American Diabetes Association) risk test, is recommended to guide health care professionals on whether performing a diagnostic test is appropriate. Approximately one-quarter of people with diabetes in the US and nearly half of Asian and Hispanic American people with diabetes are undiagnosed. Although screening of asymptomatic individuals to identify those with prediabetes or diabetes might seem reasonable, rigorous clinical trials to prove the effectiveness of such screening have not been conducted and are unlikely to occur. Clinical conditions, such as hypertension, hypertensive pregnancy and obesity, enhance risk. Additional considerations regarding testing for type 2 diabetes and prediabetes in asymptomatic individuals include the following: age, BMI (body mass index) and ethnicity, medication, HIV, testing interval, community screening and screening in dental practice.

Keywords: screening, testing, type II diabetes, prediabetes, asymptomatic

1. Introduction

In 2016 diabetes was the third leading cause of years lived with disability and the seventh leading cause of death in the United States. The number of people living with type 2 diabetes mellitus increased significantly over the past decades, going from around 151 million in 2000 to 463 million in 2019. Along with this increased prevalence, the economic health cost related to type 2 diabetes mellitus experienced a staggering increase. The expenditures related to diabetes in United States were estimated at US$232 billion and US$760 billion in 2007 and 2019, respectively [1].

This significant increase in diabetes prevalence, especially in Asia, the Middle East and North Africa (MENA), is largely attributed to changes in the living environment and lifestyles that led to declines in nutritional quality and increases in sedentary behaviors. These drastic changes in lifestyle increase the prevalence of overweight and obesity, promoting the development of insulin resistance and diabetes mellitus [1].

Prior to diabetes mellitus development and pancreatic beta-cell dysfunction, a state of prediabetes commonly preceded. Prediabetes which was defined by a fasting plasma glucose concentration of 5,6–6,9 mmol/L or hemoglobin A1c concentration of 39–46 mmol/mol, was reported to affect around 86 million adults in the United States. In a 5-year period, approximately 70% of prediabetes eventually develop type 2 diabetes mellitus.

Prediabetes state has been associated with the development of macrovascular and microvascular complication, such as nephropathy, chronic kidney disease, small fiber neuropathy, diabetic retinopathy, cognitive dysfunction and also cardiovascular disease. Despite the association of prediabetes to pathophysiological changes and morbidities, most individual with prediabetes are asymptomatic and thus unaware that they have the condition [2].

Early screening for prediabetes state and subsequent early intervention has been associated with improved all-cause mortality and morbidity caused by type 2 diabetes mellitus [3]. In this brief article, we review the need for screening for prediabetes and diabetes in the asymptomatic adult population.

2. Diabetes mellitus

Diabetes mellitus is defined as abnormal plasma glucose concentration associated with glucose metabolism disorders. Diabetes mellitus is diagnosed if fasting plasma glucose (FPG) concentration is equal or greater than 7.0 mmol/L, or a 2-h plasma glucose (2hrPG) concentration is equal or greater than 11.1 mmol/L during an oral glucose tolerance test (OGTT), or hemoglobin A1c (HbA1c) concentration is equal or greater than 47 mmol/mol.

2.1 Classification of diabetes mellitus

A new proposed classification of T2DM was based on six variables, including glutamate decarboxylate (GAD) antibodies, age at diagnosis, body mass index (BMI), HbA1c concentrations and homeostatic model assessment estimates of ß-cell function (HOMA-2B) and insulin resistance (HOMA2-IR). This novel classification divided T2DM into five groups: severe autoimmune diabetes (SAID), severe insulin-deficient diabetes (SIDD), severe insulin-resistant diabetes (SIRD), mild obesity-related diabetes (MOD) and mild age-related diabetes (MARD) [4, 5].

Cluster 1 (SAID) is characterized by early-onset disease, relatively low BMI, poor metabolic control, insulin deficiency and the presenve of GADA. Cluster 2 (SIDD) is similar to SAID but with negative GADA: low age at onset, relatively low BMI, low insulin secretion (low HOMA2-B index) and poor metabolic control. Cluster 3 (SIRD) is characterized by insulin resistance (high HOMA2-IR index) and high BMI. Cluster 4 (MOD) is characterized by obesity without insulin resistance and lastly, Cluster 5 (MARD) is similar to Cluster 4 but with older onset and milder metabolic derangements [4, 5].

This new classification identifies patients with a high risk of diabetic complications and provides information about the underlying disease mechanism. Patients in Cluster 3 (SIRD) have a higher risk for diabetic kidney disease than those in Cluster 4 and 5 patients in Cluster 2 (SIDD) have the highest risk of diabetic retinopathy. SIRD is also associated with a higher risk for diabetic ketoacidosis, diabetic retinopathy, atherosclerotic cardiovascular disease and nonalcoholic fatty liver disease [4, 5].

2.2 Prevalence of type 2 diabetes mellitus

The Global Burden of Disease (GBD) data in 2019 announced that the age-standardized global prevalence of type 2 diabetes mellitus was approximately 6.0% in men and 5.0% in women. The incidence increases with age, with the mean age of diagnosis occurring around 55 to 59 years. The highest increase in the proportion of type 2 diabetes mellitus age-standardized prevalence happens in the Middle East and North Africa (MENA) and in South Asia. Data from the International Diabetes Federation published the prevalence of people living with type 2 diabetes mellitus in 2045 will approximately increase to 700 million [1].

2.3 Risk factors for diabetes

Several factors are associated with type 2 diabetes mellitus, and they can be classified into nonmodifiable and modifiable risk factors. Nonmodifiable risk factors include age, ethnicity and genetics, while modifiable risk factors include diet, physical activity and tobacco use (**Figure 1**) [1].

Before the age of 30, type 2 diabetes incidence is typically low in most populations but rises quickly and steadily as people become older. According to prospective observational research, age is often a significant risk factor, despite the control of obesity [6, 7].

The physiological reaction to meals high in saccharides can be used to gauge the quality of dietary saccharides. The ability of particular foods to raise postprandial plasma glucose concentration is ranked by the glycemic index, which reflects the quality of saccharides. The glycemic load is the cross-product of a food's glycemic index and the number of saccharides, reflecting both the quality and quantity of the saccharides. Numerous prospective studies have assessed the relationships between glycemic index and load and risk of diabetes. These meta-analyses revealed that low glycemic index and glycemic load diets may be associated with a lower risk of developing diabetes than high glycemic index diets [6, 7].

Sedentary lifestyle choices were associated with a greater risk of type 2. According to a global assessment, physical inactivity, which the World Health Organization (2010) defines as not enough physical activity to fulfill current global standards, is responsible for 7% of type 2 diabetes mellitus burden [7].

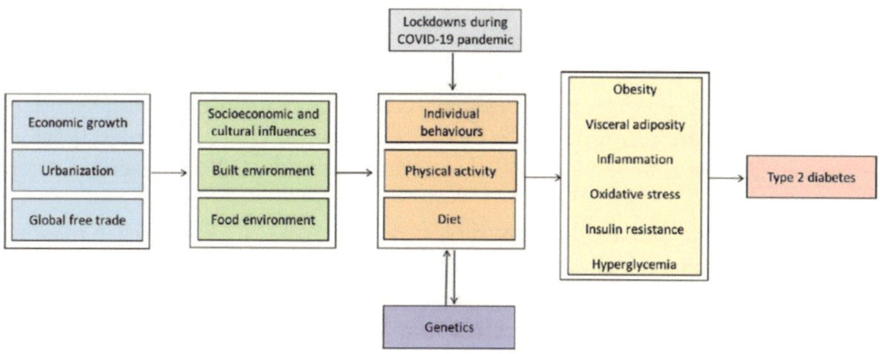

Figure 1.
Factors associated with increased prevalence of type 2 diabetes mellitus [1].

The biggest independent risk factor for type 2 diabetes is excessive body fat. The risk is connected to high body fat, indicated by BMI or anthropometric measurements like waist circumference or skinfold thickness. A dose-dependent rise in diabetes risk is linked to clinical BMI risk categories. Longer periods of maintaining a high body weight are a significant risk factor for type 2 diabetes and the degree of overweight and obesity. The Framingham Heart Study (FHS) revealed the age-adjusted relative risk per extra 2-year duration of obesity was 1.11 for men and 1.06 for women [7].

2.4 Mechanism increasing the risk of type 2 diabetes

The main pathophysiology driving the development of type 2 diabetes is impaired insulin secretion and insulin resistance in both muscle and the liver. Type 2 diabetes is commonly preceded by long-term prediabetes, in which pancreatic beta-cell dysfunction may have occurred. Type 2 diabetes is commonly diagnosed when the pancreas cannot increase insulin secretion to compensate for the insulin resistance in the peripheral insulin-sensitive tissues. Additional mechanisms affecting insulin secretion in type 2 diabetes mellitus are increasing hormone deficiency/resistance in the gastrointestinal tract and hyperglucagonemia [8].

3. Prediabetes

Prediabetes is defined as an abnormal elevation in plasma glucose concentration, but lower than needed to be diagnosed as type 2 diabetes. Prediabetes is a glycemic state between normoglycemia and diabetes mellitus and carries an increased risk for developing type 2 diabetes mellitus [9]. Prediabetes is further classified into impaired fasting glucose (IFG) and impaired glucose tolerance (IGT). There are currently two accepted definitions for IFG and IGT, either by American Diabetes Association (ADA) or by World Health Organization (WHO). ADA 2020 defined IFG as a fasting plasma glucose concentration of 5.6–6.9 mmol/L or hemoglobin A1c (HbA1c) concentration of 39–46 mmol/mol and IGT as a fasting plasma glucose concentration less than 6.9 mmol/L and 2-h plasma glucose concentration of 7.8–11.0 mmol/L. WHO 2006 defined IFG as fasting plasma glucose of 6.1–6.9 mmol/L and 2-h plasma glucose concentration less than 7.8 mmol/L (if measured) and IGT as 2-h plasma glucose concentration of 7.8–11.0 mmol/L [9].

3.1 Biological phenotypes of prediabetes

Both IFG and IGT phenotypes have various degrees of insulin resistance and beta-cell dysfunction; however, IGT is characterized with almost completely insulin resistant and has less than 20% beta-cell function, and thus IGT represents a worse glucose homeostasis disturbance.

These two phenotypes are diagnosed by fasting plasma glucose and 2-h plasma glucose concentrations which provide information on the fasting and postprandial states and, thus, on the pancreatic beta cells. HbA1c shares information about chronic hyperglycemia state and therefore may miss short-term acute hyperglycemia. Previous studies showed that HbA1c was weakly correlated with insulin resistance and beta-cell function, while FPG and 2hBG correlated better with insulin resistance and beta-cell function.

Genome-wide association studies (GWAS) revealed an overlap in the loci associated with FBG and 2hBG traits, such as MTNR1B, PCSK1 and DPYSL5, which are specific to FBG, and VPS13C, GCKR, GIPR and VPS13C which are specific to 2hBG. Some gene variants associated with HbA1c overlap with glycemia, including GCK, G6PC2 and MNTR1B, and others are specific to HbA1c.

3.2 Prediabetes burden

Differences in ADA's and WHO's criteria for prediabetes affected the number of IFG and IGT prevalence. The prevalence of IFG and IFG + IGT is estimated at 36–53% and 16–20%, respectively [9]. In 2017, the National Diabetes Statistics Report estimated around 33.9% of adult in the United States has prediabetes based on either fasting glucose or hemoglobin A1c (HbA1c) concentration, and only 103 mmol/mol adults know they have prediabetes [10].

3.3 Risk factor for prediabetes

Risk factors for prediabetes include age over 45 years, male sex, obesity, hypertension, dyslipidemia, family history of diabetes, history of gestational diabetes and Hispanic, black or Asian ethnicity [11]. According to the previous study, gaining weight results in increased insulin resistance, which may cause prediabetes. Consuming junk food with saturated fatty acids might increase weight and result in insulin resistance [12].

Changes in food habits and physical inactivity are the main causes of weight gain globally in the past decades. As mentioned before, the main independent risk factor for diabetes is excessive adiposity, which is measured by a higher body mass index (BMI). However, individuals with Asian ethnicity tend to develop diabetes at significantly lower BMIs than those with European ancestry. According to previous meta-analysis, there may be a marginally stronger association between risk of diabetes and waist size than between risk of diabetes and body mass index. Therefore, monitoring both waist circumference and BMI is crucial in clinical practice [12].

Individuals exposed to ETS (Environmental Tobacco Smoke) had an elevated risk of developing diabetes. The incidence of diabetes in prediabetic participants was also statistically affected by active smoking. The findings of this study support the notion that T2DM and smoking, whether passive or active, are related [12].

Men who drink are more likely to develop type 2 diabetes, whereas women who drink less are less likely to develop the disease. High beer intake and high booze consumption in men were associated with greater risks of prediabetes and type 2 diabetes, respectively. Women demonstrated a lower risk of prediabetes with high wine consumption and a lower risk of type 2 diabetes with medium intakes of both wine and spirits, but prediabetes risk rose with high spirits consumption. In summary, males who drink a lot are more likely to have impaired glucose regulation. The relationships are more nuanced in women, with risk decreasing with low to moderate alcohol use and rising with high consumption [12].

3.4 Progression to prediabetes

The onset of prediabetes is influenced by several factors, comprising genetics, peripheral insulin resistance, defects in insulin secretion, glucotoxicity, lipotoxicity, impaired incretin release, amylin accumulation, inflammation, oxidative stress and decreased beta cell mass, and eventually beta cell dysfunction [11].

Previous studies pointed out several predictors of transition from normal glucose regulation to prediabetes, consisting of demographic and adiposity (older age, male sex, higher body mass index, higher waist circumference, higher total and abdominal fat), glucoregulatory (upper-normal fasting plasma glucose and 2-h plasma glucose concentration, low insulin sensitivity, impaired insulin secretion and lower disposition index), plasma lipid and amino acid levels (higher triglycerides, higher LDL or lower HDL cholesterol, higher asparagine or aspartic acid, higher glutamine or glutamic acid and lower histidine) and miscellaneous factors (higher plasma pressure, lower adiponectin, higher hematocrit and higher alanine aminotransferase) [13].

Prediabetes condition is strongly associated with an increased risk of diabetes development. A previous meta-analysis showed that HbA1c concentration of 42–47 mmol/mol was associated with a 25 to 50% higher risk of incident diabetes over 5 years. The cumulative probability of progression to diabetes in patients diagnosed with HbA1c alone and IFG was 53 and 73 mmol/mol, respectively, over a 4.7-year follow-up period. In a pooled analysis, the annual incidence rate of diabetes was 3.6% in patients with HbA1c concentrations of 42–47 mmol/mol, while in patients with ADA-defined IFG, the annual rate was 3.6% [14].

Prediabetes shares a similar pathophysiology pathway as type 2 diabetes mellitus that, include insulin resistance, pancreatic beta-cell dysfunction and insulin resistance in organs. Insulin resistance will cause hyperinsulinemia in prediabetic patients, characterized by alteration of the insulin signaling pathway, reduced concentration, phosphorylation and activity of insulin receptors and decreased intracellular translocation of glucose transporter 4 (GLUT-4) [15].

Both IFG and IGT share a similar state of insulin resistance; however, the former is associated with hepatic insulin resistance, while the latter is associated with muscle insulin resistance. IFG has moderate hepatic insulin resistance and impaired early (1–30 min) insulin response exocytosis of insulin during OGTT. The intact late-phase plasma insulin response and normal to near-normal muscle sensitivity in IFG will return 2-h plasma glucose concentration to the initial fasting plasma glucose concentration. On the other hand, IGT is associated with impaired early and also late insulin (60–120 min) response during OGTT [15].

Pancreatic beta-cell dysfunction occurs along with insulin resistance in prediabetic patients. The sensitivity of pancreatic beta-cells in responding to changes in glucose concentration is impaired in prediabetes. Normally, as long as beta-cells can secrete insulin to overcome the insulin resistance, the body's tolerance to glucose remains normal; however, as the beta-cells fail to overcome the insulin resistance, the individual will develop prediabetes state and then eventually develop type 2 diabetes mellitus [15].

Physiologically, the secretion of insulin occurs in a biphasic pattern. This biphasic pattern may aid in differentiating IFG from IGT. The first phase of insulin secretion inhibits the endogenous hepatic glucose production in postprandial period, which maintain glucose concentrations at 150–160 g/dL in the first hour of OGTT. The second half is responsible for the gradual decrease in plasma glucose concentration. IFG will show a reduction in the first phase of insulin secretion and a greater increase in glucose concentrations at 60 and 30 min, as normally, the response following glucose ingestion is late. Changes in the second phase of insulin secretion are associated with muscle insulin resistance in IGT and showed through constant concentration of plasma glucose concentrations after 60–120 min during OGTT [15].

3.5 Prediabetes screening

Screening is defined as the utilization of tests to identify unrecognized diseases among apparently healthy populations. Screening is used for early identification of disease in the population and thus leads to early intervention to reduce the individual risk of the disease. Screening for undiagnosed diabetes is not recommended in the general population as the screening may be poorly targeted and may fail to reach the intended group at risk of diabetes; therefore, screening should be done in high-risk individuals to increase the likelihood of diabetes detection and to maximize the cost-effectiveness of screening testing [3].

There are currently two widely used screening tests to identify people with prediabetes and to diagnose type 2 diabetes, CDC and ADA screening tools [11]. These include the oral glucose tolerance test and the fasting glucose concentration.

After the food ingested is broken down into sugars, glucose molecules will then be absorbed into the plasma stream and transported to the cells in the body. In response to the elevated glucose concentration, pancreatic beta cells will secrete insulin. Insulin facilitates the transportation of glucose from the plasma stream into cells. Insulin also inhibits gluconeogenesis in the liver and facilitates the storage of glucose in the form of glycogen (glycogenesis) and fats (de novo lipogenesis (DNL)), which serve as short- and long-term stores of energy, respectively [16].

Plasma glucose homeostasis is maintained at 4–6 mmol/L. This homeostasis is influenced by several factors, such as the functional capacity of pancreatic beta-cells and cellular (skeletal muscles, liver and adipose tissue) sensitivity to insulin. In diabetes mellitus, there is either insulin deficiency or insulin resistance. Dysfunction in the production or uptake of insulin may disturb the plasma glucose homeostasis [16].

The oral glucose tolerance test (OGTT) is considered the gold standard for diabetes and prediabetes diagnosis. OGTT provides a serial measurement of plasma glucose after a specific amount of glucose is given orally to evaluate the individuals. OGTT may help distinguish IFG grom IGT and is reported to have a higher sensitivity than fasting plasma glucose measurement. However, the regular use of OGTT is limited by the need for an overnight fast, a lengthy testing time, higher cost, intra-individual variability, differences in glucose absorption rate and low reproducibility [17, 18].

OGTT should be avoided in hospitalized, acutely ill or inactive patients. Before starting the test, the discontinuation of medications that affect glucose tolerance should be confirmed. The test should be done in the morning with 75-gram glucose load orally in nonpregnant adults and 15 grams in children (1.75 g/kg up to 75 grams). The glucose should be dissolved in 300 mL water and ingested within 5 min period [17, 18].

Theoretically, fasting insulin and glucose concentration could differentiate beta-cell dysfunction from insulin resistance; however, in homeostasis model assessment (HOMA), there exists a feedback loop from fasting insulin which hinders the precision and interpretation of assay results. Overnight basal plasma glucose concentrations are lower than stressed fasting glucose concentrations. As hyperglycemia results from the combination of beta-cell dysfunction and insulin resistance, the degree of hyperglycemia does not directly associate with either degree of beta-cell dysfunction or insulin resistance. Therefore, the fasting plasma insulin concentration should be measured in a 15-min period from a rested patient to avoid confounding effects of oscillatory release and stress [19].

HOMA index (Insulin * glycemia in µmol/L/22.5) has been used widely in epidemiological studies for insulin sensitivity assessment. The beta-cell function was estimated from responses to a hyperglycemic clamp and intravenous glucose tolerance test. In 2000, the QUICKY index (1/log insulin + log glycemia in mg/dL) was introduced and compared with the HOMA index for measuring insulin sensitivity. HOMA index was able to discriminate the increase in insulin resistance in diabetic patients with impaired glucose tolerance and healthy person; however, the QUICKI index was shown to be more sensitive and more straightforward in discriminating the two [19, 20].

Random plasma glucose concentration is reported to have 63% sensitivity and 87% specificity in detecting diabetes disease. Individuals with glucose concentrations indicative of diabetes should then undergo a second confirmatory test. On the other hand, fasting plasma glucose has modest sensitivity for prediabetes screening, with 56% sensitivity and 97.7% specificity [17].

Glycated hemoglobin with a 48 mmol/mol cutoff has 68.4% sensitivity and 95.9% specificity for diabetes diagnosis; however, its use in prediabetes screening is complicated by the varying definitions from ADA and the International Expert Committee (IEC). A previous meta-analysis has shown that HbA1c was neither sensitive nor specific in detecting prediabetes, with a mean sensitivity of 49% and specificity of 79% [17].

Previous studies evaluated the reproducibility of both IGT and IFG and showed that the kappa coefficient for IGT indicated a poor-to-fair agreement (0.04 to 0.56), while it indicated a moderate agreement for IFG (0.22 to 0.56). The reproducibility of IGT was reported at 33–48%, whereas IFG was 51–64%. These results suggested that the reproducibility of prediabetes defined by FPG or 2hBG (~50%) is lower than that for diabetes (> 70%). However, there is limited data on the reproducibility of HbA1c for prediabetes [14].

Studies have found biological variability of glycemic markers, which drove the ADA diagnostic recommendation to repeat glycemic marker testing (glucose or/and HbA1c) on two different occasions to minimalize a false-positive diagnosis. However, the latest study suggested that the diagnosis of diabetes based on HbA1c and FBG tested on a single plasma test had a high positive predictive value for subsequent diagnosis and thus strongly associated with clinical endpoints. Therefore, the use of a single simple confirmatory test may limit the effect of biological variability in individual tests and the collection of a second plasma sample, and thus decrease the rate of false-positive diagnosis and increase its specificity [14].

ADA recommendations for diabetes and prediabetes screening in asymptomatic adults include adults aged over 45 years and any overweight adults with at least one risk factor for diabetes. The risk factors include previously tested hemoglobin A1c concentration over 39 mmol/mol, impaired glucose tolerance test (> 7.8 mmol/L), or impaired fasting glucose concentration (> 5.6 mmol/L), first-degree relative with type 2 diabetes, high-risk ethnicity (black, Hispanic, Native American, Alaska Native, Asian, Pacific Islander, or Native Hawaiian), gestational diabetes in women, history of cardiovascular disease, hypertension, high-density lipoprotein cholesterol level of 1.9 mmol/L or less, or triglyceride level of 2.8 mmol/L or more, polycystic ovarian syndrome in women, physical inactivity and other clinical conditions associated with insulin resistance (severe obesity and acanthosis nigricans) [11].

Tinajero and Malik suggested that prediabetes screening should be done earlier (≥ 30 years old) in groups with higher risk of type 2 diabetes and at lower BMI levels (≥ 23 kg/m^2). Screening should include the measurement of visceral adiposity (waist circumference) with ethnic-specific cutoff values. Pregnant women should be screened for gestational diabetes early in the second trimester, while high-risk women should be screened earlier [1].

If the fasting glucose concentration, 2-h plasma glucose concentration and/or hemoglobin A1c concentration are within the normal limit, ADA recommended repeated testing at 3-year intervals and annually for individuals with prediabetes [1].

The US Preventive Services Task Force (USPTF) recommended screening for overweight or obese adults aged 40–70 years and adults with at least one of the following risk factors: family history of diabetes, history of gestational diabetes or polycystic ovarian syndrome and high-risk ethnicity. If results are within the normal range, the testing should be repeated at 3-year intervals [21, 22].

Special consideration is needed for ethnic/racial minorities with higher prevalence and complications. Population with African American, American Indians or Alaskan Natives, Asian Americans, Hispanic or Latinos, or Native Hawaiians or Pacific Islanders ethnicity should be considered for screening at a younger age or at a lower BMI cutoff [17].

3.6 Intervention

Management for prediabetic patients may delay or prevent the development of diabetes mellitus. Both ADA and European Society of Cardiology (ESC) recommended a combination of lifestyle modifications and pharmacotherapy for the management of prediabetes [2]. These include optimal glycemic control, lipid-lowering therapy for cardiovascular disease prevention, anti-hypertensive treatment and aspirin therapy for cardiovascular disease prevention if needed [17].

There are currently four approved medications for prediabetes state: Metformin, Pioglitazone, Acarbose and Liraglutide. The American Association of Clinical Endocrinologists (AACE) has also proposed three weight loss therapies: orlistat, lorcaserin and phentermine/topiramate ER; and lastly, the American College of Surgeons Bariatric Surgery Center Network (ACS-BSCN) has also proposed bariatric surgery as a possible intervention for type 2 diabetes and also prediabetes in order to aid body mass loss (**Figure 2**) [10].

A long-term adherence to lifestyle modification is required in order to ensure the benefits of preventing overt diabetes. Motivational therapy is needed to ensure timely and optimal management of prediabetes and should be personalized based on the patient's needs, preferences and values. The American Association of Diabetes Educators encouraged the primary care physician to utilize a comprehensive framework for healthy behaviors in the prediabetic population. Common elements in these approaches include digital education program, professional health coaching, tracking and group therapy support [23].

3.7 Reversal of prediabetes to Normal glucose regulation

Several studies on diabetes prevention have reported cases where subjects experienced a restoration of normal glucose regulation. Lifestyle modification with supervision from a physiotherapist was reported to have declines in body weight (2.3–3.7%) and experienced glycemic improvements accompanied by favorable changes in plasma pressure, lipids and hyperinsulinemia and restoration of acute insulin secretory response to glucose [13].

Bariatric surgery has been associated with the reversal or prevention of type 2 diabetes through weight loss, improved insulin sensitivity and alteration in inflammatory cytokines. A previous study showed a ~ 90% reduction in type 2 diabetes incidents during a 15 years period in subjects who underwent bariatric surgery [13].

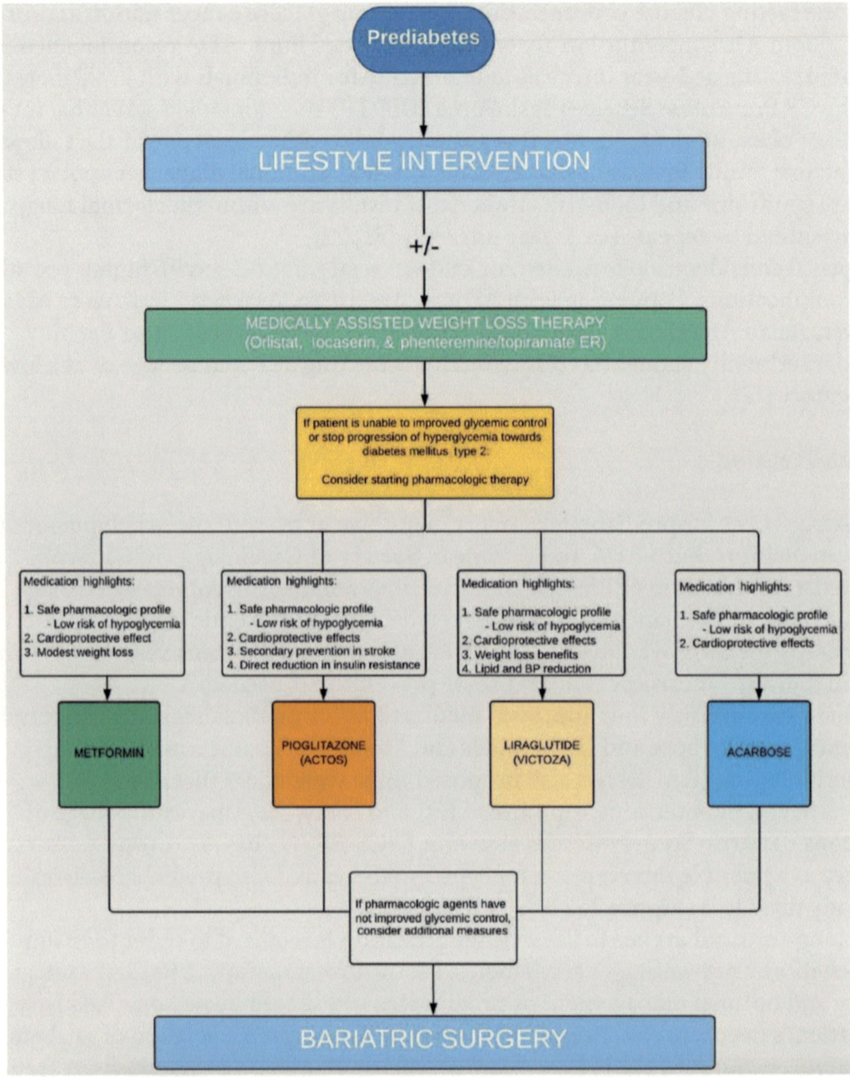

Figure 2.
Management algorithm for people without overt diabetes [10].

Prediabetes state has long been associated with micro- and macrovascular complications. A previous study showed that the reversal of prediabetes to normal glucose regulation was associated with lower risk (~56%) of incident diabetes mellitus. The number of times a patient achieved normoglycemic was shown to have a direct association with the risk reduction in the diabetes incidence: 47% if normoglycemia was performed once, 61% if achieved twice and 67% if achieved thrice. This risk reduction was independent of the prior treatment group [13].

The decreased incidence of diabetes mellitus in patients experiencing the reversal to normal glucose regulation had been associated with the corresponding reduction in the prevalence of microvascular disease after a 15-years follow-up. Regression of the prediabetes state into normal glucose regulation was also associated with a reduction in macrovascular risk. The reversion from 2hPG-defined prediabetes to normoglycemia was associated with a reduced risk of cardiovascular disease and mortality [13].

In a previous meta-analysis, the annual relative risk of regression of IGT to normoglycemia was estimated at 33%. This study also mentioned the high variability of the regression based on 2hBG concentrations. In the British Whitehall study, individuals with prediabetes (defined by HbA1c) were less likely to regress to normoglycemia than individuals with isolated IFG or IGT or a combination of both in a 5 years follow-up [14].

4. Conclusion

Prior to the onset of diabetes mellitus, a state known as prediabetic precedes. Similar to diabetes, prediabetes is also associated with macro- and microvascular complications and carries a higher risk for the development of diabetes. Early and effective screening may aid in earlier intervention and result in the delay and even prevention of overt diabetes. Studies have shown that prediabetes individuals may revert to normal glucose regulation with effective interventions and therefore may help reduce the burden of diabetes disease in the general population. Screening for prediabetes, either with fasting glucose concentration, 2-h plasma glucose concentration or hemoglobin A1c concentration, should be done in a high-risk population instead of the general population to maximize the cost-effectiveness of screening tests.

Acknowledgements

No financial support was received for this article.

Conflict of interest

There are no conflicts of interest regarding the publication of this article.

Author details

Loudry Amsal Elfa Gustanar* and Nanang Miftah Fajari
Endocrinology Division, Department of Internal Medicine, Faculty of Medicine, Lambung Mangkurat University, Ulin General Hospital Banjarmasin, Indonesia

*Address all correspondence to: loudryaeg@gmail.com

References

[1] Tinajero MG, Malik VS. An update on the epidemiology of type 2 diabetes. Endocrinology and Metabolism Clinics of North America. 2021;**50**(3):337-355. DOI: 10.1016/j.ecl.2021.05.013

[2] Rett K, Gottwald-Hostalek U. Understanding prediabetes: Definition, prevalence, burden and treatment options for an emerging disease. Current Medical Research and Opinion. 2019;**35**(9):1529-1534. DOI: 10.1080/03007995.2019.1601455

[3] Peer N, Balakrishna Y, Durao S. Screening for type 2 diabetes mellitus. Cochrane Database of Systematic Reviews. 2020;(6):5. DOI: 10.1002/14651858.CD005266.pub2

[4] Ahlqvist E, Storm P, Käräjämäki A, Martinell M, Dorkhan M, Carlsson A, et al. Novel subgroups of adult-onset diabetes and their association with outcomes: A data-driven cluster analysis of six variables. The Lancet Diabetes & Endocrinology. 2018;**6**(5):361-369. DOI: 10.1016/S2213-8587(18)30051-2

[5] Toledano Y, Knobler H. Not all patients with type 2 diabetes are equal. The American Journal of Medicine. 2021;**134**(6):707-709. DOI: 10.1016/j.amjmed.2021.02.005

[6] Ley SH, Schulze MB, Hivert M, Meigs JB, Hu FB. Diabetes in America. 3rd ed. Vol 1. National Library of Medicine's Bookshelf. Chapter 13 Risk Factors for Type 2 Diabetes. 2017

[7] Ismail L, Materwala H, Al Kaabi J. Association of risk factors with type 2 diabetes: A systematic review. Computational and Structural Biotechnology Journal. 2021;**19**:1759-1785. DOI: 10.1016/j.csbj.2021.03.003

[8] Laakso M. Biomarkers for type 2 diabetes. Molecular Metabolism. 2019;**27**:S139-S146. DOI: 10.1016/j.molmet.2019.06.016

[9] Davarpasand T, Hosseinsabet A. Prediabetes, heart mechanics, and echocardiography: A narrative review. Echocardiography. 2021;**38**(2):304-313. DOI: 10.1111/echo.14929

[10] Zand A, Ibrahim K, Patham B. Prediabetes: Why should we care? Methodist DeBakey Cardiovascular Journal. 2018;**14**(4):289. DOI: 10.14797/mdcj-14-4-289

[11] Dugan J, Cantillep A, Newberry K, Shubrook J. A call to action on prediabetes. Journal of the American Academy of Physician Assistants. 2018;**31**(10):26-30. DOI: 10.1097/01.JAA.0000545064.33107.8f

[12] Janet Mary G, Karthiga KA. Prediabetes: Prevalence, screening, risk factors, and interventions: A review. IP Journal of Nutrition, Metabolism and Health Science. 2020;**2**(1):8-13. DOI: 10.18231/j.ijnmhs.2019.002

[13] Sallar A, Dagogo-Jack S. Regression from prediabetes to normal glucose regulation: State of the science. Experimental Biology and Medicine. 2020;**245**(10):889-896. DOI: 10.1177/1535370220915644

[14] Echouffo-Tcheugui JB, Kengne AP, Ali MK. Issues in defining the burden of prediabetes globally. Current Diabetes Reports. 2018;**18**(11):105. DOI: 10.1007/s11892-018-1089-y

[15] Mahat RK, Singh N, Arora M, Rathore V. Health risks and interventions in prediabetes: A review. Diabetes &

Metabolic Syndrome: Clinical Research & Reviews. 2019;**13**(4):2803-2811. DOI: 10.1016/j.dsx.2019.07.041

[16] Mathew TK, Zubair M, Tadi P. Blood Glucose Monitoring. 2023 Apr 23. In: StatPearls [Internet]. Treaseure Island (FL): StatPearls Publishing; 2023 Jan. PMID: 32310436

[17] Duan D, Kengne AP, Echouffo-Tcheugui JB. Screening for diabetes and prediabetes. Endocrinology and Metabolism Clinics of North America. 2021;**50**(3):369-385. DOI: 10.1016/j.ecl.2021.05.002

[18] Gurung P, Zubair M, Jialal I. Plasma Glucose. 2023 Jan 18. In: StatPearls [Internet]. Treasure Island (FL): StatPearls Publishing; 2023 Jan. PMID: 31082125

[19] Matthews DR, Hosker JR, Rudenski AS, Naylor BA, Treacher DF, Turner RC, et al. Homeostasis model assessment: Insulin resistance and fl-cell function from fasting plasma glucose and insulin concentrations in man. Diabetologia. 1985;**28**(7):412-419. DOI: 10.1007/BF00280883

[20] Hrebícek J, Janout V, Malincíková J, Horáková D, Cízek L. Detection of insulin resistance by simple quantitative insulin sensitivity check index QUICKI for epidemiological assessment and prevention. The Journal of Clinical Endocrinology and Metabolism. 2002;**87**(1):144-147. DOI: 10.1210/jcem.87.1.8292

[21] Jonas DE, Crotty K, Yun JDY, Middleton JC, Feltner C, Taylor-Phillips S, et al. Screening for prediabetes and type 2 diabetes: Updated evidence report and systematic review for the US Preventive Services Task Force. JAMA-Journal of The American Medical Association. 2021;**326**(8):744-760. DOI: 10.1001/jama.2021.10403

[22] US Preventive Services Task Force. Screening for prediabetes and type 2 diabetes: US Preventive Services Task Force Recommendation Statement. JAMA-Journal of The American Medical Association. 2021;**326**(8):736-743. DOI: 10.1001/jama.2021.12531

[23] Kalra S, Singal A, Kapoor N. Prediabetes: A pragmatic approach to counselling and coaching. Journal of the Pakistan Medical Association. 2022;**72**(4):771-772. DOI: 10.47391/JPMA.22-29

Chapter 3

Fuelling Life and Managing Surplus: Revisiting Type 2 Diabetes

Uwe Gudat

"The narrative is biology, the language is chemistry, the alphabet is physics."

Abstract

Type 2 Diabetes (T2D) is becoming an increasing global health challenge. Despite intensive efforts to understand its pathophysiology we seem still to be scratching on the surface. Starting from first principles this essay attempts to explore new ways to approach T2D. The premise is that a prolonged nutrient surplus lies at the heart of T2D. Given that homeostasis relies on steady states that require a balance between in- and efflux to maintain the milieu interieur, imbalances between energy uptake and utilisation can only be reconciled by storing unused energy. This explains the link between obesity and T2D. But putting on unlimited reserves is impractical. This is the dilemma the body faces. The natural conclusion is to reduce energy intake or increase expenditure to regain balance. The essay further explores rates of change of fluxes as the medium through which homeostatic control occurs. Steady states are maintained by resisting perturbations and in that way create corridors of control. In closing the essay advocates a pluralistic integrated approach to studying the multi-faceted phenomena that underlie T2D.

Keywords: type 2 diabetes, glucose, fatty acids, ketone bodies, steady state, flux rates, adipocytes, buffers, insulin, rates of change, exercise, diet

1. Introduction

The purpose of this chapter is to revisit the disease mechanisms and dynamics underlying T2D starting from first principles to come closer to an understanding of what is causing the condition and how best to approach it therapeutically. Nutrition therapy or "diet" that is limiting energy intake and being more physically active, thereby increasing energy expenditure are widely considered cornerstones in the treatment of women and men with type 2 diabetes mellitus (T2D) [1]. These interventions also delay the onset of T2D in patients with pre-diabetes [2, 3]. Why is this so? Why do they work? What can we learn from them as we make therapeutic choices as we care for women and men with T2D?

2. Fuelling life

"The alphabet is physics" – on the energetics of life itself.

To find answers to these questions it helps to remind ourselves of the energetics of life itself. Life is a self-organising energy dissipative system driven by the flow of energy and entropy [4–6]. Common to all autonomously living organisms is proton flux [7]. In photoautotrophic organisms such as plants photon energy from the sun is translated into a proton flux which is converted into chemical bond energy. Non-photosynthetic or heterotrophic organisms release bond energy via molecular rearrangement and electron transfer onto oxygen as the final electron acceptor to generate a proton gradient and flux. This then transfers the bond energy (releases Gibbs free energy) into smaller energy units such as high energy phosphate bonds of ATP in a process we call oxidative phosphorylation. This is the common fate of all substrates utilised for energy production: catabolic breakdown and liberation of Gibbs free energy as outer electrons of carbon and hydrogen atoms are "donated" to oxygen [8]. The energetics of life are firmly anchored in bond energy and quantum physics [9]. The various substrate classes carbohydrates, lipids and ketone bodies are all carriers of bond energy, and regarding them in isolation when considering energy balance in humans with T2D is probably misleading (**Figure 1**).

"I believe seeing biology as a thermodynamic process governed by the most fundamental laws of physics brings clarity and an understanding of life, its structures, evolution and meaning, which cannot be obtained from other perspectives." [6]

"The language is chemistry" – chemical bonds hold the energy.

Aside from the interchangeability of the various bond-energy sources at the most fundamental level, biochemical pathways that allow the interconversion of energy rich metabolites also propose a wholistic perspective when contemplating energy balance. Of particular importance is the synthesis of fatty acids from carbohydrate precursors as well as the interplay between fatty acid flux and glucose utilisation [10]. The interdependency between carbohydrate and lipid metabolism is also given credence by ectopic lipid deposits characteristic of chronic hyperglycaemia [11].

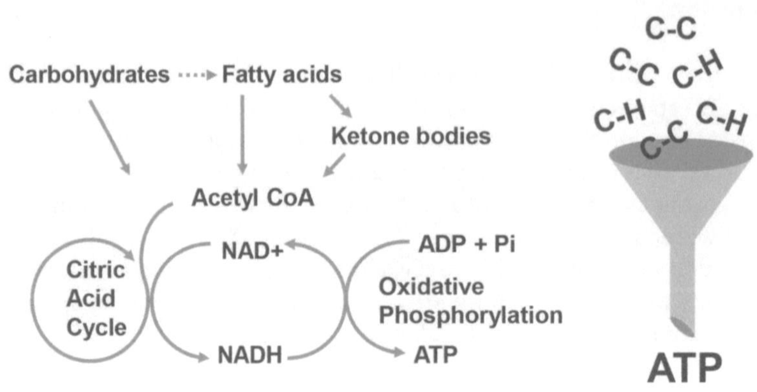

Figure 1.
Turning bond energy into ATP.

Three substrate classes stand out with respect to energy provision in humans: the hexose or pentose sugars and their polymers, the fatty acids and their glycerol esters, and ketone bodies derived from the latter.

Glucose is the molecule that has received the most attention with respect to the syndrome we call T2D. A PubMed search for the term "type 2 diabetes mellitus and glucose" yielded more than 72,000 records whereas a query for "type 2 diabetes and fatty acids" just under 7000. (July 2023) Why does glucose receive so much more attention? One possible explanation is that historically it has been easy to detect the sweet taste of glucosuria [12]. Chemically glucose has a 6-carbon skeleton with alcohol groups attached to every aside from the terminal carbon, which carries an aldehyde group. The molecule combines non-polar C-C and C-H bonds with polar side groups. These readily form hydrogen bonds rendering glucose water soluble. The carbon backbone can fold back upon itself to form a ring structure, in which the oxygen of the aldehyde group links up with the terminal carbon at its other end. The ring persists upon polymerisation of glucose to starch, cellulose, or glycogen.

> *Glucose combines water solubility with energy content, reactivity, compact packaging (ring form) and an avidity for polymer formation. With this catalogue of features, it is indeed a remarkable molecule. Unsurprisingly, it is one of the most represented molecular entities in nature.*

The remarkable features of glucose bring with it intriguing challenges. Glucose is osmotically active, requiring cells to store it intracellularly as a polymer: glycogen in animals or starch in plants. Glucose is not inert as a molecule and attaches itself spontaneously to proteins (why glycosylated haemoglobin can be used to monitor metabolic control) [13]. Finally, chronically elevated plasma glucose concentrations predict the complications of long-standing T2D [14–16].

Carbohydrates including glucose are not the major contributor to energy supply. Only an estimated 2% of total on-body energy reserves in humans are stored as carbohydrate. Lipids constitute the principal energy store [17]. This preponderance suggests that focussing only on glucose when contemplating energy utilisation in women and men with T2D may be inappropriate. The advantages of lipids as energy sources stem from a combination of density and metabolic efficiency. Due to their hydrophobic nature lipids are stored in a non-hydrated form. Accordingly, most of the mass of adipocytes is derived from pure triacylglycerol. Free fatty acids (FFA) carry fewer partially oxidised carbon atoms (e.g., OH functional groups) when compared to carbohydrates thus carrying more energy normalised per carbon. Glycogen, the predominant carbohydrate storage form in animal cells is hydrophilic. More than half of the mass of hydrated cellular glycogen is water that does not provide utilizable bond energy. Furthermore, glucose carbons are partially oxidised carrying oxygen bearing functional groups. In terms of the terminal pathway, the products of both FFA and glucose catabolism enter the citric-acid cycle as acetyl-CoA, from whence on they share a common fate. From an energy balance point of view carbohydrates are important but lipids perhaps more so (**Figure 2**).

Triacylglycerols (TAG) and their component FFA chains are not without issues. Long-chain FFA are not water soluble and must be transported attached to albumin in the blood stream, or when conjugated to TAG in lipoprotein transport vehicles. Long-chain FFA do not pass readily through the blood brain barrier and cannot be used by the brain as an energy source [18]. Unlike glucose that is amenable to glycolysis FFA cannot be metabolised anaerobically. Finally, not all tissues can utilise FFA, e.g., erythrocytes which lack mitochondria.

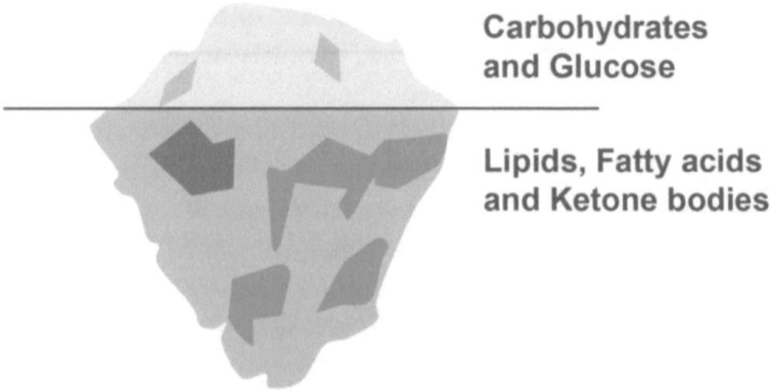

Figure 2.
Carbohydrates above and lipids below the "iceberg" waterline.

The limitations of long chain fatty acids are not prohibitive, as nature has found a work around in the form of ketone bodies. Acetoacetate, beta-hydroxybutyrate and acetone are small soluble molecules synthesised by partial oxidation of fatty acids in hepatic mitochondria. Production and utilisation correspond to a continuation of the catabolic lipid pathway: triacylglycerols to fatty acids to ketone bodies to acetyl-CoA [17]. In clinical practice ketone bodies signal a prolonged catabolic state or the life-threatening complication of ketoacidosis. A focus that does not give credit to their beneficial role in human energy supply, making lipid energy more accessible [19]. Beta-hydroxybutyrate that represents 70% of the blood borne ketone bodies provides an alternative source of energy for tissues when glucose concentrations are low, or tissue function is compromised [20]. In healthy subjects ketonemia is in the range of 0.1–0.4 mmol/l after an overnight fast, accompanied by a high synthesis rate and flux of 0.2–0.4 mmol/min. During a prolonged fast of 5 days ketone body flux rises to 1.5–2.5 mmol/min with concentrations reaching 7–10 mmol/l [21]. Ketone bodies exemplify again how closely carbohydrate and lipid metabolism are linked and interdependent.

Energy in human catabolism is derived to a large part from the oxidation of C−C and C−H bonds, which may be sourced from a variety of substrates [22]. If energy needs are met through the catabolism of one substrate, there is less demand for another. As both the oxidation of glucose and fatty acids delivers acetyl-CoA for the citric acid cycle they are competitive providers of bond energy in many tissues. Energy sourced from one, need no longer be supplied by the other. When enjoying a set menu that involves a choice of the main dish, after having selected and eaten the preferred dish one is satiated and will not wish to eat another. Once a need has been met, the demand abates. Focussing on glucose in isolation without accounting for energy sourced from FFA (or ketones) ignores the fundamentals of supply and demand (**Figure 3**).

"The narrative is biology" – of fluxes and buffers.

Flux drives the motor of life [9]. It is the throughput of bond energy providing substrates that keeps cells running, just as the flow of petrol through a combustion engine keeps a motor running. Catabolic pathways capture free energy released from continuous biological combustion. This continuity of throughput requires that at least one step in a catabolic pathway is sufficiently removed from chemical equilibrium [23]. Let us consider a series of connected ponds as an analogy. When all ponds are at the same height the water levels in the individual ponds are the same (at equilibrium). Water moves back and forth at random between the ponds, but there is no net

DOI: http://dx.doi.org/10.5772/intechopen.1002613

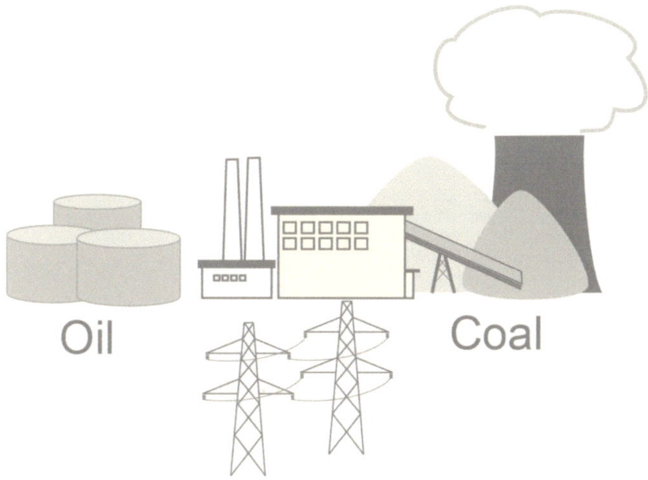

Figure 3.
Competing sources of primary energy: Carbohydrates and lipids.

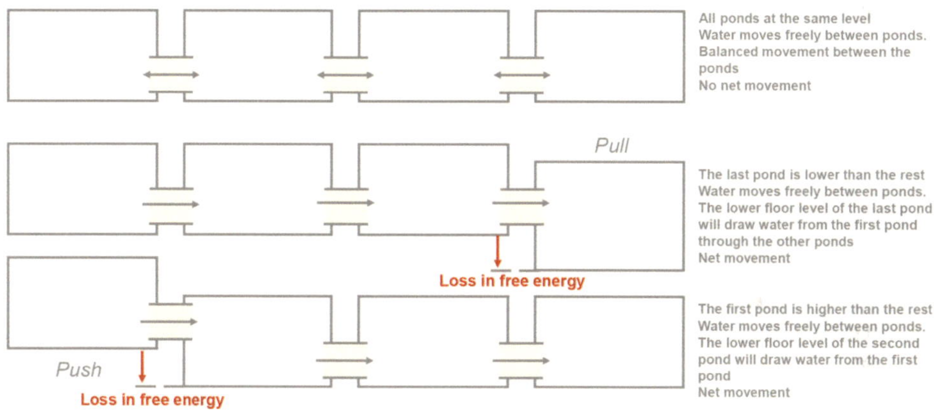

Figure 4.
Connected ponds analogy.

movement of water in any one direction. However, if the first pond in the series is elevated or the last pond is lowered there is a directed flow of water (**Figure 4**).

A directed flux as seen in catabolic pathways requires non-equilibrium states. Non equilibrium states are achieved either by a "push"- (provision of reactants or substrates) or a "pull"-mechanism (removal of reactants) so that a balance cannot set in and there is constant flow through the pathway. Modifying the pond analogy by introducing an inflow into the first and an outflow from the last pond results in a steady stream of water through the ponds. Introducing mill wheels that are turned by the directed flow of water creates a system that captures the flow energy to do work. This is very similar to how a hydroelectric power plant works and resembles the logic of a metabolic pathway (**Figure 5**).

The essential role of flux through metabolic pathways as emphasized by Eric Newsholme at Oxford half a century ago reflects a fundamental understanding of biology itself. An understanding that has been more recently echoed in a chapter title

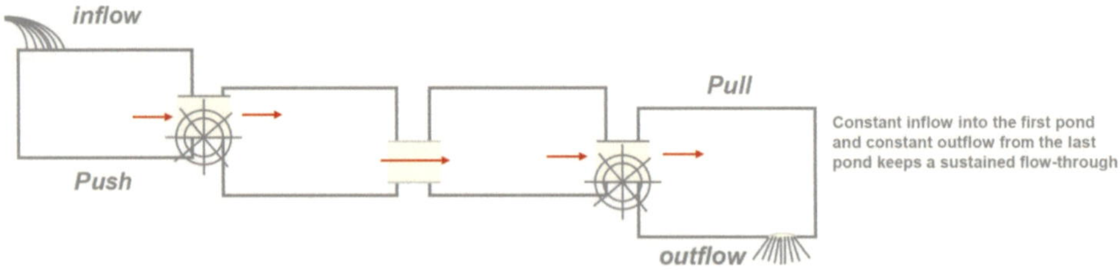

Figure 5.
Modified connected ponds analogy.

"Reconceptualizing the organism: From complex machine to flowing stream" from the book "Everything flows: Toward a processual philosophy of biology [23, 24]". The dissipative nature of biological systems requires a constant flow of energy. Just as the wind, the movement of air allows boats to sail and drives wind turbines, movement of substrates through catabolic pathways fuels life [25].

In medical practice we are often looking at absolute concentrations (e.g., of glucose in the blood) rather than flux rates or throughput. This is also true when considering T2D. In doing so we may be missing important information. For similar concentrations of metabolites in the blood stream may be associated with different flux rates and thus provision of energy [26]. A steady state level is an expression of a balance between in- and outflow. It is not an expression of a specific flux rate. This may be illustrated by a bathtub. If water inflow from a tap and the outflow into the drain are in balance the level in the bathtub remains the same and a steady state is maintained. At the same time the volumes of water entering and leaving may differ considerably: the same level associated with very different flow rates (**Figure 6**). If energy supply to cells follows nutrient flux, focussing on steady state levels (e.g., blood glucose concentrations) may miss important relevant information with respect to the dynamics of T2D (e.g., plausibly altered fluxes in the pre-diabetic state).

There is a fundamental connection between flux, the milieu interieur, and homeostasis. Homeostasis serves to assure an internal environment regulated within bounds, the milieu interieur. Balanced flux rates create the steady states which constitute homeostasis [27]. The milieu interieur represents a network of steady states, each kept within boundaries by balancing as much as necessary respective in- and outflows so controlled levels can be maintained (**Figure 7**).

As noted with the bathtub analogy however, balanced flux rates underlying a given steady state may be very different. In- and outflow through a system may not be comparable although on the surface in terms of concentrations everything looks the same. This is a critical idea to hold onto for the further discussion.

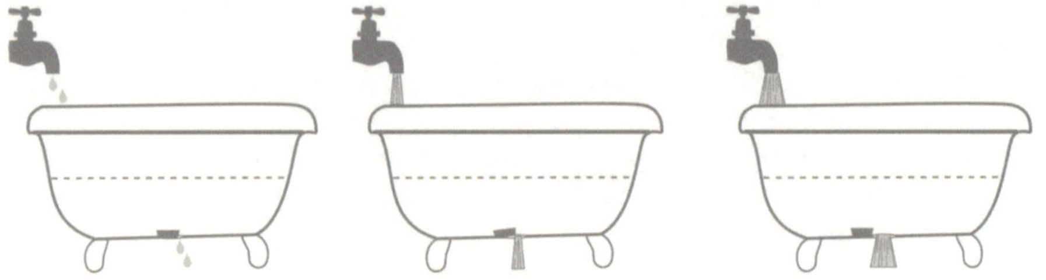

Figure 6.
Different possible flux rates underlying a common steady state level.

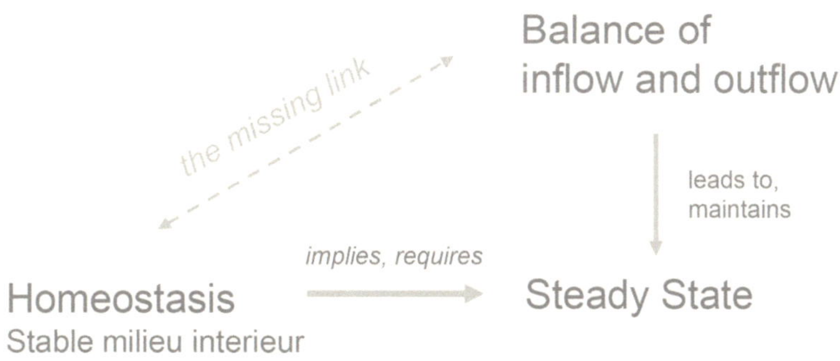

Figure 7.
Balanced flux rates create the steady states of homeostasis.

Cells are the principal organisational unit of biology that must be supplied with sufficient energy to sustain the energy dissipative system of life [28]. Cellular energy demands are continuous and variable. Coordinative efforts are directed at enabling uninterrupted cellular fluxes of substrates under the caveat that whole body uptake of nutrients is discontinuous and that energy demands are variable. This implicates buffers that can absorb and supply substrate on demand (**Figure 8**). The movement in and out of buffers playing an essential role in securing adaptive flux continuity. A network of substrate depots that stockpile nutrients and subsequently release them is intuitive from a systems design perspective. Glycogen and triglyceride depots at the cellular level and the liver and adipocytes at the organ level qualify as dynamic substrate buffers.

Human biology qualifies as a complex system of systems [29, 30]. In which component systems organise into self-regulating sub-systems. The flux of energy, the supply and provision of matter (from which structure evolves), the exchange of information within and between systems (allowing for cooperation and adaptation) etc., requires coordination. Metabolic pathways self-regulate via the concentrations of the reactants and products of the chemical reactions, the flow rates through the system, availability and activities of enzymes and the availability of co-factors [31]. These in turn are modifiable by mechanisms such as hormone signalling induced de-or phosphorylation of a rate limiting enzyme or gene expression. Information may be encoded in constellations and relationships of molecules

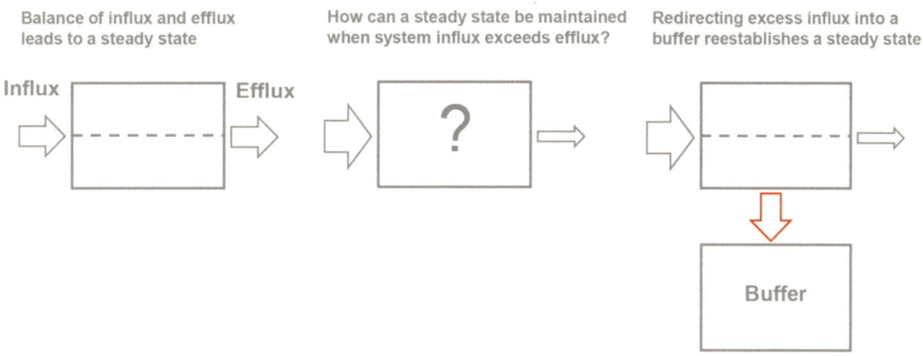

Figure 8.
The critical role of buffers in maintaining steady states.

to one another and their synchronous shifts (rates of change) rather than individual concentrations. In an adaptive self-correcting system, dynamics and rates of change carry the relevant information. Synchronicity or coordination of rates of change being the actual control medium. Homeostatic set points in biology are plausibly phenomena of counter-regulation to perturbations of the internal environment and system inertia rather than the directed attainment of a defined set point. It is the resistance to perturbation that results in convergence toward set points. Response lag times and overshoot manifest as a control interval or homeostatic corridor representing performance characteristics of a self-correcting system. In this understanding rates of change define biological regulation. What we observe when measuring plasma glucose or serum insulin are the cumulative effects of ongoing instantaneous rate adjustments. Figuratively, as we are looking at the water level in a bathtub biology is turning the taps to adjust the inflows and playing with the drains to manipulate the outflows. The water level is an expression of the net effects of these ongoing adjustments.

Multicellular organisms represent collaborative communities. With increasing organisational complexity more sophisticated mechanisms are applied to facilitate their cooperation. Signalling molecules such as hormones and the information flow they support serve this purpose. Homeostatic substrate regulation serves to assure that all the cells of the body are adequately supplied with energy rich metabolites. In this understanding the purpose of blood glucose regulation is a "means to end, and not an end in itself". The controlled variable is the provision of nutrient to critical tissues. If this understanding is applied what is regulated are not substrate concentrations rather adequate cellular substrate fluxes. These must suffice to meet energy demands, accounting for differential substrate utilisation by diverse cell populations. The system provides a flow of energy rich metabolites that allows cells to meet their needs. Human biology follows a multi-fuel model in which a mix of substrates is on offer. Homeostatic adaptation involves adjusting the blend of circulating energy rich substrates at the flux level, which reflects itself in their circulating concentrations.

Glucose is the by far the preferred substrate of the central nervous system. The selfish brain hypothesis gives priority to the brain's substrate needs proposing that prevention of neuroglycopenia is the objective of blood glucose homeostasis [32]. Coordinating access to systemic glucose supply between tissues that can clear large quantities of glucose from the blood stream is intuitive in the light of the threat that neuroglycopenia represents. Loss of consciousness when escaping from a predator due to increased muscle glucose uptake is unlikely to confer an evolutionary advantage. Following this line of reasoning one or more fuel gauges that monitor and inform of substrate availability in the central compartment and signal glucose surplus above the limits needed to secure brain function carries engineering elegance (**Figure 9**). The pancreatic islet qualifies as such a device. If structure follows function, then anatomical location can point to functional purpose. Islets of Langerhans are found in the tail of the pancreas in proximity to the aorta. Blood perfusing the pancreatic artery can be considered providing an informative sample of central aortic blood representative of that flowing through the carotids. Sensing glucose content in these samples and sharing this information through the systemic circulation provides a means to synchronize supply and demand; to coordinate between major actors in the regulation of substrate availability liver, muscle and adipose tissue. This in such a way that it assures adequate substrate availability for the brain. It informs cells of systemic substrate availability, for example, glucose available to the brain [33–35]. Plausibly, a well-fed brain is at the heart of glucose homeostasis and insulin helps

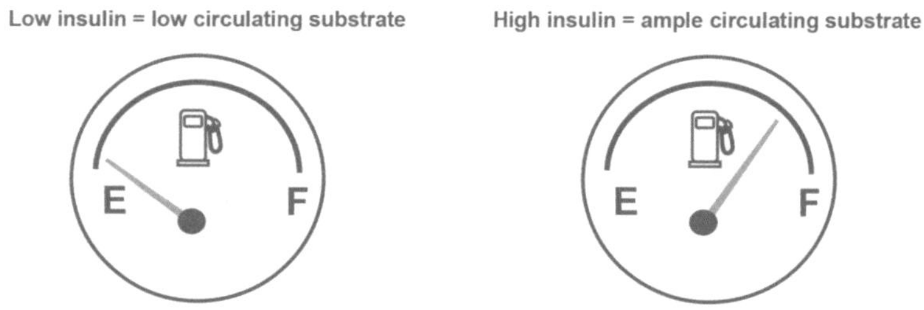

Figure 9.
Insulin a figurative fuel gauge?

to make this happen. Insulin concentrations constituting the permissive signal for glucose uptake. Rates of change in glucose availability may be the pertinent signal that is responded to directly by changing rates of glucose uptake correspondingly. The concept deserving consideration is that substrate regulation is more appropriately represented by calculus (rates of change) than by algebra (absolute concentrations). Computationally the coordination and callibration of rates of change may be more straight forward than working with concentrations. As in the former only the direction of change and proportionality suffice to engineer a tailored response [36].

Cellular signalling serves the receipt, integration, and distribution of information. Intercellular communication involves attachment of a ligand to a molecular docking site on target cells resulting in a conformational change of the latter. Binding alters the spatial arrangement of atoms in the target changing its properties by exposing or hiding a catalytic site, opening or closing a channel, etc. These conformational changes alter the molecule's behaviour modifying its catalytic activity, allowing or preventing in- or outflow of ions etc. Such effects subsequently trigger downstream events resulting in the multi-step relay of information, culminating in a terminal effector step for example, the phosphorylation of an enzyme, changing the site at which a molecule is found (translocation of GLUT 4 to the plasma membrane), or initiation of gene expression and subsequent synthesis of a peptide or protein. All regulation traces back to arrangements and associations of atoms and resulting alterations in molecular behaviour.

This is relevant when contemplating one of T2D's hallmarks, insulin resistance. If insulin is contended to "mandate" glucose uptake, as is suggested by the concept of "insulin resistance" there must be a corresponding molecular mechanism in place. The argument deserving consideration is that insulin provides a permissive rather than mandatory signal. Metabolic flux rates are generally regulated by a "push-pull". The "push" represented by the concentrations of reactants and the "pull" by the passing on of products to the next step in a sequence. The additive effects of push and pull driving the flux rate subject to bottlenecks such as the activities of rate limiting enzymes or availability of transporters. Similarly cellular nutrient uptake can be envisaged to respond to a push-pull logic, subject to bottlenecks [37, 38]. Research in T2D has emphasised the push side of this logic, represented by blood glucose concentrations and the ambient concentrations of insulin. An example of modifying pull given by improvements of insulin-mediated glucose uptake in muscle following exercise. The logic of fluxes proposes a "pull me - push you" analogous to the fable animal "pushmi-pullyu" in Hugh Lofting's Doctor Dolittle. Why should cells take up glucose if their energy requirements are met and their buffers full? The construct of insulin resistance hints that glucose uptake at the cellular level is independently regulated by insulin without accounting for cellular substrate needs or storage capacity. This may represent a too narrow view.

3. Managing surplus

The increasing prevalence of obesity in many parts of the world provides indirect evidence that energy intake for many of us is above our requirements. How much energy do we really need? Resting energy expenditure (REE) which corresponds to the energy consumed when inactive equates to approximately 4.2 KJ/kg (1 Kcal/kg) per hour in humans. For a sedentary 70 kg male an intake of approximately 7000 kJ (1700 kcal) balances daily resting energy needs with expenditure [39]. The same energy is contained in 3 Big Mac Hamburgers (590 Kcal or 2468 KJ). (McDonalds) [40] For a sedentary woman of 58 kg about 5800 kJ (1400 kcal) per day suffice [39]. The energy contained in the main nutrient classes are 37 kJ/g (9 kcal/g) for fat, 3.75 kcal (16 kJ)/g for carbohydrates and 17 kJ/g (4 kcal/g) for protein [41]. Thus about 200 g of fat meet the daily requirements of a sedentary 70 kg male. A handful of peanuts (about 300 g) at 2400 kJ/g (570 kcal/g) meet these energy needs for a day [42].

In parallel to an increasing availability of nutrients in many regions the need to be physically active decreases. It is estimated that labour saving household devices alone decrease domestic energy expenditure by about 110 kcal/day [43].

Assuring an adequate energy flux is essential to maintaining life. What if energy supply exceeds demand? The dilemma facing human biology in many regions of the world today is a persistent positive energy balance. The energy content of ingested nutrients exceeds energy expenditure. A situation resembling a bathtub where inflow is greater than outflow. If maintained for long enough the bathtub will overflow (**Figure 10**).

Applied to T2D, homeostatic mechanisms strive to maintain a controlled milieu interieur by balancing influxes and effluxes to create steady states. Critical herein are holding devices. When nutrient intake consistently exceeds demand transient buffers are repurposed to provide permanent storage. Energy assimilated in the form of nutrients must either be consumed by doing work (e.g., thermoregulation, anabolic synthesis, locomotion, fuelling of host defences etc.) or stored. With a more sedentary life-style energy expenditure declines. If coupled with an unchanged or even greater intake of nutrients a surplus sets in. Energy not used must be excreted (e.g., glucosuria) or stored. In humans with T2D renal glucose loss is usually modest. Most of the excess in energy providing substrates must be stored. Adipocytes are the principal energy storing cells. Consequently, adipose tissue mass increases, as reflected in the increasing global prevalence of obesity (**Figure 11**) [44].

Storing excess energy for times of lack is essential for survival. However, there comes a point where the benefits of securing reserves are plausibly offset by the cost

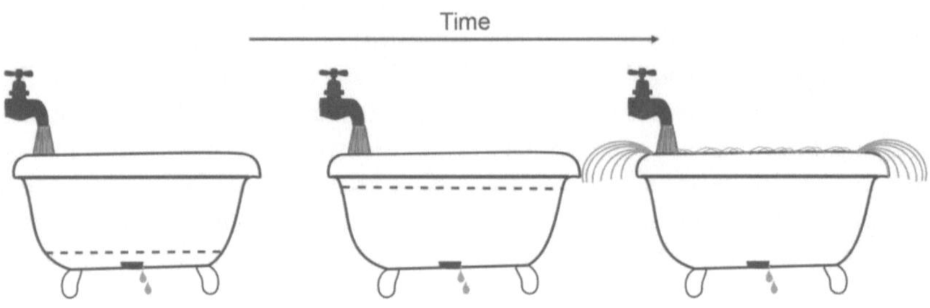

Figure 10.
Persistent surplus leads to overflow.

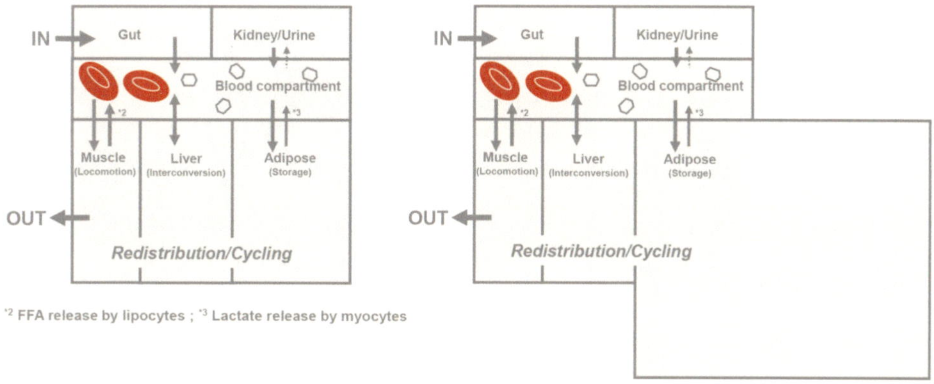

Figure 11.
Expansion of adipose tissue.

of warehousing, as illustrated by the Pickwick Syndrome. For an ambulatory species large on-body energy reserves compromise the ability to hunt and forage or escape from predators. Accordingly, from an evolutionary point of view a case can be made for putting a limit on long-term stockpiling. The evolutionary objective lying in finding a compromise, that secures reserves for times of lack, while not putting survival at risk. This reminds of the children's story of Goldilocks and the 3 Bears, in which the moral of the story was to get it "just right"; to avoid excesses to either side of too much or not enough. Extending this line of thought, the additional functions that more recently are being attributed to adipose tissue also suggest that expanding total body fat mass limitlessly is not expected to be otherwise innocuous. Also when accounting for the heterogeneity of fat depots [28].

The focus in seeking to understand T2D often concentrates on the triumvirate pancreatic islet, liver, and muscle. In 1994 at the EASD meeting in Düsseldorf Gerald Reaven proposed that in so doing a major tissue showing GLUT4 insulin mediated glucose uptake, was being under-represented [45]. Adipocytes represent the body's principal energy warehouse, holding about 4500 kcal/19000 kJ (men) and about 5500 kcal/23200 kJ (women) of energy per kg [46]. The total amount of stockpiled energy depending on the fat mass. Adipose tissue is *the* "energy buffer" of the body. This deserves to be kept in mind when reflecting upon chronic energy surplus.

Let us consider the following thought experiment. What if adipocytes behaved similarly to balloons? When a balloon is empty and there is no wall tension, no resistance is encountered when blowing air into it. As the balloon fills and its walls stretch resistance increases, and it may become impossible to blow it up further (without bursting it). The resistance of balloons to further stretching depending on their natural size, the properties of the materials used and the wall thickness. In practice we need to blow harder to fill more air into a progressively more filled balloon (**Figure 12**).

If human adipocytes were to show similar properties, long-standing nutrient surplus over time would be expected to lead to increasing resistance to the uptake of further nutrients (mirroring a balloon's resistance to further distension) [47]. In this situation the balance between FFA uptake and esterification versus hydrolysis and FFA release by adipocytes shifts. The driving force for the shift is a property of the adipocyte itself and its willingness to store additional substrate. The increase in the proportion of large abdominal adipocytes seen in patients with T2DM matches these

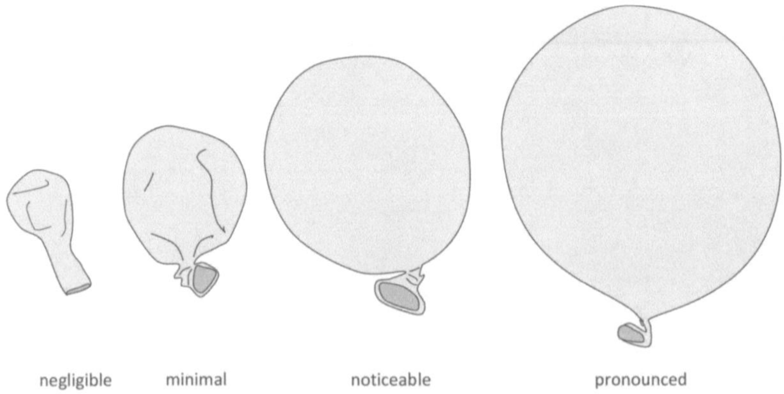

Figure 12.
As a balloon inflates blowing it up becomes more difficult.

considerations [48]. As does data linking enlarged subcutaneous abdominal adipocytes with hyperinsulinaemia, insulin resistance, glucose intolerance and an increase in *in vitro* lipolysis [49, 50].

To draw on a related analogy. If a parking lot is full the next car can only enter once a car leaves. Storage facilities generally show a maximal uptake capacity. In a biological system this may be a probabilistic rather than a deterministic limit. The preponderance to to take up and store further nutrients depending on a variety of variables including cross-membrane concentration gradients. Beyond the carrying capacity of adipocytes with increasing body-mass other organs also increase in size leading to a further increase in stockpiling ability. Resting energy expenditure also increases leading to a greater tolerance for energy surplus [46]. However, despite a catalogue of noteworthy adaptive mechanisms the ability to deal with a chronic excess in nutrients is likely to show limits. Limits that differ between individuals [51].

If the above thought experiment has merits, with a prolonged surplus in energy intake and a progressive unwillingness of adipocytes to take up additional energy rich substates, clearance of these substrates from the blood stream decreases. Until now we have considered adipocytes in isolation and ignored any signals concerning systemic substrate availability. Let us continue to do so. As the figurative lorries laden with supply are turned away from the warehouses, they go back on the road eventually returning to the dispatcher. In the human body this is the liver, which is confronted with an increase in returning uncleared energy rich substrate, primarily FFA. FFA are the principle aerobic energy substrate at the whole-body level at rest. This increased FFA supply does not leave glucose uptake unaffected [52]. If energy requirements remain unchanged glucose utilisation is expected to decrease [53]. Implicitly it becomes more difficult to maintain the steady state in blood glucose and blood glucose concentrations rise. Insulin concentrations which track blood glucose also rise. This constellation of increased blood glucose and insulin concentrations reminds of T2D.

Circumstantial evidence suggests that T2D may qualify as an unwillingness to warehouse high energy substrates to the extent needed to assure normoglycaemia [54]. Maintaining a steady state requires that efflux balances influx. If nutrient influx increases and energy utilisation decreases, balance can only be secured by shunting surplus into buffers. Once the storage capacity of these is reached or they otherwise throttle uptake a steady state can no longer be maintained, as clearance no longer matches inflow. Such an aetiological scenario is supported by epidemiological data demonstrating a strong correlation between T2D and adiposity. While not all obese women and men develop T2D with increasing excess body fat the proportion rises.

The natural history frequently shown by humans when moving from impaired glucose tolerance (IGT) to frank T2D is consistent with such a model. In healthy individuals ingested glucose is rapidly cleared from the blood stream and stored. In settings of IGT analogous to trying to find a parking spot in peak times, complete storage of a glucose load is delayed. Finally, in frank T2D not all ingested substrates can be removed before the next meal. This is not unlike the situation in populated metropolitan areas where the availability of parking is chronically below demands. Cars that cannot find a regular place to park either continue circling looking for an empty spot or park illegally (**Figure 13**). While the trivial nature of this analogy is recognised it may be illustrative of what we are facing when contending T2D.

At the heart of T2D is plausibly an attenuated tendency to expand fat cell mass in an environment of chronic nutrient surplus [55].

This thought experiment anticipates observations seen in T2D and is consistent with much of the evidence that has been published concerning insulin resistance and hyperglycaemia [56]. It also explains why decreasing energy intake and/or increasing energy expenditure are effective in managing women and men with T2D [47]. In the former the storage demands on adipocytes decrease and in the latter storage space is freed up as more energy rich substrate is being consumed.

A wealth of data has been published showing numerous alterations in patients with T2D. Many of these showing associative or correlative phenomena that seem to be coupled with chronically increased blood glucose. A putative mechanism to limit on-body storage of energy rich substrate that puts a cap on body fat depots is consistent with much of this evidence (**Figure 14**).

While the diagnostic criteria for T2D are widely agreed upon, biology may have a different perspective on the matter. The diagnostic limits are possibly historically motivated, influenced by the thresholds for glucosuria. Epidemiological evidence however suggests that the increase in risk of macrovascular complications begins at a lower threshold, in the realm of pre-diabetes [57]. Additional support also comes from interventions directed at post-prandial glucose in patients with pre-diabetes that reduced cardiovascular events [58, 59]. Observations that agree with a role of fluxes in the pathophysiology of T2D. The prediabetic state being indicative of altered substrate fluxes, leading to difficulties in maintaining the steady state.

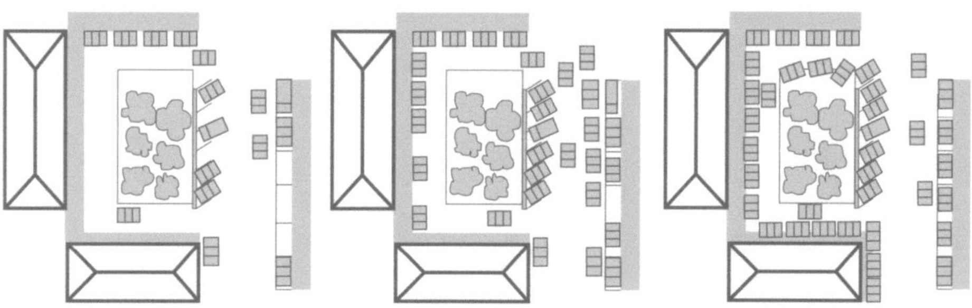

Figure 13.
No where to park: Keep circling or park illegally.

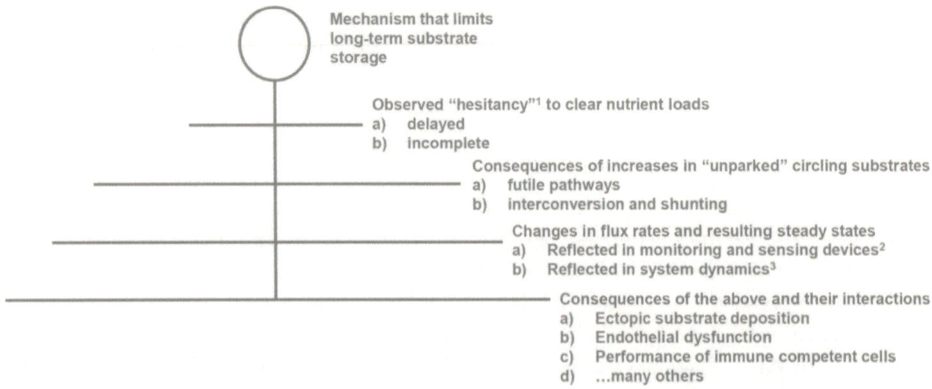

Figure 14.
A systems biology perspective on limiting substrate storage.

As an aside, the current discussion intentionally does not include the gut, – islet – liver axis and the complex distributed biocomputing realised therein. The role of the gut, pancreatic islet, liver network is understood as primarily to secure efficient nutrient absorption. It lies upstream of dealing with an established chronic surplus of nutrients.

Looking now at the other end of the disease lifecycle. With increasing duration of chronic nutrient surplus, the glucoregulatory system seems to be adversely affected [55, 56, 60]. If homeostatic control is achieved through synchronicity of rates of change, then a signalling system would need to maintain a dynamic range that allows for rate changes to be monitored and relayed when the baseline shifts. Increases in serum insulin in response to chronic rises in blood glucose concentrations may not passively follow blood glucose, but rather be actively readjusted to maintain a dynamic range. Such a mechanism would allow ongoing signalling of rates of change of blood glucose concentrations despite a shift in baseline blood glucose concentrations. Beta cell failure in such an understanding represents less the inability of insulin secretion to keep up with rising blood glucose, rather blood glucose concentrations moving out of the physiological insulin response curve. Unless the glucose-insulin response curve adjusts as blood glucose rises chronically, insulin secretion will concentrate on the top of the dose response curve. The result is a compromised ability to effectively signal changes (**Figure 15A**). If the whole curve moves right to adjust for the change in baseline the dynamic range for insulin would be regained (**Figure 15B**). However, only shifting the same curve horizontally does not account for the greater spread of blood glucose

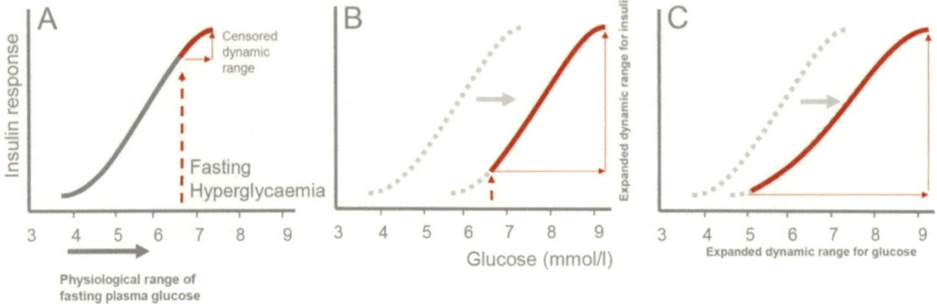

Figure 15.
Maintaining the dynamic range of insulin signalling.

concentrations seen in T2D. Which is achieved by stretching the curve (**Figure 15C**). These adjustments in insulin secretion kinetics moving from normal glucose tolerance to T2D are what is observed experimentally [61]. There is one more aspect to consider. To draw on the analogy of travelling in a vehicle, the faster one is travelling the more difficult it becomes to accelerate. Plausibly, the beta cell is facing the same dilemma. While it is striving to signal the dynamics in blood glucose, the adjusted high baseline insulin secretion needed to calibrate to the shifted dynamic range of blood glucose makes it difficult to secrete even more insulin. What we paraphrase with "beta cell failure" in patients with T2D may have less to do with failing of the beta cell as such than with blood glucose concentrations moving out of the physiological response range of the glucose sensor. To draw on another analogy. When using a thermometer to measure temperature, not one size fits all. An oven thermometer will measure at a different temperature interval than a freezer thermometer. Using a freezer thermometer to measure body temperature cannot give the desired read-out as the dynamic range is unsuited. This is not a failing of the thermometer.

4. Conclusions

The discussion above reemphasizes the merits of restoring energy balance by reducing energy uptake or increasing energy expenditure when striving to prevent or delay progression of T2D. This is most promising in pre- or early diabetes before long-standing hyperglycaemia has taken its toll on the glucoregulatory apparatus. All the while it must be recognised that eating less and moving more is a lot easier said than done. Energy expenditure while walking equates on average to about 4.8 kJ (1.15 kcal) /kg/1600 m, running expends about 7.15 kJ (1.71 kcal) /kg/1600 m and cycling about 2.5 kJ (0.6 kcal) kg/1600 m [62]. To lose 500 g of adipose tissue by jogging alone requires running for about 16 km. For many this is neither attractive nor feasible. To include bouts of physical activity in our everyday lives such as walking a stop when taking a bus, climbing one or two flights of stairs rather than taking an elevator or escalator and parking the car a little further away from the shops is practical and in the long run adds up. Physical activity used in this way serves to reduce energy surplus and not primarily to acutely lower blood glucose concentrations. The latter has repeatedly been shown to have only modest and short-lived effects in adults with T2D [63].

If a patient is unable reduce energy input or increase energy output directly, pharmacological support should be considered. If the above reasoning is followed, agents that emulate diet and exercise have the greatest theoretical footing. In this respect, the merits of overriding a stipulated hesitancy to store additional surplus energy, as suggested by the gain in body mass during therapy with sulfonylureas and thiazolidinediones seems counterintuitive. With progressive beta cell failure blood glucose control in patients with T2D is no longer as amenable to "diet and exercise", other therapeutic concepts must be adapted [64]. In practical terms, when endogenous insulin secretion is no longer able to replicate glucose dynamics extending the range of the insulin signal by exogenous insulin supplementation should not be unduly delayed.

Returning to the onset of our journey. Could we look at glucose and the other high-energy substrates and their interrelationships differently? Could revisiting the physiological role of insulin help us come closer to answers to the open questions we still face concerning the enigma of T2D? Could a revised understanding of the mechanisms leading to the increasing number of glucose molecules circulating in the blood stream (looking for a place to park) bring us closer to treatments that halt the progression of

T2D seen in many patients. Could such a perspective bring us closer to treatments that put an end to the complications that result from persistent exposure of blood vessels to uncleared glucose moeities? Is it only glucose or not the overall balance of energy-rich substrates that deserves consideration in humans with T2D? Does glucose not only represent the tip of an iceberg of energy rich substrates, in which lipids make up much of what is under the water line? Are not fluxes and flows at the heart of metabolic control rather than concentrations? Does insulin serve to inform more than to command? Are not rates of change the medium through which homeostatic control is negotiated?

Biological organisms are system of systems, within which structure, function, energy, and information flow are intertwined and mutually interdependent [65]. To fully appreciate an organism's dynamics these interrelated aspects deserve to be considered simultaneously. Regarding each aspect in isolation can provide valuable insights, but often provides only an approximative cut-out. As we study T2D further holding multiple lines of thought in parallel may be needed to solve the puzzles we still face. The life mission of the polymath Edward de Bono, who is most famously known for coining the term "lateral thinking", was to develop and teach thinking techniques. Aside from lateral thinking he also advocated parallel thinking. In two popular books *six thinking hats* or *six action shoes* he emphasised the merits of regarding issues simultaneously from multiple perspectives [66, 67]. By looking at T2D from multiple complementary vantage points simultaneously such as supply chain, energy balance, information exchange, control logic, etc. insights may become apparent that remain hidden when each aspect is considered in isolation.

The purpose of this essay is to remind of the fundamentals of energy metabolism when considering T2D. This leads naturally to the merits of matching energy intake to expenditure as has been repeatedly advocated over decades. The goal is also to encourage an unorthodox look at the condition. Rather than provide ready-made answers this essay hopes to stimulate exploration down the road less travelled. By questioning generally accepted facts and revisting taken for granted premises we may come to a revised understanding of a syndrome that is increasing in prevalance globally due to a greater availability of nutrients, a more widespread sedentary lifestyle and aging populations. An understanding that will help us better tackle this insidious syndrome that threatens to become an unsurmountable public health challenge world-wide in terms of the condition itself and its long term complications.

Author details

Uwe Gudat
Aretaeus sàrl, Geneva, Switzerland

*Address all correspondence to: uwe.gudat@aretaeus.ch

References

[1] Davies MJ, Aroda VR, Collins BS, Gabbay RA, Green J, Maruthur NM, et al. Management of hyperglycaemia in type 2 diabetes, 2022. A consensus report by the American Diabetes Association (ADA) and the European Association for the Study of diabetes (EASD). Diabetologia. 2022;**65**(12):1925-1966

[2] Tuomilehto J, Lindstorm J, Eriksson JG, Valle TT, Hamalainein H, Ilanne-Parikka P, et al. Prevention of type 2 diabetes mellitus by changes in lifestyle among subjects with impaired glucose tolerance. The New England Journal of Medicine. 2001;**333**:1343-1350

[3] Knowler WC, Barrett-Connor E, Fowler SE, Hamman RF, Lachin JM, Walker EA, et al. Diabetes prevention program research group. Reduction in the incidence of type 2 diabetes with lifestyle intervention or metformin. The New England Journal of Medicine. 2002;**346**(6):393-403. DOI: 10.1056/NEJMoa012512

[4] Schrödinger E. What Is Life? Cambridge, UK: Cambridge University Press; 1944

[5] Kondepudi DK, De Bari B, James A, Dixon JA. Dissipative structures, organisms and evolution. Entropy. 2020;**22**:1305. DOI: 10.3390/e22111305

[6] Cushman SA. Entropy, ecology, and evolution: Toward a unified philosophy of evolution. Entropy. 2023;**25**:405. DOI: 10.3390/e250300405

[7] Lane N. The vital question. Why is life the way it is? Chapter 3. In: Energy at life's Origin. London, UK: Profile books London; 2015. pp. 89-12

[8] Newsholme EA, Leech TR. Functional Biochemistry. Chichester: Wiley-Blackwell; 2010

[9] Yang X, Heinemann M, Howard J, Greg G, Iyer-Biswas S, Le Treut G, et al. Physical bioenergetics: Energy fluxes, budgets, and constraints in cells. Proceedings of the National Academy of Sciences of the United States of America. 2021;**118**(26):e2026786118. DOI: 10.1073/pnas.2026786118

[10] Hue L, Taegtmeyer H. The Randle cycle revisited: A new head for an old hat. American Journal of Physiology. Endocrinology and Metabolism. 2009;**297**(3):E578-E591

[11] Levelt E, Pavlides M, Banerjee R, Mahmod M, Kelly C, Sellwood J, et al. Ectopic and visceral fat deposition in lean and obese patients with type 2 diabetes. Journal of the American College of Cardiology. 2016;**68**(1):53-63

[12] Raza SI, Raza SA, Kazmi M, Saad M, Hussain I. 100 years of glucose monitoring in diabetes management. Journal of Diabetes Mellitus. 2021;**11**:221-233

[13] Pischetsrieder M. Chemistry of glucose and biochemical pathways of biological interest. Peritoneal Dialysis International. 2000;**20**(Suppl. 2):S26-S30

[14] Pirart J. Diabetes mellitus and its degenerative complications: A prospective study of 4,400 patients observed between 1947 and 1973. Diabetes Care. 1978;**1**(4):252-263

[15] Hadden DR, Patterson CC, Atkinson AB, Kennedy L, Bell PM, McCance DR, et al. Macrovascular disease and hyperglycaemia:

10-year survival analysis in type 2 diabetes mellitus: The Belfast diet study. Diabetic Medicine. 1997;**14**(8):663-672. DOI: 10.1002/(SICI)1096-9136(199708)14:8<663::AID-DIA450>3.0.CO;2-Y

[16] Stratton IM, Adler AI, Neil HA, Matthews DR, Manley SE, Cull CA, et al. Association of glycaemia with macrovascular and microvascular complications of type 2 diabetes (UKPDS 35): Prospective observational study. BMJ. 2000;**321**(7258):405-412. DOI: 10.1136/bmj.321.7258.405

[17] Newsholme EA, Leech TR. Biochemistry for the Medical Sciences. Chichester, UK: John Wiley and Sons; 1983

[18] Schönfeld P, Reiser G. Why does brain metabolism not favor burning of fatty acids to provide energy? - reflections on disadvantages of the use of free fatty acids as fuel for brain. Journal of Cerebral Blood Flow & Metabolism. 2013;**33**:1493-1499

[19] Kolb H, Kempf K, Röhling M, Lenzen-Schulte M, Schloot NC, Martin S. Ketone bodies: From enemy to friend and guardian angel. BMC Medicine. 2021;**19**(1):313. DOI: 10.1186/s12916-021-02185-0

[20] Manolis AS, Manolis TA, Manolis AA. Ketone bodies and cardiovascular disease: An alternate fuel source to the rescue. International Journal of Molecular Sciences. 2023;**24**(4):3534. DOI: 10.3390/ijms24043534

[21] Balasse EO, Fery F. Ketone body production and disposal: Effects of fasting, diabetes, and exercise. Diabetes/Metabolism Reviews. 1989;**5**:247-270

[22] Galgani JE, Moro C, Ravussin E. Metabolic flexibility and insulin resistance. American Journal of Physiology. Endocrinology and Metabolism. 2008;**295**(5):E1009-E1017. DOI: 10.1152/ajpendo.90558.2008 Epub 2008 Sep 2

[23] Curi R, Newsholme P, Marzuca-Nassr GN, Takahashi HK, Hirabara SM, Cruzat V, et al. Regulatory principles in metabolism-then and now. The Biochemical Journal. 2016;**473**(13):1845-1857

[24] Nicholson DJ. Reconceptualizing the organism. From complex machine to flowing stream. In: Nicholson DJ, Dupré J, editors. Everything Flows: Towards a Processual Philosophy of Biology. Oxford, UK: Oxford University Press; 2018

[25] Nicholson DJ. In: Dupré J, editor. Everything Flows. Towards a Processual Philosophy of Biology. Oxford: Oxford University Press; 2018

[26] Hameri T, Fengos G, Ataman M, Miskovic L, Hatzimanikatis V. Kinetic models of metabolism that consider alternative steady-state solutions of intracellular fluxes and concentrations. Metabolic Engineering. 2019;**52**:29-41. DOI: 10.1016/j.ymben.2018.10.005 Epub 2018 Oct 26

[27] Dai Z, Locasale JW. Understanding metabolism with flux analysis: From theory to application. Metabolic Engineering. 2017;**43**(Pt B):94-102. DOI: 10.1016/j.ymben.2016.09.005

[28] Roth J, Szulc AL, Danoff A. Energy, evolution, and human diseases: An overview. The American Journal of Clinical Nutrition. 2011;**93**(4):875S-8783S. DOI: 10.3945/ajcn.110.001909

[29] Lemberger T. Systems biology in human health and disease. Molecular Systems Biology. 2007;**3**:136

[30] Ma'ayan A. Complex systems biology. Journal of the Royal Society Interface. 2017;**14**(134):20170391. DOI: 10.1098/rsif.2017.0391

[31] Newsholme EA, Start C. Regulation in Metabolism. London: John Wiley and Sons; 1973

[32] Peters A, Schweiger U, Pellerin L, Hubold C, Oltmanns KM, Conrad M, et al. The selfish brain: Competition for energy resources. Neuroscience and Biobehavioral Reviews. 2004;**28**(2):143-180. DOI: 10.1016/j.neubiorev.2004.03.002

[33] Rorsman P. The pancreatic beta-cell as a fuel sensor: An electrophysiologist's viewpoint. Diabetologia. 1997;**40**(5):487-495. DOI: 10.1007/s001250050706

[34] MacDonald PE, Joseph JW, Rorsman P. Glucose-sensing mechanisms in pancreatic beta-cells. Philosophical Transactions of the Royal Society of London. Series B, Biological Sciences. 2005;**360**(1464):2211-2225. DOI: 10.1098/rstb.2005.1762

[35] Lu M, Li C. Nutrient sensing in pancreatic islets: Lessons from congenital hyperinsulinism and monogenic diabetes. Annals of the New York Academy of Sciences. 2018;**1411**(1):65-82. DOI: 10.1111/nyas.13448 Epub 2017 Oct 16

[36] Hughes-Hallett D, Lock PF, Gleason AM, Flath DE, Gordon SP, Lomen DO, et al. Applied Calculus. 6th ed. Hoboken: John Wiley and Sons; 2018

[37] Oakes ND, Furler SM. Evaluation of free fatty acid metabolism *in vivo*. Annals of the New York Academy of Sciences. 2002;**967**:158-175. DOI: 10.1111/j.1749-6632.2002.tb04273.x

[38] Peters A. The selfish brain: Competition for energy resources. American Journal of Human Biology. 2011;**23**(1):29-34. DOI: 10.1002/ajhb.21106

[39] Heymsfield SB, Smith B, Dahle J, Kennedy S, Fearnbach N, Thomas DM, et al. Resting energy expenditure: From cellular to whole-body level, a mechanistic historical perspective. Obesity (Silver Spring). 2021;**29**(3):500-511. DOI: 10.1002/oby.23090

[40] Available from: https://www.mcdonalds.com/us/en-us/product/big-mac.html#accordion-c921f9207b-item-842cb18782

[41] Available from: https://www.nutrition.org.uk/health-conditions/overweight-obesity-and-weight-loss/energy-balance-and-weight/?level=Health%20professional

[42] Arya SS, Salve AR, Chauhan S. Peanuts as functional food: A review. Journal of Food Science and Technology. 2016;**53**(1):31-41. DOI: 10.1007/s13197-015-2007-9

[43] Lanningham-Foster L, Nysse LJ, Levine JA. Labor saved, calories lost: The energetic impact of domestic labor-saving devices. Labor saved, calories lost: The energetic impact of domestic labor-saving devices. Obesity Research. 2003;**11**(10):1178-1181. DOI: 10.1038/oby.2003.162

[44] Chooi YC, Ding C, Magkos F. The epidemiology of obesity. Metabolism. 2019;**92**:6-10. DOI: 10.1016/j.metabol.2018.09.005

[45] Reaven GM. The fourth musketeer – From Alexandre dumas to Claude Bernard. Diabetologia. 1995;**38**:3-13

[46] Hwaung P, Bosy-Westphal A, Muller MJ, Geisler C, Heo M,

Thomas DM, et al. Obesity tissue: Composition, energy expenditure, and energy content in adult humans. Obesity (Silver Spring). 2019;**27**(9):1472-1481. DOI: 10.1002/oby.22557

[47] Larson-Meyer DE, Heilbronn LK, Redman LM, Newcomer BR, Frisard MI, Anton S, et al. Effect of calorie restriction with or without exercise on insulin sensitivity, beta-cell function, fat cell size, and ectopic lipid in overweight subjects. Diabetes Care. 2006;**29**(6):1337-1344. DOI: 10.2337/dc05-2565

[48] Pasarica M, Xie H, Hymel D, Bray G, Greenway F, Ravussin E, et al. Lower total adipocyte number but no evidence for small adipocyte depletion in patients with type 2 diabetes. Diabetes Care. 2009;**32**(5):900-902. DOI: 10.2337/dc08-2240 Epub 2009 Feb 19

[49] Weyer C, Foley JE, Bogardus C, Tataranni PA, Pratley RE. Enlarged subcutaneous abdominal adipocyte size, but not obesity itself, predicts type II diabetes independent of insulin resistance. Diabetologia. 2000;**43**(12):1498-1506. DOI: 10.1007/s001250051560

[50] Frankl J, Piaggi P, Foley JE, Krakoff J, Votruba SB. *In vitro* lipolysis is associated with whole-body lipid oxidation and weight gain in humans. Obesity (Silver Spring). 2017;**25**(1):207-214. DOI: 10.1002/oby.21670 Epub 2016 Nov 21

[51] Galgani J, Ravussin E. Energy metabolism, fuel selection and body weight regulation. International Journal of Obesity. 2008;**32**(Suppl 7):S109-S119. DOI: 10.1038/ijo.2008.246

[52] Fryk E, Olausson J, Mossberg K, Strindberg L, Schmelz M, Brogren H, et al. Hyperinsulinemia and insulin resistance in the obese may develop as part of a homeostatic response to elevated free fatty acids: A mechanistic case-control and a population-based cohort study. eBioMedicine. 2021;**65**:103264. DOI: 10.1016/j.ebiom.2021.103264

[53] Roden M. How free fatty acids inhibit glucose utilization in human skeletal muscle. News in Physiological Sciences. 2004;**19**:92-96. DOI: 10.1152/nips.01459.2003

[54] Heilbronn L, Smith SR, Ravussin E. Failure of fat cell proliferation, mitochondrial function and fat oxidation results in ectopic fat storage, insulin resistance and type II diabetes mellitus. International Journal of Obesity and Related Metabolic Disorders. 2004;**28**(Suppl. 4):S12-S21. DOI: 10.1038/sj.ijo.0802853

[55] Dubois SG, Heilbronn LK, Smith SR, Albu JB, Kelley DE, Ravussin E, et al. Decreased expression of adipogenic genes in obese subjects with type 2 diabetes. Obesity. 2006;**14**(9):1543-1552. DOI: 10.1038/oby.2006.178

[56] Boden G. Obesity, insulin resistance and free fatty acids. Current Opinion in Endocrinology, Diabetes, and Obesity. 2011;**18**(2):139-143. DOI: 10.1097/MED.0b013e3283444b09

[57] Schnell O, Standl E. Impaired glucose tolerance, diabetes, and cardiovascular disease. Endocrine Practice. 2006;**12**(Suppl. 1):16-19. DOI: 10.4158/EP.12.S1.16

[58] Chiasson J-L, Josse RG, Gomis R, Hanefeld M, Karasik A, Laakso M, et al. Acarbose treatment and the risk of cardiovascular disease and hypertension in patients with impaired glucose tolerance: The STOP-NIDDM trial. JAMA. 2003;**290**(4):486-494. DOI: 10.1001/jama.290.4.486

[59] Hanefeld M, Schaper F. Acarbose: Oral anti-diabetes drug with additional cardiovascular benefits. Expert Review of Cardiovascular Therapy. 2008;**6**(2):153-163. DOI: 10.1586/14779072.6.2.153

[60] Bagust A, Beale S. Deteriorating beta-cell function in type 2 diabetes: A long-term model. QJM. 2003;**96**(4):281-288. DOI: 10.1093/qjmed/hcg040

[61] Ferrannini E, Gastaldelli A, Miyazaki Y, Matsuda M, Mari A, DeFronzo RA. Beta-cell function in subjects spanning the range from normal glucose tolerance to overt diabetes: A new analysis. The Journal of Clinical Endocrinology and Metabolism. 2005;**90**(1):493-500. DOI: 10.1210/jc.2004-1133 Epub 2004 Oct 13

[62] Franklin BA, Rubinfire M. Losing weight through exercise. Journal of the American Medical Association. 1980;**244**(4):377-379

[63] Gudat U, Berger M, Lefebvre PJ. Physical activity, fitness, and non-insulin dependent (type II) diabetes mellitus. In: Bouchard C, Shepard RJ, editors. Physical Activity and Health: International Proceedings and Consensus Statement. Champaign IL: Human Kinetics Publishers; 1994. pp. 669-684

[64] Levy J, Atkinson AB, Bell PM, McCance DR, Hadden DR. Beta-cell deterioration determines the onset and rate of progression of secondary dietary failure in type 2 diabetes mellitus: The 10-year follow-up of the Belfast diet study. Diabetic Medicine. 1998;**15**(4):290-296. DOI: 10.1002/(SICI)1096-9136(199804)15:4<290::AID-DIA570>3.0.CO;2-M

[65] Newman JC, Verdin E. Ketone bodies as signaling metabolites. Trends in Endocrinology and Metabolism. 2014;**25**(1):42-52. DOI: 10.1016/j.tem.2013.09.002 Epub 2013 Oct 18

[66] De Bono E. Six Action Shoes. London: Harper Collins; 1992

[67] De Bono E. Six Thinking Hats. London: Penguin Books; 1985

Chapter 4

Paradigm of Insulin Resistance, Type 2 Diabetes, Obesity, Fatty Liver and Atherosclerosis in Metabolic Syndrome

Adina Mitrea, Ionela Mihaela Vladu, Maria Magdalena Rosu, Diana Clenciu, Eugen Mota and Maria Mota

Abstract

Insulin resistance is the most important characteristic of both metabolic syndrome (MetS) and type 2 diabetes mellitus (T2D). It is estimated that MetS has a prevalence of up to 35% in the general population, rising up to 72% in individuals with T2D. Furthermore, insulin resistance promotes lipotoxicity through an increased free fatty acids flux, leading to both liver and heart disorders. Thus, recent studies have proven the association of metabolic dysfunction-associated fatty liver disease (MAFLD) with MetS and T2D. Interestingly, recent data incriminate the same mechanism for the development of metabolic cardiomyopathy, also known as cardiometabolic heart failure. The aim of this paper is to review the most important data regarding the association of T2D with the classic and the newer elements of the MetS, as well as to emphasize the molecular mechanisms that are accountable for this linkage and the possible therapeutic prospects that could influence these pathologies.

Keywords: type 2 diabetes, metabolic syndrome, insulin resistance, fatty liver disease, metabolic cardiomyopathy, atherogenic dyslipidemia, cardiovascular risk

1. Introduction

Metabolic syndrome (MetS) is a condition that associates metabolically related traits, that increase the risk of type 2 diabetes (T2D) as well as atherosclerotic cardiovascular disease [1, 2]. The components of MetS are central obesity, high blood pressure, dyslipidemia (elevated triglycerides, decreased levels of high-density lipoprotein (HDL) cholesterol) and carbohydrate intolerance, the presence of at least 3 of these impairments defining MetS [3]. MetS is considered a major public health issue, both for its complications and high prevalence. Although worldwide there are several definitions still in use, regardless of the criteria used for the diagnosis, the global estimated prevalence of MetS in the adult population is 20–45%, with a predicted prevalence of 53% by 2035 [4, 5]. A more worrisome problem is the increase in obesity observed in children and adolescents, which was associated with a prevalence of MetS in the pediatric population of about 16% [6, 7].

The prevalence of overweight, obesity and T2D have also reached epidemic proportions. The World Health Organization (WHO) appreciated that the prevalence of obesity worldwide has nearly tripled since 1975, with an estimated prevalence of overweight of 39%, respectively 13% in the adult population in 2016 [8]. The International Diabetes Federation estimated that in 2021 537 million adults were living with diabetes, number that is projected to increase to 643 million by 2030, respectively to 783 million by 2045 [9].

Persons with MetS have a significantly higher risk of developing T2D, insulin resistance (IR) playing an important role in this association. Insulin is the main hormone involved in maintaining the glucose homeostasis. In addition to promoting glycogen synthesis, downregulating gluconeogenesis and glucose uptake through GLUT-4 receptor, insulin is an active participant in promoting nitric oxide and endothelin release in the endothelial cells, leading to vasodilation and/or vasoconstriction, in order to improve the blood glucose uptake of different organs [10]. In insulin resistant states, such as obesity, MetS and T2D, the insulin-dependent tissues undergo an inadequate response to insulin, with a decreased activation of endothelial nitric oxide synthase at the level of endothelial cells, with impaired insulin signaling pathways [10]. Due to the role played by IR in many noncommunicable disease (T2D, MetS, fatty liver, cardiovascular disease, Alzheimer's disease, etc.), many fundamental and clinical studies have tried to assess the molecular mechanisms of this impairment [10].

The first author that has thoroughly studied IR was Reaven [11]. He suggested that IR, revealed by hyperinsulinemia, is the main factor responsible for both atherogenic dyslpidemia and dysfunctional glucose metabolism, as well as for an increase in arterial blood pressure [11, 12]. The clinical evaluation of IR and insulin sensitivity in vivo is a delicate issue, as the gold standard method is considered the euglycemic-hyperinsulinemic clamp, which in the clinical practice has limited use do to its sophisticated and technical nature [12, 13]. This is the reason why in the clinical practice other markers of insulin resistance are currently utilized. Among these, the homeostasis model assessment of insulin resistance (HOMA-IR) [14] is the main index used for estimating IR.

Another index that was proposed for assessing insulin sensibility/IR is the quantitative insulin sensitivity check index (QUICKI), which presents significantly lower values in persons that present insulin resistant states, such as MetS, prediabetes and T2D [15].

A biomarker which is easy to calculate, the triglyceride-glucose (TyG) index was also proposed for the assessment of IR [16]. A recent study, performed in over 15,000 subjects, concluded that although both HOMA-IR and TyG index were predictors of incident MetS, the TyG index had a higher predictive power [16]. Many other biomarkers are proposed as tools for assessing IR. However, there is still need for further studies in order to conclude the utility of these equations in the clinical practice, in order to improve the early diagnosis of metabolic complications such as fatty liver disease, obstructive sleep apnea, metabolic cardiomyopathy, neoplasms, etc.

Subjects with T2D that present MetS are at a higher risk of developing metabolic complications, as well as at higher risk for all-cause mortality [17]. The association of MetS and T2D is a frequent occurrence in the clinical practice, both disorders having as important risk factors the unhealthy lifestyle and obesity [18]. The aim of this paper is to gather information about the complications of MetS and T2D, in order to improve the early diagnosis and the therapeutic options for these persons.

2. From metabolic syndrome to type 2 diabetes: physiopathological mechanisms

MetS is one of the most common risk factors for developing T2D, these subjects having a 5 times higher risk than the general population [18]. One of the most important physiopathological mechanism that leads to the development of T2D in individuals with MetS is the pancreatic β-cell dysfunction [1]. The metabolic impairments (increased free fatty acids (FFA) and blood glucose) present in MetS, together with the proinflammatory status that characterizes this disorder, represent an adverse environment to β cells [1, 19].

Under these conditions, two possible scenarios might happen. In the first instance, the β cell must undergo compensatory functional changes, respectively insulin hypersecretion, to respond to the increased metabolic demands [1]. However, sometimes this hypersecretion of insulin may lead to IR, in the end resulting in impaired β cells (loss of β cell function and β cell mass) [1, 20]. On the other side, the metabolic stressor may first diminish insulin response in insulin – dependent tissues (liver), leading to IR which will promote insulin hypersecretion that may progress towards β cell dysfunction [1]. The exact mechanism involved in these two scenarios are not completely elucidated, however the ethnic factor seems to play an important role, the dysfunction of the β cells being more pronounced in individuals with Asian origins compared to Caucasians [1, 21]. In order to develop viable therapeutic intervention to prevent the progression from MetS to T2D, it is important to try to understand the intracellular mechanisms that are responsible for the shift in β cell adaptive response responsible for this progression, regardless if IR and/or nutrient response set off this complex process.

Subjects with MetS that in time develop T2D present only transient compensatory adaptation of the pancreatic β cells. The hypersecretion at cellular level leads to dysfunctions of the endoplasmic reticulum, translated into improper synthesis, folding, trafficking and, in the end, decreased insulin secretion, the β cells being unable to further sustain the enlarged workload necessary for maintaining normal blood glucose level. Animal and human studies [1, 22–28] likewise have described these same molecular endoplasmic reticulum and mitochondria defects, that over time result in β cells apoptosis.

However, it also must be noted that emerging studies have described two mechanisms through which the pancreatic β cells respond to environmental stress, respectively dedifferentiation and transdifferentiation, in order to avoid significant islet cell mass loss [1, 29]. In a 2012 study by Talchai et al. [30] aiming to assess the role of decreased β cell mass or impaired β cell function in animal models with diabetes, concluded that under stress conditions, not all dysfunctional cells were eliminated through apoptosis, some of the β cells suffering dedifferentiation process, reverting to a progenitor-like state. Interestingly, this study demonstrated that some of the differentiated cells are able to produce pancreatic hormones [30]. In a recent review, Bensellam et al. [31] proposed a novel hypothesis, concluding that dedifferentiation of β cells is a protective mechanism under stress conditions, such as MetS. This theory supported by the results obtained in many other animal and human models of prolonged insulin demand [32–36] is still incompletely understood, the characterization of both the trigger and the molecular pathways involved in β cells dedifferentiation requiring further studies [1, 31].

Recent studies [1, 37–39] have proposed transdifferentiation of β cells, defined as the loss of the β cell identity and converting into cell expressing different hormones, suggesting that these cells are prone to reprogramming. Furthermore, in the anatomopathological study by Sun et al. [34] on islet samples from both type 2 and type 1 diabetes, it was evidenced that β cells can express multiple hormones, which suggests their ability to lose their cell identity. Nonetheless, there is need for lineage analysis in order to demonstrate that these polymorphal cells emerged from mono-hormonal pancreatic β cells [1]. **Figure 1** summarizes the pathological mechanisms leading to the development of T2D in persons with obesity and MetS.

IR is universally accepted as the central trait of MetS. However, animal and human studies have proposed hyperinsulinism as the initiating event leading to MetS [40–42]. In one of these studies [42] it was postulated that basal insulin secretion is

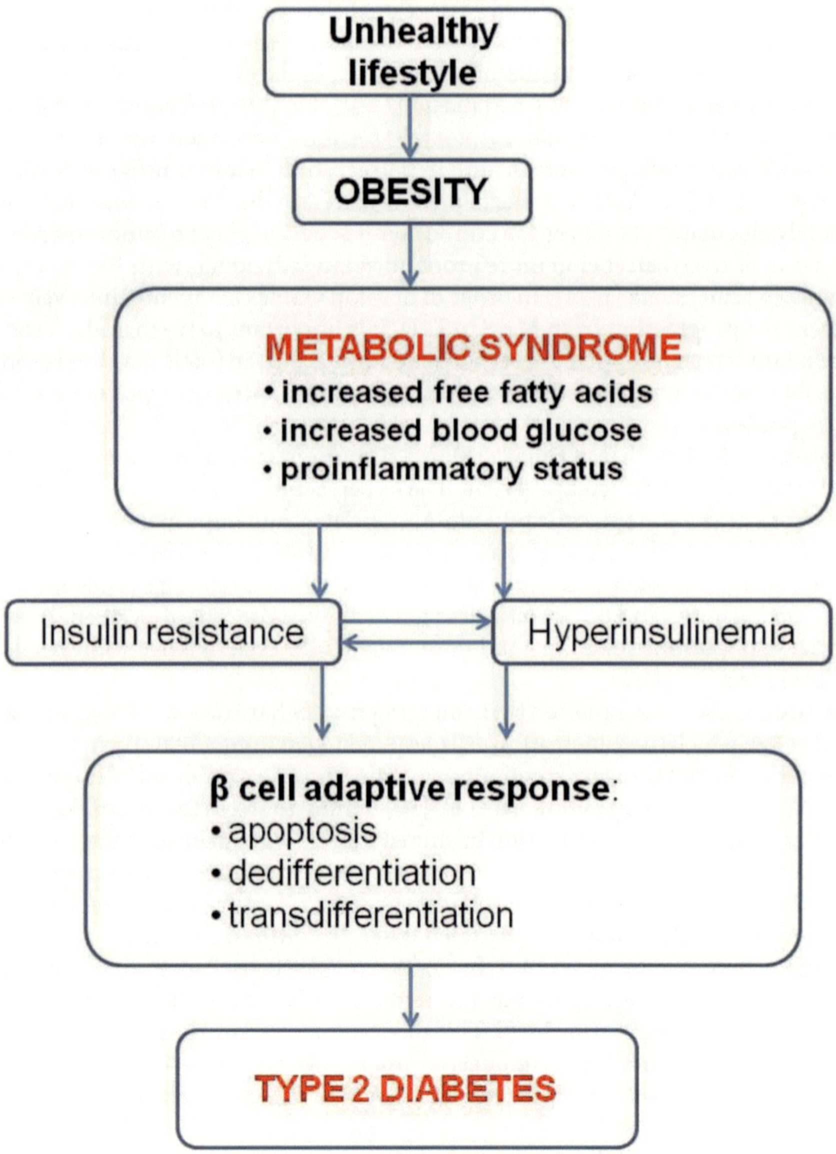

Figure 1.
Dysfunctions of pancreatic β cells that lead from MetS to T2D (adapted from [1]).

increased while glucose stimulated insulin secretion is decreased as the subjects move from normal glucose tolerance (lean individuals) to obesity to impaired glucose tolerance, with glucose stimulated insulin secretion being less than half of total insulin secretion in persons with T2D [1].

All these data support the concept of early intervention in terms of lifestyle optimization in individuals with MetS and prediabetes. Indeed, two recent interventional studies [43, 44] have proved the role of diet and physical activity in regulating β cell function and preventing T2D in populations at risk.

3. Insulin resistance: the link between metabolic syndrome, type 2 diabetes and fatty liver disease

With a worldwide prevalence estimated at 25%, nonalcoholic fatty liver disease (NAFLD) is the most common liver disease, representing a major public health concern [45, 46]. From an anatomopathological point of view, the term NAFLD includes a diversity of hepatic lesions, such as steatosis, nonalcoholic steatohepatitis (NASH), fibrosis and cirrhosis, in subjects that have as a common trait the absence of alcohol consumption [47–49].

Studies [48, 50, 51] have revealed the association between NAFLD and metabolic disorders, a meta-analysis performed by Ballestri et al. demonstrating that persons with NAFLD have a 2-fold increased risk for the development of MetS and T2D over a median follow-up of 5 years [50]. Another meta-analysis form 2016 demonstrated that NAFLD was associated with MetS in 42.54% of the cases and with T2D in 22.51% of the cases, while obesity was the metabolic disease with the highest frequency in subjects with NAFLD (51.34%) [52]. In a study [53] that aimed to assess the frequency of steatosis and NASH in individuals with MetS or T2D that presented elevated liver enzymes, it was demonstrated that NAFLD had a prevalence of 94.82% in persons with MetS, while all the persons with T2D presented NAFLD. Furthermore, NASH was present in 58.52% in the case of people with MetS, while it had a prevalence of 96.82% in the individuals with T2D. This study concluded that NASH might be an early complication of T2D, IR being the link between the two pathologies [53].

Taking into consideration the high frequency of NAFLD in subjects with metabolic diseases, in 2020, an international panel of experts proposed the new terminology, metabolic dysfunction-associated fatty liver disease (MAFLD) [54]. This definition no longer restricts alcohol consumption or other secondary liver diseases, while introducing an important diagnosis criterion: the presence of a metabolic disorder [55–57]. This new term emphasizes the importance of metabolic factors in fatty liver pathophysiology, as well as facilitates patient – physician communication, making easier for the patient to understand the relationship between this syndrome and metabolic health [58].

IR is the main mechanism linking NAFLD/MAFLD and metabolic disorders. It is well documented the fact that systemic IR present in MetS and T2D is responsible for an increase in the flux of FFA from the visceral adipose cells towards the liver, followed by increased lipogenesis, that on one hand leads to fatty liver disease and on the other hand aggravates liver IR [59]. Moreover, continuous body of evidence supports the association of MAFLD with increased cardiovascular risk [59]. A possible explanation for this association comes from the fact that in MAFLD the hepatic tissue releases bioactive mediators that further increase liver and systemic IR, while also promoting atherogenic dyslipidemia and low grade inflammation [59–61]. It is important for the individuals with MetS and T2D to be screened for the presence of MAFLD, as these people have three major mortality causes: cardiovascular disease, extrahepatic malignancies and liver related complications (cirrhosis and hepatocellular carcinoma) [59, 60, 62, 63].

Among the etipathogenic factors involved in MAFLD, the most important remain lifestyle (unhealthy diet, increased alcohol consumption, etc.), microbiota dysregulations, ethnicity and genetic predisposition [64]. The role of unhealthy diet in the development of both MAFLD and metabolic disease is well recognized. High sugar and fructose intake as well as increased hepatic diacylglycerols levels lead to liver fat accumulation [59]. At the level of the hepatocyte, unhealthy dietary choices are translated into hepatic IR, oxidative stress and chronic inflammation, with subsequent development and progression of fatty liver [59].

Gut microbiota is another important factor for the maintenance of metabolic health. Intestinal dysbiosis was associated with both fatty liver and metabolic disorders development [65]. The analysis of gut microbiota in subjects with MAFLD showed a decrease in Ruminococcaceae family compared to healthy controls, while subjects with NASH presented an increase in *Clostridium coccoides*, with decreased Bacteroides species [66, 67].

One of the mechanisms proposed to explain the role of impaired gut microbiota in fatty liver disease is the type and amount of short chain fatty acids (SCFAs), precursors of both gluconeogenisis and lipogenesis, which are produced by the fermentation of carbohydrates at the level of the gut, and therefore, are directly affected by gut dysbiosis [59]. SCFAs can regulate gluconeogenesis and lipogenesis, as they have a short bowel transit and increase the rate of nutrient absorption [59, 68].

Dysbiosis is also responsible for an increased intestinal permeability as well as for flaws in intestinal tight junctions, impairments described in individuals with MAFLD [69]. Other proposed mechanisms involve dysfunctions regarding choline, fasting-induced adypocite factor secretion (which induces fat accumulation in both adipocytes and hepatocytes), as well as increased lipopolysaccharide and bile acid production (which promote low grade inflammation) [59]. In summary, impaired gut microbiota is a promoter of MetS, T2D and MAFLD through all these pathways.

4. Cardiovascular risk in persons with insulin resistance, metabolic syndrome and type 2 diabetes

Cardiovascular disease (CVD) accounts for 46.2% of deaths due to non-communicable diseases, being the primary cause of disability and premature death [70]. CVD is the main cause of death in persons with MetS and T2D [71]. By definition, the individuals with MetS have an increased cardiovascular risk, as all components of this disorder are independent risk factors for CVDs; what is more, in MetS the combination of these risk factors further increases both the rates and the severity of CVDs [72]. So, it is not surprising that subjects with MetS and T2D are at risk for coronary atherosclerosis, myocardial infarction, microvascular dysfunctions, cardiac dysfunction and heart failure [72, 73].

Studies showed that persons with MetS often present CVDs. In a study from 2005 [74], it was observed that MetS was a frequent comorbidity in patients with acute myocardial infarction (46%). However, although the medical literature recognizes the high cardiovascular risk of individuals with MetS, there still exists controversy regarding the impact of this syndrome on subjects with CVDs [70]. In this regard, some studies concluded that persons with MetS remain at high cardiovascular risk independent of active management [75], other researches evidenced that the main prognosis factor for myocardial infarction in individuals with MetS is the presence of heart failure [76], while the study by van Kuijk et al. [77] concluded that MetS is not associated with an increase in mortality in individuals with CVDs. Starting from these premises and taking into account that the majority of the studies have assessed the impact of MetS on the prognosis and progression of CVDs, a meta-analysis from 2022 aimed to evaluate the associations between MetS, using different definitions, and the risk of cardiovascular events, cardiovascular death and all cause mortality [70]. The analysis of cardiovascular events in persons with MetS was analyzed based on the results reported by 23 studies totalizing a number of 77,125 subjects and proved that the risk of myocardial infarction is statistically significant higher in individuals with MetS [RR = 1.460, 95% CI (1.242, 1.716), P = 0.000] [70]. The risk of stroke, analyzed in 60,297 subjects, was also higher for the persons with MetS (RR = 1.435, 95% CI (1.131, 1.820), P = 0.000) [70]. Regarding all cause mortality, the results of this meta-analysis including over 145,000 subjects with MetS demonstrated an increase of all cause mortality in these individuals (RR = 1.220, 95% CI (1.103, 1.349), P = 0.000) [70].

Persons with T2D have a high risk of developing CVDs, that have higher prevalence rates in T2D compared with the general population and, what is more, there is an increase in the cardiovascular risk parallel to the fasting plasma glucose levels, starting from the stage of prediabetes/impaired fasting glucose [78, 79]. Fortunately, although the prevalence of T2D is increasing, in the last two decades there was observed a decrease in the incidence of CVDs and cardiovascular mortality in these individuals, compared to the general population [78]. A declining pattern was observed in many countries (Canada, United States, Sweden, United Kingdom, Korea) [80–85]. However, even though the overall prevalence of CVDs in persons with T2D is decreasing, a new phenomenon was observed in these subjects, an increase in the prevalence of heart failure [78, 86]. A possible explanation might be the increase in life expectancy that came with the advances in diabetes therapeutic options [78, 86, 87].

The physiopathological mechanisms that link MetS, T2D and CVDs are complex and multifactorial, including IR, low grade inflammation and neurohormonal activation [88, 89]. The epicardial fat accumulation observed in persons with obesity is accountable for lipolysis, FFA release and reactive inflammation [88]. Additionally, obesity is also associated with increased oxidative stress, mitochondria being the main source of reactive oxygen species (ROS), mechanisms through which MetS leads to the development and progression of T2D, atherosclerosis and CVDs [90, 91]. MetS is characterized by a chronic increase in adiposity which can lead to important neuro-hormonal changes in the cardiovascular system, including activation of the renin-angiotensin-aldosterone system, increased proinflammatory cytokines, altered adipokines levels, as well as activation of the sympathetic nervous system [72]. The latter can lead to vasoconstriction, tachycardia, as well as metabolic abnormalities, such as excess lipolysis with an increase in FFA, peripheral and hepatic IR [72].

The relationship between IR and cardiovascular risk is well recognized by many studies, being considered as a major predictor of atherosclerotic disease [78, 92–94]. Recent studies [95] describe the role of IR at the myocyte level as a main contributor to the appearance of cardiomyopathy in persons with MetS and T2D, giving this way a possible explication to the increase in heart failure observed in persons with T2D.

Insulin signaling is mainly described in insulin dependent cells, as the activation of these pathways play important roles in cell metabolism, as well as cell growth and survival. Although the myocytes are not insulin dependent, insulin signaling is involved in maintaining normal heart functions, as studies have shown that these pathways are important under stress conditions, transcending the metabolic effects of insulin [95, 96]. Systemic IR, increased circulating FFA, both characteristic of MetS and T2D are described as major contributors to metabolic cardiomyopathy [97–100]. Metabolic cardiomyopathy is characterized by hypertrophy and diastolic dysfunction that can progress to overt heart failure, the most frequent being heart failure with preserved ejection fraction (HFpEF) [97–99]. Although diabetic cardiomyopathy makes the object of many studies, the fact that at the moment there is no accurate definition for this disease, makes the interpretation of different studies more difficult; however, the prevalence of heart failure in persons with T2D was estimated at 10–30%, compared to 12% in the general population [101, 102]. Furthermore, in subjects with heart failure, the prevalence of diabetes was estimated at about 30% and it was observed that these people are generally younger and also the presence of T2D is associated with a worse prognosis in the case of heart failure with reduced ejection fraction (HFrEF), having a 75% higher mortality and increased risk of hospitalization [101–104]. For the clinical practice it is very important to know that a good metabolic control can reduce the risk of developing heart failure, studies showing that a reduction of HbA1c of only 1% can lead to a 16% reduction of developing heart failure in persons with T2D [105].

5. Prevention strategies and therapeutic options

The main cause for the continuous increase in the prevalence of metabolic diseases (obesity, MetS, T2D) is the unhealthy lifestyle, consisting of high caloric intake and sedentarism. Therefore, the optimization of lifestyle can be an effective tool in preventing or delaying the onset of metabolic diseases. In individuals with T2D, weight loss of about 3–10% can bring benefits on the glycemic control [106]. Furthermore, weight loss can be associated with T2D remission, which makes dietary intervention very important for the correct managing of T2D [107]. Currently, many diets were proposed for weight control, amidst them Mediterranean diet, continuous energy-restricted diet (CERD), low carbohydrate diet, ketogenic diet, vegetarian diet, intermittent fasting (IF), etc. A type of diet still controversial in persons with T2D, despite studies showing improvements in metabolism, is CERD, as most guidelines recommend balanced diets with moderate calorie restriction [108–110].

One of the most discussed diets in chronic non-communicable disease is calorie restriction (CR), without malnutrition, this type of diet has increased life span and has impeded the development of age-related disorders in many animal models, including primates [111]. CR is defined by the reduction of caloric intake by 25–30%, maintaining all the essential nutrients [111]. In humans, moderate CR studies assessing longevity are still ongoing, while many other benefits are already recognized [112, 113]. **Table 1** summarizes the benefic effects of CR in subjects with metabolic disorders.

In a recent meta-analysis that compared the safety of IF and CERD in subjects with MeTS and T2D, including four studies with a total of 355 individuals, it was demonstrated that the two diets had similar effects in term of glycemic control, while IF had a better effect on weight loss [107]. The authors concluded that IF represents a safe diet pattern for persons with MetS and T2D, which could be implemented as a part of these individuals' management [107].

Parameter	Effects
Body mass	• Significant weight loss • Weight maintenance
Body composition	• Decrease in visceral fat mass • Significant reduction in subcutaneous adipocyte size • Significant reduction in deposition of lipid in the liver
Glycemic metabolism	• Improved insulin sensitivity • Improvements in fasting insulin concentration
Lipid metabolism	• Improved lipid profile • Decreased LDL-cholesterol
Inflammation	• Decline in markers of oxidative stress • Decreased C-reactive protein
Other benefits	• 29% reduction in the 10-year risk for CVD • Increased adiponectin • Reduced leptin serum concentrations

Table 1.
Benefits of CR in persons with MetS and T2D [112, 113].

Lifestyle optimization must also address sedentarism. Observational and interventional studies alike have proved the importance of physical activity in mitigating MetS, as each of its components can be favorably influenced by physical exercise [114]. Regular physical activity can induce weight loss, together with a decrease in arterial blood pressure and improvements of lipid and glycemic profiles, through a reduction of IR [115–118]. Due to all these benefits, persons with MetS and T2D should be encouraged to practice physical activity on a regular basis.

For subjects that require more than lifestyle interventions, there are two more therapeutic options that can help with weight loss and reduction in metabolic complication: bariatric surgery and pharmacological agents. Newer antidiabetic drugs, such as SGLT2 inhibitors and GLP-1 receptor agonists have demonstrated cardiovascular benefits beyond glycemic control in these persons [119, 120].

6. Conclusion

Metabolic diseases, particularly MetS and T2D have continuous increasing prevalence rates and have negative impact on the individual's quality of life, bearing in the same time an important social and economic burden for the society. Therefore, it is imperious that prevention measures must be taken globally, as well as developing new strategies for the better control and delayed progression of these disorders, through lifestyle optimization and, when necessary, pharmacologic interventions.

Conflict of interest

The authors declare no conflict of interest.

Author details

Adina Mitrea[1,2], Ionela Mihaela Vladu[1,3*], Maria Magdalena Rosu[3], Diana Clenciu[1,2], Eugen Mota[4] and Maria Mota[4]

1 Department of Diabetes, Nutrition and Metabolic Diseases, University of Medicine and Pharmacy of Craiova, Craiova, Romania

2 Department of Diabetes, Nutrition and Metabolic Diseases, Clinical Municipal Hospital "Philanthropy" of Craiova, Craiova, Romania

3 Department of Diabetes, Nutrition and Metabolic Diseases, County Clinical Emergency Hospital of Craiova, Craiova, Romania

4 Doctoral School, University of Medicine and Pharmacy of Craiova, Craiova, Romania

*Address all correspondence to: ionela.vladu@umfcv.ro

References

[1] Hudish LI, Reusch JE, Sussel L. β cell dysfunction during progression of metabolic syndrome to type 2 diabetes. The Journal of Clinical Investigation. 2019;**129**:4001-4008. DOI: 10.1172/JCI129188

[2] Gemeda D, Abebe E, Duguma A. Metabolic syndrome and its associated factors among type 2 diabetic patients in Southwest Ethiopia, 2021/2022. Journal Diabetes Research. 2022;**2022**:8162342. DOI: 10.1155/2022/8162342

[3] Alberti KG, Eckel RH, Grundy SM, Zimmet PZ, Cleeman JI, Donato KA, et al. Harmonizing the metabolic syndrome: A joint interim statement of the international diabetes federation task force on epidemiology and prevention; National Heart, Lung, and Blood Institute; American Heart Association; world heart federation; international atherosclerosis society; and International Association for the Study of obesity. Circulation. 2009;**120**:1640-1645. DOI: 10.1161/CIRCULATIONAHA.109.192644

[4] de Siqueira Valadares LT, de Souza LSB, Salgado Júnior VA, de Freitas BL, de Macedo LR, Silva M. Prevalence of metabolic syndrome in Brazilian adults in the last 10 years: A systematic review and meta-analysis. BMC Public Health. 2022;**22**:327. DOI: 10.1186/s12889-022-12753-5

[5] Engin A. The definition and prevalence of obesity and metabolic syndrome. Advances in Experimental Medicine and Biology. 2017;**960**:1-17. DOI: 10.1007/978-3-319-48382-5_1

[6] Weihe P, Weihrauch-Blüher S. Metabolic syndrome in children and adolescents: Diagnostic criteria, therapeutic options and perspectives. Current Obesity Reports. 2019;**8**:472-479. DOI: 10.1007/s13679-019-00357-x

[7] Weghuber D, Zelzer S, Stelzer I, Paulmichl K, Kammerhofer D, Schnedl W, et al. "metabolically healthy" phenotype in juvenile obesity - neck subcutaneous adipose tissue and serum uric acid are clinically relevant. Experimental and Clinical Endocrinology & Diabetes. 2013;**121**:384-390. DOI: 10.1055/s-0033-1341440

[8] World Health Organization. Obesity and Overweight [Internet]. 2021. Available from: https://www.who.int/news-room/fact-sheets/detail/obesity-and-overweight [Accessed: June 6, 2023]

[9] International Diabetes Federation. IDF Diabetes Atlas. 10th ed. Brussels, Belgium: International Diabetes Federation; 2021

[10] Onyango AN. Cellular stresses and stress responses in the pathogenesis of insulin resistance. Oxidative Medicine and Cellular Longevity. 2018;**2018**:4321714. DOI: 10.1155/2018/4321714

[11] Reaven GM. Pathophysiology of insulin resistance in human disease. Physiological Reviews. 1995;**75**:473-486. DOI: 10.1152/physrev.1995.75.3.473

[12] Ighbariya A, Weiss R. Insulin resistance, prediabetes, metabolic syndrome: What should every pediatrician know? Journal of Clinical Research in Pediatric Endocrinology. 2017;**9**:49-57. DOI: 10.4274/jcrpe.2017.S005

[13] Kim JK. Hyperinsulinemic-euglycemic clamp to assess insulin sensitivity in vivo. Methods in

Molecular Biology. 2009;**560**:221-238. DOI: 10.1007/978-1-59745-448-3_15

[14] Matthews DR, Hosker JP, Rudenski AS, Naylor BA, Treacher DF, Turner RC. Homeostasis model assessment: Insulin resistance and beta-cell function from fasting plasma glucose and insulin concentrations in man. Diabetologia. 1985;**28**:412-419. DOI: 10.1007/BF00280883

[15] Hrebícek J, Janout V, Malincíková J, Horáková D, Cízek L. Detection of insulin resistance by simple quantitative insulin sensitivity check index QUICKI for epidemiological assessment and prevention. The Journal of Clinical Endocrinology and Metabolism. 2002;**87**:144-147. DOI: 10.1210/jcem.87.1.8292

[16] Son DH, Lee HS, Lee YJ, Lee JH, Han JH. Comparison of triglyceride-glucose index and HOMA-IR for predicting prevalence and incidence of metabolic syndrome. Nutrition, Metabolism, and Cardiovascular Diseases. 2022;**32**:596-604. DOI: 10.1016/j.numecd.2021.11.017

[17] Earnest CP, Johannsen NM, Swift DL, Gillison FB, Mikus CR, Lucia A, et al. Aerobic and strength training in concomitant metabolic syndrome and type 2 diabetes. Medicine and Science in Sports and Exercise. 2014;**46**:1293-1301. DOI: 10.1249/MSS.0000000000000242

[18] Regufe VMG, Pinto CMCB, Perez PMVHC. Metabolic syndrome in type 2 diabetic patients: A review of current evidence. Porto Biomedical Journal. 2020;**5**:e101. DOI: 10.1097/j.pbj.0000000000000101

[19] Gupta D et al. Temporal characterization of β cell-adaptive and -maladaptive mechanisms during chronic high-fat feeding in C57BL/6NTac mice. The Journal of Biological Chemistry. 2017;**292**:12449-12459. DOI: 10.1074/jbc.M117.781047

[20] Halban PA et al. β-Cell failure in type 2 diabetes: Postulated mechanisms and prospects for prevention and treatment. Diabetes Care. 2014;**37**:1751-1758. DOI: 10.2337/dc14-0396

[21] Yabe D, Seino Y, Fukushima M, Seino S. β cell dysfunction versus insulin resistance in the pathogenesis of type 2 diabetes in east Asians. Current Diabetes Reports. 2015;**15**:602. DOI: 10.1007/s11892-015-0602-9

[22] Prentki M, Nolan CJ. Islet beta cell failure in type 2 diabetes. The Journal of Clinical Investigation. 2006;**116**:1802-1812. DOI: 10.1172/JCI29103

[23] Chen C, Cohrs CM, Stertmann J, Bozsak R, Speier S. Human beta cell mass and function in diabetes: Recent advances in knowledge and technologies to understand disease pathogenesis. Molecular Metabolism. 2017;**6**:943-957. DOI: 10.1016/j.molmet.2017.06.019

[24] Rabhi N, Salas E, Froguel P, Annicotte JS. Role of the unfolded protein response in beta cell compensation and failure during diabetes. Journal Diabetes Research. 2014;**2014**:795171. DOI: 10.1155/2014/795171

[25] Eizirik DL, Cardozo AK, Cnop M. The role for endoplasmic reticulum stress in diabetes mellitus. Endocrine Reviews. 2008;**29**:42-61. DOI: 10.1210/er.2007-0015

[26] Marchetti P, Bugliani M, De Tata V, Suleiman M, Marselli L. Pancreatic beta cell identity in humans and the role of type 2 diabetes. Frontiers in Cell and Development Biology. 2017;5:55. DOI: 10.3389/fcell.2017.00055

[27] Supale S, Li N, Brun T, Maechler P. Mitochondrial dysfunction in pancreatic β cells. Trends in Endocrinology and Metabolism. 2012;**23**:477-487. DOI: 10.1016/j.tem.2012.06.002

[28] Gerber PA, Rutter GA. The role of oxidative stress and hypoxia in pancreatic beta-cell dysfunction in diabetes mellitus. Antioxidants & Redox Signaling. 2017;**26**:501-518. DOI: 10.1089/ars.2016.6755

[29] Remedi MS, Emfinger C. Pancreatic β-cell identity in diabetes. Diabetes, Obesity & Metabolism. 2016;**18**:110-116. DOI: 10.1111/dom.12727

[30] Talchai C, Xuan S, Lin HV, Sussel L, Accili D. Pancreatic β cell dedifferentiation as a mechanism of diabetic β cell failure. Cell. 2012;**150**:1223-1234. DOI: 10.1016/j.cell.2012.07.029

[31] Bensellam M, Jonas JC, Laybutt DR. Mechanisms of β-cell dedifferentiation in diabetes: Recent findings and future research directions. The Journal of Endocrinology. 2018;**236**:R109-R143. DOI: 10.1530/JOE-17-0516

[32] Ediger BN et al. LIM domain-binding 1 maintains the terminally differentiated state of pancreatic β cells. The Journal of Clinical Investigation. 2017;**127**:215-229. DOI: 10.1172/JCI88016

[33] Neelankal John A, Ram R, Jiang FX. RNA-Seq analysis of islets to characterise the dedifferentiation in type 2 diabetes model mice db/db. Endocrine Pathology. 2018;**29**:207-221. DOI: 10.1007/s12022-018-9523-x

[34] Sun J et al. β-Cell dedifferentiation in patients with T2D with adequate glucose control and nondiabetic chronic pancreatitis. The Journal of Clinical Endocrinology and Metabolism. 2019;**104**:83-94

[35] Diedisheim M et al. Modeling human pancreatic beta cell dedifferentiation. Molecular Metabolism. 2018;**10**:74-86. DOI: 10.1016/j.molmet.2018.02.002

[36] Cinti F et al. Evidence of β-cell dedifferentiation in human type 2 diabetes. The Journal of Clinical Endocrinology and Metabolism. 2016;**101**:1044-1054. DOI: 10.1210/jc.2015-2860

[37] Gutierrez GD, Gromada J, Sussel L. Heterogeneity of the pancreatic beta cell. Frontiers in Genetics. 2017;**8**:22. DOI: 10.3389/fgene.2017.00022

[38] Swisa A et al. PAX6 maintains β cell identity by repressing genes of alternative islet cell types. The Journal of Clinical Investigation. 2017;**127**:230-243. DOI: 10.1172/JCI88015

[39] Gao T et al. Pdx1 maintains β cell identity and function by repressing an α cell program. Cell Metabolism. 2014;**19**:259-271. DOI: 10.1016/j.cmet.2013.12.002

[40] Nolan CJ, Prentki M. Insulin resistance and insulin hypersecretion in the metabolic syndrome and type 2 diabetes: Time for a conceptual framework shift. Diabetes & Vascular Disease Research. 2019;**16**:118-127. DOI: 10.1177/1479164119827611

[41] Erion K, Corkey BE. β-Cell failure or β-cell abuse? Frontiers in Endocrinology (Lausanne). 2018;**9**:532. DOI: 10.3389/fendo.2018.00532

[42] Ferrannini E, Gastaldelli A, Miyazaki Y, Matsuda M, Mari A, DeFronzo RA. β-Cell function in subjects spanning the range from normal glucose tolerance to overt diabetes: A new analysis. The Journal of Clinical Endocrinology and Metabolism. 2005;**90**(1):493-500. DOI: 10.1210/jc.2004-1133

[43] Malin SK, Kullman EL, Scelsi AR, Godin JP, Ross AB, Kirwan JP. A whole-grain diet increases glucose-stimulated insulin secretion independent of gut hormones in adults at risk for type 2 diabetes. Molecular Nutrition & Food Research. 2019;**63**:e1800967. DOI: 10.1002/mnfr.201800967

[44] Malin SK et al. Impact of short-term exercise training intensity on β-cell function in older obese adults with prediabetes. Journal of Applied Physiology. 2018;**125**:1979-1986. DOI: 10.1152/japplphysiol.00680.2018

[45] Kaya E, Yilmaz Y. Metabolic-associated fatty liver disease (MAFLD): A multi-systemic disease beyond the liver. Journal of Clinical and Translational Hepatology. 2022;**10**:329-338. DOI: 10.14218/JCTH.2021.00178

[46] Younossi Z, Tacke F, Arrese M, Chander Sharma B, Mostafa I, Bugianesi E, et al. Global perspectives on nonalcoholic fatty liver disease and nonalcoholic Steatohepatitis. Hepatology. 2019;**69**:2672-2682. DOI: 10.1002/hep.30251

[47] Amzolini AM, Forţofoiu MC, Barău Abu-Alhija A, Vladu IM, Clenciu D, Mitrea A, et al. Triglyceride and glucose index: A useful tool for non-alcoholic liver disease assessed by liver biopsy in patients with metabolic syndrome? Romanian Journal of Morphology and Embryology. 2021;**62**:475-480. DOI: 10.47162/RJME.62.2.13

[48] Davis TME. Diabetes and metabolic dysfunction-associated fatty liver disease. Metabolism. 2021;**123**:154868. DOI: 10.1016/j.metabol.2021.154868

[49] Micu ES, Amzolini AM, Barău Abu-Alhija A, Forţofoiu MC, Vladu IM, Clenciu D, et al. Systemic and adipose tissue inflammation in NASH: Correlations with histopathological aspects. Romanian Journal of Morphology and Embryology. 2021;**62**:509-515. DOI: 10.47162/RJME.62.2.17

[50] Ballestri S, Zona S, Targher G, Romagnoli D, Baldelli E, Nascimbeni F, et al. Nonalcoholic fatty liver disease is associated with an almost twofold increased risk of incident type 2 diabetes and metabolic syndrome. Evidence from a systematic review and meta-analysis. Journal of Gastroenterology and Hepatology. 2016;**31**:936-944. DOI: 10.1111/jgh.13264

[51] Muzurović E, Mikhailidis DP, Mantzoros C. Non-alcoholic fatty liver disease, insulin resistance, metabolic syndrome and their association with vascular risk. Metabolism. 2021;**119**:154770. DOI: 10.1016/j.metabol.2021.154770

[52] Younossi ZM, Koenig AB, Abdelatif D, Fazel Y, Henry L, Wymer M. Global epidemiology of nonalcoholic fatty liver disease-meta-analytic assessment of prevalence, incidence, and outcomes. Hepatology. 2016;**64**:73-84. DOI: 10.1002/hep.28431

[53] Masarone M, Rosato V, Aglitti A, Bucci T, Caruso R, Salvatore T, et al. Liver biopsy in type 2 diabetes mellitus: Steatohepatitis represents the sole feature of liver damage. PLoS One. 2017;**12**:e0178473. DOI: 10.1371/journal.pone.0178473

[54] Eslam M, Sanyal AJ, George J. International consensus panel. MAFLD: A consensus-driven proposed nomenclature for metabolic associated fatty liver disease. Gastroenterology. 2020;**158**:1999-2014.e1

[55] Efrem IC, Moţa M, Vladu IM, Mitrea A, Clenciu D, Timofticiuc DCP,

et al. A study of biomarkers associated with metabolic dysfunction-associated fatty liver disease in patients with type 2 diabetes. Diagnostics (Basel). 2022;**12**:2426. DOI: 10.3390/diagnostics12102426

[56] Sakurai Y, Kubota N, Yamauchi T, Kadowaki T. Role of insulin resistance in MAFLD. International Journal of Molecular Sciences. 2021;**22**:4156. DOI: 10.3390/ijms22084156

[57] Eslam M, Newsome PN, Sarin SK, Anstee QM, Targher G, Romero-Gomez M, et al. A new definition for metabolic dysfunction-associated fatty liver disease: An international expert consensus statement. Journal of Hepatology. 2020;**73**:202-209

[58] Yilmaz Y, Byrne CD, Musso G. A single-letter change in an acronym: Signals, reasons, promises, challenges, and steps ahead for moving from NAFLD to MAFLD. Expert Review of Gastroenterology & Hepatology. 2021;**15**:345-352. DOI: 10.1080/17474124.2021

[59] Lim S, Kim JW, Targher G. Links between metabolic syndrome and metabolic dysfunction-associated fatty liver disease. Trends in Endocrinology and Metabolism. 2021;**32**:500-514. DOI: 10.1016/j.tem.2021.04.008

[60] Lim S, Taskinen MR, Borén J. Crosstalk between nonalcoholic fatty liver disease and cardiometabolic syndrome. Obesity Reviews. 2019;**20**: 599-611. DOI: 10.1111/obr.12820

[61] Lim S, Meigs JB. Links between ectopic fat and vascular disease in humans. Arteriosclerosis, Thrombosis, and Vascular Biology. 2014;**34**:1820-1826. DOI: 10.1161/ATVBAHA.114.303035

[62] Vilar-Gomez E, Calzadilla-Bertot L, Wai-Sun Wong V, Castellanos M, Aller-de la Fuente R, Metwally M, et al. Fibrosis severity as a determinant of cause-specific mortality in patients with advanced nonalcoholic fatty liver disease: A multi-National Cohort Study. Gastroenterology. 2018;**155**:443-457.e17. DOI: 10.1053/j.gastro.2018.04.034

[63] Anstee QM, Reeves HL, Kotsiliti E, Govaere O, Heikenwalder M. From NASH to HCC: Current concepts and future challenges. Nature Reviews. Gastroenterology & Hepatology. 2019;**16**:411-428. DOI: 10.1038/s41575-019-0145-7

[64] Cotter TG, Rinella M. Nonalcoholic fatty liver disease 2020: The state of the disease. Gastroenterology. 2020;**158**:1851-1864. DOI: 10.1053/j.gastro.2020.01.052

[65] Sharpton SR, Schnabl B, Knight R, Loomba R. Current concepts, opportunities, and challenges of gut microbiome-based personalized medicine in nonalcoholic fatty liver disease. Cell Metabolism. 2021;**33**:21-32. DOI: 10.1016/j.cmet.2020.11.010

[66] Raman M, Ahmed I, Gillevet PM, Probert CS, Ratcliffe NM, Smith S, et al. Fecal microbiome and volatile organic compound metabolome in obese humans with nonalcoholic fatty liver disease. Clinical Gastroenterology and Hepatology. 2013;**11**:868-75.e1-3. DOI: 10.1016/j.cgh.2013.02.015

[67] Mouzaki M, Comelli EM, Arendt BM, Bonengel J, Fung SK, Fischer SE, et al. Intestinal microbiota in patients with nonalcoholic fatty liver disease. Hepatology. 2013;**58**:120-127. DOI: 10.1002/hep.26319

[68] Aguirre M, Bussolo de Souza C, Venema K. The gut microbiota from lean and obese subjects contribute differently to the fermentation of arabinogalactan and inulin. PLoS One. 2016;**11**:e0159236. DOI: 10.1371/journal.pone.0159236

[69] Mao JW, Tang HY, Zhao T, Tan XY, Bi J, Wang BY, et al. Intestinal mucosal barrier dysfunction participates in the progress of nonalcoholic fatty liver disease. International Journal of Clinical and Experimental Pathology. 2015;**8**(4):3648-3658

[70] Li X, Zhai Y, Zhao J, He H, Li Y, Liu Y, et al. Impact of metabolic syndrome and It's components on prognosis in patients with cardiovascular diseases: A meta-analysis. Frontiers in Cardiovascular Medicine. 2021;**8**:704145. DOI: 10.3389/fcvm.2021.704145

[71] Bornachea O, Vea A, Llorente-Cortes V. Interplay between epicardial adipose tissue, metabolic and cardiovascular diseases. Clinic and Research in Arteriosclerosis. 2018;**30**:230-239. DOI: 10.1016/j.arteri.2018.03.003

[72] Tune JD, Goodwill AG, Sassoon DJ, Mather KJ. Cardiovascular consequences of metabolic syndrome. Translational Research. 2017;**183**:57-70. DOI: 10.1016/j.trsl.2017.01.001

[73] Bajaj NS, Osborne MT, Gupta A, Tavakkoli A, Bravo PE, Vita T, et al. Coronary microvascular dysfunction and cardiovascular risk in obese patients. Journal of the American College of Cardiology. 2018;**72**:707-717. DOI: 10.1016/j.jacc.2018.05.049

[74] Zeller M, Steg PG, Ravisy J, Laurent Y, Janin-Manificat L, L'Huillier I, et al. Prevalence and impact of metabolic syndrome on hospital outcomes in acute myocardial infarction. Archives of Internal Medicine. 2005;**165**:1192-1198. DOI: 10.1001/archinte.165.10.1192

[75] Boulon C, Lafitte M, Richeboeuf V, Paviot B, Pradeau V, Coste P, et al. Prevalence of metabolic syndrome after acute coronary syndrome and its prognostic significance. The American Journal of Cardiology. 2006;**98**:1429-1434. DOI: 10.1016/j.amjcard.2006.07.025

[76] Selcuk H, Temizhan A, Selcuk MT, Sen T, Maden O, Tekeli S, et al. Impact of metabolic syndrome on future cardiovascular events in patients with first acute myocardial infarction. Coronary Artery Disease. 2009;**20**:370-375. DOI: 10.1097/MCA.0b013e32832ed31e

[77] van Kuijk JP, Flu WJ, Chonchol M, Bax JJ, Verhagen JM, Poldermans HD. Metabolic syndrome is an independent predictor of cardiovascular events in high-risk patients with occlusive and aneurysmatic peripheral arterial disease. Atherosclerosis. 2010;**210**:596-601. DOI: 10.1016/j.atherosclerosis.2009.12.018

[78] Yun JS, Ko SH. Current trends in epidemiology of cardiovascular disease and cardiovascular risk management in type 2 diabetes. Metabolism. 2021;**123**:154838. DOI: 10.1016/j.metabol.2021.154838

[79] Danaei G, Lawes CM, Vander Hoorn S, Murray CJ, Ezzati M. Global and regional mortality from ischaemic heart disease and stroke attributable to higher-than-optimum blood glucose concentration: Comparative risk assessment. Lancet. 2006;**368**:1651-1659. DOI: 10.1016/S0140-6736(06)69700-6

[80] Rawshani A, Rawshani A, Franzén S, Eliasson B, Svensson AM, Miftaraj M, et al. Mortality and cardiovascular disease in type 1 and type 2 diabetes. The New England Journal of Medicine. 2017;**376**:1407-1418. DOI: 10.1056/NEJMoa1608664

[81] Booth GL, Kapral MK, Fung K, Tu JV. Recent trends in cardiovascular complications among men and women

with and without diabetes. Diabetes Care. 2006;**29**:32-37. DOI: 10.2337/diacare.29.01.06.dc05-0776

[82] Gregg EW, Cheng YJ, Srinivasan M, Lin J, Geiss LS, Albright AL, et al. Trends in cause-specific mortality among adults with and without diagnosed diabetes in the USA: An epidemiological analysis of linked national survey and vital statistics data. Lancet. 2018;**391**:2430-2440. DOI: 10.1016/S0140-6736(18)30314-3

[83] Lind M, Garcia-Rodriguez LA, Booth GL, Cea-Soriano L, Shah BR, Ekeroth G, et al. Mortality trends in patients with and without diabetes in Ontario, Canada and the UK from 1996 to 2009: A population-based study. Diabetologia. 2013;**56**:2601-2608. DOI: 10.1007/s00125-013-3063-1

[84] Jung CH, Chung JO, Han K, Ko SH, Ko KS, Park JY, et al. Improved trends in cardiovascular complications among subjects with type 2 diabetes in Korea: A nationwide study (2006-2013). Cardiovascular Diabetology. 2017;**16**:1. DOI: 10.1186/s12933-016-0482-6

[85] Park JH, Ha KH, Kim BY, Lee JH, Kim DJ. Trends in cardiovascular complications and mortality among patients with diabetes in South Korea. Diabetes and Metabolism Journal. 2021;**45**:120-124. DOI: 10.4093/dmj.2020.0175

[86] Cheng YJ, Imperatore G, Geiss LS, Saydah SH, Albright AL, Ali MK, et al. Trends and disparities in cardiovascular mortality among U.S. adults with and without self-reported diabetes, 1988-2015. Diabetes Care. 2018;**41**:2306-2315. DOI: 10.2337/dc18-0831

[87] Wright AK, Suarez-Ortegon MF, Read SH, Kontopantelis E, Buchan I, Emsley R, et al. Risk factor control and cardiovascular event risk in people with type 2 diabetes in primary and secondary prevention settings. Circulation. 2020;**142**:1925-1936. DOI: 10.1161/CIRCULATIONAHA.120.046783

[88] Martinelli I, Tomassoni D, Moruzzi M, Roy P, Cifani C, Amenta F, et al. Cardiovascular changes related to metabolic syndrome: Evidence in obese Zucker rats. International Journal of Molecular Sciences. 2020;**21**:2035. DOI: 10.3390/ijms21062035

[89] Rochlani Y, Pothineni NV, Kovelamudi S, Mehta JL. Metabolic syndrome: Pathophysiology, management, and modulation by natural compounds. Therapeutic Advances in Cardiovascular Disease. 2017;**11**:215-225. DOI: 10.1177/1753944717711379

[90] Marseglia L, Manti S, D'Angelo G, Nicotera A, Parisi E, Di Rosa G, et al. Oxidative stress in obesity: A critical component in human diseases. International Journal of Molecular Sciences. 2014;**16**:378-400. DOI: 10.3390/ijms16010378

[91] Steven S, Frenis K, Oelze M, Kalinovic S, Kuntic M, Bayo Jimenez MT, et al. Vascular inflammation and oxidative stress: Major triggers for cardiovascular disease. Oxidative Medicine and Cellular Longevity. 2019;**2019**:7092151. DOI: 10.1155/2019/7092151

[92] Koenen M, Hill MA, Cohen P, Sowers JR. Obesity, adipose tissue and vascular dysfunction. Circulation Research. 2021;**128**:951-968. DOI: 10.1161/CIRCRESAHA.121.318093

[93] Franks PW, Hanson RL, Knowler WC, Sievers ML, Bennett PH, Looker HC. Childhood obesity, other cardiovascular risk factors, and premature death. The New England Journal of Medicine. 2010;**362**:485-493. DOI: 10.1056/NEJMoa0904130

[94] Lee MJ, Wu Y, Fried SK. Adipose tissue heterogeneity: Implication of depot differences in adipose tissue for obesity complications. Molecular Aspects of Medicine. 2013;**34**:1-11. DOI: 10.1016/j.mam.2012.10.001

[95] Abel ED. Insulin signaling in the heart. American Journal of Physiology. Endocrinology and Metabolism. 2021;**321**:E130-E145. DOI: 10.1152/ajpendo.00158.2021

[96] Belke DD, Betuing S, Tuttle MJ, Graveleau C, Young ME, Pham M, et al. Insulin signaling coordinately regulates cardiac size, metabolism, and contractile protein isoform expression. The Journal of Clinical Investigation. 2002;**109**:629-639. DOI: 10.1172/JCI13946

[97] Capone F, Vettor R, Schiattarella GG. Cardiometabolic HFpEF: NASH of the heart. Circulation. 2023;**147**:451-453. DOI: 10.1161/CIRCULATIONAHA.122.062874

[98] Nakamura M, Sadoshima J. Cardiomyopathy in obesity, insulin resistance and diabetes. The Journal of Physiology. 2020;**598**:2977-2993. DOI: 10.1113/JP276747

[99] Jia G, Whaley-Connell A, Sowers JR. Diabetic cardiomyopathy: A hyperglycaemia- and insulin-resistance-induced heart disease. Diabetologia. 2018;**61**:21-28. DOI: 10.1007/s00125-017-4390-4

[100] Jia G, DeMarco VG, Sowers JR. Insulin resistance and hyperinsulinaemia in diabetic cardiomyopathy. Nature Reviews. Endocrinology. 2016;**12**:144-153. DOI: 10.1038/nrendo.2015.216

[101] Seferović PM, Petrie MC, Filippatos GS, Anker SD, Rosano G, Bauersachs J, et al. Type 2 diabetes mellitus and heart failure: A position statement from the heart failure Association of the European Society of cardiology. European Journal of Heart Failure. 2018;**20**:853-872. DOI: 10.1002/ejhf.1170

[102] Lorenzo-Almorós A, Cepeda-Rodrigo JM, Lorenzo Ó. Diabetic cardiomyopathy. Revista Clínica Española (Barc). 2022;**222**:100-111. DOI: 10.1016/j.rceng.2019.10.012

[103] Nichols GA, Hillier TA, Erbey JR, Brown JB. Congestive heart failure in type 2 diabetes: Prevalence, incidence, and risk factors. Diabetes Care. 2001;**24**:1614-1619. DOI: 10.2337/diacare.24.9.1614

[104] Sarma S, Mentz RJ, Kwasny MJ, Fought AJ, Huffman M, Subacius H, et al. Association between diabetes mellitus and post-discharge outcomes in patients hospitalized with heart failure: Findings from the EVEREST trial. European Journal of Heart Failure. 2013;**15**:194-202. DOI: 10.1093/eurjhf/hfs153

[105] Stratton IM, Adler AI, Neil HA, Matthews DR, Manley SE, Cull CA, et al. Association of glycaemia with macrovascular and microvascular complications of type 2 diabetes (UKPDS 35): Prospective observational study. BMJ. 2000;**321**:405-412. DOI: 10.1136/bmj.321.7258.405

[106] Reber E, Norman K, Endrich O, Schuetz P, Frei A, Stanga Z. Economic challenges in nutritional management. Journal of Clinical Medicine. 2019;**8**:1005. DOI: 10.3390/jcm8071005

[107] Wang X, Li Q, Liu Y, Jiang H, Chen W. Intermittent fasting versus continuous energy-restricted diet for patients with type 2 diabetes mellitus and metabolic syndrome for glycemic control: A systematic review and meta-analysis

of randomized controlled trials. Diabetes Research and Clinical Practice. 2021;**179**:109003. DOI: 10.1016/j.diabres.2021.109003

[108] Colman RJ, Anderson RM, Johnson SC, Kastman EK, Kosmatka KJ, Beasley TM, et al. Caloric restriction delays disease onset and mortality in rhesus monkeys. Science. 2009;**325**:201-204. DOI: 10.1126/science.1173635

[109] Das SK, Roberts SB, Bhapkar MV, Villareal DT, Fontana L, Martin CK, et al. Body-composition changes in the comprehensive assessment of long-term effects of reducing intake of energy (CALERIE)-2 study: A 2-y randomized controlled trial of calorie restriction in nonobese humans. The American Journal of Clinical Nutrition. 2017;**105**:913-927. DOI: 10.3945/ajcn.116.137232

[110] Johnson ML, Distelmaier K, Lanza IR, Irving BA, Robinson MM, Konopka AR, et al. Mechanism by which caloric restriction improves insulin sensitivity in sedentary obese adults. Diabetes. 2016;**65**:74-84. DOI: 10.2337/db15-0675

[111] Pignatti C, D'Adamo S, Stefanelli C, Flamigni F, Cetrullo S. Nutrients and pathways that regulate health span and life span. Geriatrics. 2020;**5**:95. DOI: 10.3390/geriatrics5040095

[112] Fontana L. The scientific basis of caloric restriction leading to longer life. Current Opinion in Gastroenterology. 2009;**25**:144-150. DOI: 10.1097/MOG.0b013e32831ef1ba

[113] Redman LM, Fontana L. Calorie restriction in humans: An update. Ageing Research Reviews. 2017;**39**:36-45. DOI: 10.1016/j.arr.2016.08.005

[114] Myers J, Kokkinos P, Nyelin E. Physical activity, cardiorespiratory fitness, and the metabolic syndrome. Nutrients. 2019;**11**:1652. DOI: 10.3390/nu11071652

[115] Pucci G. Sex- and gender-related prevalence, cardiovascular risk and therapeutic approach in metabolic syndrome: A review of the literature. Pharmacological Research. 2017;**120**:34-42. DOI: 10.1016/j.phrs.2017.03.008

[116] Sallis RE, Matuszak JM, Baggish AL, Franklin BA, Chodzko-Zajko W, Fletcher BJ, et al. Call to action on making physical activity assessment and prescription a medical standard of care. Current Sports Medicine Reports. 2016;**15**:207-214. DOI: 10.1249/JSR.0000000000000249

[117] Berra K, Rippe J, Manson JE. Making physical activity counseling a priority in clinical practice: The time for action is now. Journal of the American Medical Association. 2015;**314**:2617-2618. DOI: 10.1001/jama.2015.16244

[118] Omura JD, Bellissimo MP, Watson KB, Loustalot F, Fulton JE, Carlson SE. Primary care providers' physical activity counseling and referral practices and barriers for cardiovascular disease prevention. Preventive Medicine. 2018;**108**:115-122. DOI: 10.1016/j.ypmed.2017.12.030

[119] Brown E, Heerspink HJL, Cuthbertson DJ, Wilding JPH. SGLT2 inhibitors and GLP-1 receptor agonists: Established and emerging indications. Lancet. 2021;**398**:262-276. DOI: 10.1016/S0140-6736(21)00536-5

[120] Cowie MR, Fisher M. SGLT2 inhibitors: Mechanisms of cardiovascular benefit beyond glycaemic control. Nature Reviews. Cardiology. 2020;**17**:761-772. DOI: 10.1038/s41569-020-0406-8

Section 2

Diabetes Complications and Companions

Chapter 5

From a Glycocentric Approach to Prevention of Multi-Organ Damage in Type 2 Diabetes

Fernando Grover-Páez, Arantza Maya Gómez,
Alejandra Hernández Suárez and Andrea Martínez Echauri

Abstract

Nowadays, we are seeing radically interesting and promising changes in the treatment of patients with type-2 diabetes mellitus (T2 D), which favorably modify the prognosis related to fundamentally neuro-nephro and cardiorenal outcomes. Since no more than two decades ago, the pharmacological armamentarium for the treatment of people with T2D has basically consisted of the use of biguanides, sulfonylureas, insulin sensitizers, and insulins. A great amount of information has been accumulated through the results of new molecules such as sodium/glucose co-transporter type-2 inhibitors (SGLT2i), based on robust data arising from the experience of numerous studies, both clinical and experimental, as well as the glucagon-like peptide 1 receptor agonists (GLP-1ra), that has clearly shown multisystem benefits that improve the function of target organs and delay the onset of complications that ultimately impact the quality of life and the neuro-nephro-cardiovascular outcomes. In this review chapter, we not only highlight the different strategies for glucose control through SGLT2i, GLP-1ra or insulin, including even some fixed combinations, but also some information on different studies with GIP/GLP1 biagonist tirzepatide and on GIP/GLP1/Glucagon triagonist retatrutide primarily focused on weight loss, even though today, they are neither FDA approved nor a part of routine treatment.

Keywords: type 2 diabetes mellitus, Glycocentric, SGLT2i, glucagon like peptide-1 analog, tirzepatide, retatrutide, Nephro-protection, cardio-protection, neuroprotection

1. Introduction

Diabetes is a chronic, metabolic syndrome affecting about 537 million people worldwide, without considering those with undiagnosed diabetes. Type 2 diabetes (T2D) is the most common, and it represents around 80–90% of the cases [1].

Type 2 diabetes is characterized by chronic high blood glucose levels due to a deficiency in insulin production, a peripheral body's resistance to it, or both. The phenotypic expression of genetic defects in diabetogenic genes conditions alterations in insulin secretion, while peripheral insulin resistance is a consequence of the interaction of environmental risk factors (type of diet, sedentary lifestyle, etc.) [2].

IntechOpen

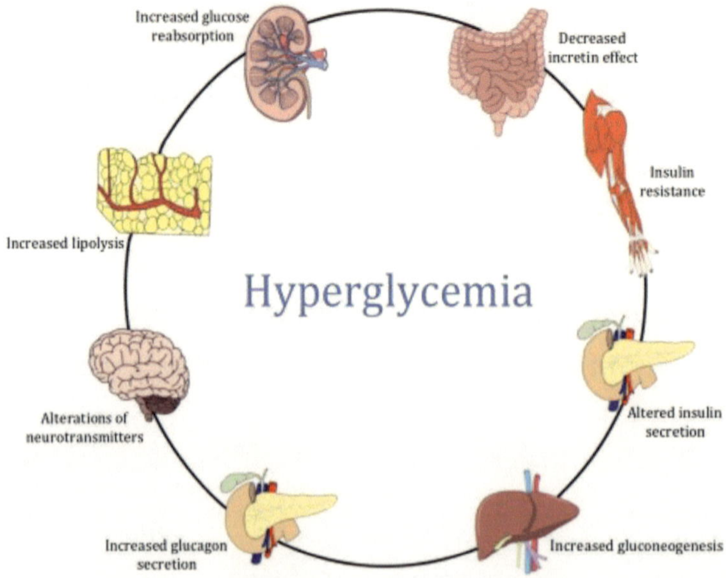

Figure 1.
The ominous octet summarizes the different mechanisms that lead to hyperglycemia.

The pathogenesis of diabetes has changed over time, from a unique approach collectively, from the insulin resistance in muscle and liver and β-cell failure referred to as the triumvirate (triumvirate), to the interaction of several phenomena as explained in the ominous octet. This ominous octet refers to the interaction of different pathways and organs related to the pathophysiology of T2D, including pancreatic β-cell failure, increased glucagon secretion, increased gluconeogenesis, increased lipolysis, insulin resistance, decreased incretin effect, decreased peripheral glucose uptake, increased renal glucose reabsorption, and alterations of neurotransmitters. All these leads are called the ominous octet (**Figure 1**) [3–5].

2. Macrovascular complications

Type 2 diabetes is related to accelerating atherosclerosis and is a leading cause of macrovascular complications, which include coronary heart disease, heart failure, cerebrovascular disease, and peripheral artery disease [6].

2.1 Coronary heart disease

As the prevalence of obesity and diabetes is increasing, the incidence of coronary heart disease (CHD) is also increasing, and it is reported as the leading cause of morbidity and mortality in people with diabetes. T2D is related to an increased risk of angina pectoris and asymptomatic ischemic episodes [7].

2.2 Heart failure

The prevalence of heart failure in people with diabetes is high, and it is a factor with a high impact on cardiovascular mortality and morbidity. Observations over the years have shown that myocardial dysfunction can occur in the absence of other cardiovascular diseases such as CHD, valvular heart disease, or hypertrophy [8].

An important characteristic observed in diabetic myocardium by imaging studies is the left ventricular concentric remodeling, and it is possibly attributed to impaired myocardial energetics and reduced systolic strain. Myocardial hypertrophy is attributed to hyperinsulinemia, myocardial triglyceride deposition, and an increased extracellular volume, which promotes collagen deposition and fibrosis. Mortality and hospitalization due to heart failure are higher in people with diabetes compared with non-diabetics [9].

2.3 Cerebrovascular disease

People with diabetes are highly susceptible to suffering a cerebrovascular event, and they are 12 times more likely to be hospitalized due to those events. Diabetes is a high-risk factor syndrome for ischemic stroke due to a group of events that include excessive oxidation, formation of advanced glycation end products, increased platelet aggregation, endothelial dysfunction, insulin resistance, impaired fibrinolysis, and hypercoagulability; these factors increase the risk for large artery atherosclerotic occlusive disease, facilitating an ischemic event [10].

2.4 Peripheral vascular disease

Peripheral vascular disease (PVD) is a common complication in people with diabetes, and it is usually a predictive factor for generalized artery dysfunction, including the prediction of cardiovascular events. Unfortunately, PVD is a disorder that occurs asymptomatic in many patients due to the presence of peripheral neuropathy; therefore, PVD is noticed until a complication like gangrene or ischemic ulcer appears, which inevitably leads to amputation [11].

3. Microvascular complications

The duration of the hyperglycemic state and genetic predisposition interacts and eventually affects the microvasculature, leading to complications in organs such as kidneys and eyes, as well as diabetic neuropathy [12].

3.1 Retinopathy

The most common cause of blindness worldwide is diabetic retinopathy (DR), and it appears in approximately 25.16% of the diabetic population. DR early signs are usually asymptomatic, so it is important to keep a regular eye examination in people with diabetes. DR is classified into two categories, non-proliferative DR and proliferative DR. It is important to identify early signs of DR to reduce the risk of visual loss [11].

3.2 Nephropathy

Diabetic nephropathy is defined as impaired kidney function in diabetic patients. This disease affects approximately 25% of people with diabetes. The diabetic nephropathy diagnosis is important because not all kidney alterations should be attributed to diabetes [11].

The American Diabetes Association (ADA) established that the diagnosis should be based upon the findings of decreased glomerular filtration rate (<60 ml/min/1.73 m^2) and/or an increased urinary albumin excretion (≥30 mg/g creatinine) for at least 3 months [12].

4. Current treatment of type 2 diabetes mellitus

Despite the successful generation of a major difference in glycemic control between the intensive and conventional treatment arms, the well-known United Kingdom Prospective Diabetes Study (UKPDS) did not demonstrate the benefits on macrovascular disease, including the Action to Control Cardiovascular Risk in Diabetes (ACCORD), the Action in Diabetes and Vascular Disease (ADVANCE), and the Veterans Affairs Diabetes Trial (VADT) [13–15]. Even the ACCORD caused alarm when the trial was terminated prematurely at 3.5 years in response to an unexpected—and to date unexplained—22% increased mortality in the intensive glycemic control group [13, 16, 17]. The ACCORD investigators concluded that even though intensive glycemic control reduced non-fatal myocardial infarctions, this approach could not be recommended for high-risk patients with advanced type 2 diabetes [16].

On the other hand, in epidemiological studies, it is well known that cardiovascular risk rises with worsening glycemic control, defined by fasting glucose or HbA 1c [18]. For this reason, we must remember the essential role of insulin in glycemic control, which remains the therapy of choice, particularly when the patient is metabolically uncontrolled as reported in a meta-analysis and meta-regression in five RCTs involving 590 participants with type 2 diabetes, that insulin pump therapy continuous subcutaneous insulin infusion (CSII; insulin pump therapy) achieves better glycemic control than multiple daily insulin injections (MDI) in participants with poor diabetes control at baseline; even more, CSII therapy safely and significantly improved metabolic control with less insulin usage and with no sustainable reduction of BM, blood pressure, and lipid profile, in insulin-resistant T2D people, with excellent treatment adherence and satisfaction [19, 20]. Besides, it is worth noting the importance played by insulin analogs such as insulin glargine or degludec, as well as fixed combinations with glucagon-like peptide-1 receptor agonists such as liraglutide, where in a study carried out to demonstrate the efficacy and safety of a fixed-ratio combination of insulin degludec and liraglutide (IDegLira) compared with its components given alone, IDeLira reduced 1.9% HbA1c, and no clinically relevant differences between treatments with respect to standard safety assessments were noted, and the safety profile of IDegLira reflected those of its component parts [21]. However, recent landmark cardiovascular outcome trials (CVOTs) in patients with T2D have revealed major benefits of certain glucose-lowering medications in terms of reduction of cardiovascular events [18]. Trials of agents from two classes of novel glucose-lowering drugs, that is, sodium-glucose cotransporter-2 inhibitors (SGLT2i) and glucagon-like peptide receptor agonists (GLP-1ra), have shown statistically significant and clinically meaningful reductions in three- or four-point major adverse cardiovascular events (MACE), both in patients with established cardiovascular diseases and in those at high risk for such disease [13–16]. These results stand in marked contrast to earlier trials trying to primarily lower HbA1c, by using combinations of antihyperglycemic agents that failed to show any benefit of lowering HbA1c in reducing macrovascular events.

In this regard, the ADA/EASD consensus report "Management of Hyperglycemia in Type 2 Diabetes, 2022" [22–24] recommends a holistic, multifactorial, person-centered approach accounting for the lifelong nature of type 2 diabetes. Person-specific factors that affect the choice of treatment include individualized glycemic and weight goals, impact on weight, hypoglycemia and cardiorenal protection, underlying physiologic factors, side effect profiles of medications, complexity of regimen, regimen choice to optimize medication use and reduce treatment discontinuation, and access, cost, and availability of medication. Lifestyle modifications and health behaviors that improve health should be emphasized along with any pharmacologic therapy. This chapter will broadly address the benefits of preventing or delaying the progression of complications, particularly at the cardiovascular and renal level, and in less detail the effects on the central nervous system observed in experimental studies with these pharmacological classes, such as SGLT2i, as well as GLP-1ra, which have shown a favorable impact, especially on cardiovascular and renal outcomes.

5. The role of glucose/sodium cotransporter type 2 (ISGLT2) inhibitors

Sodium-glucose cotransporter-2 inhibitors (SGLT2i), also known as gliflozins or flozins, are relatively new glucose-lowering drugs that include empagliflozin, dapagliflozin, canagliflozin, and ertugliflozin; they are used as a T2D treatment. By inhibiting the SGLT2 expressed in the proximal convoluted tubule of the nephron (responsible for 90% of glucose reabsorption), these drugs favor glycosuria and hence lower glycemia levels. Although they are believed to cause smaller HbA1C reductions (between 0.5 and 0.7%) than other antidiabetics, the multi-organic benefits addressed in this section, which comprehend neuro, cardio, and nephroprotective effects, are simply outstanding [25] (**Figure 2**).

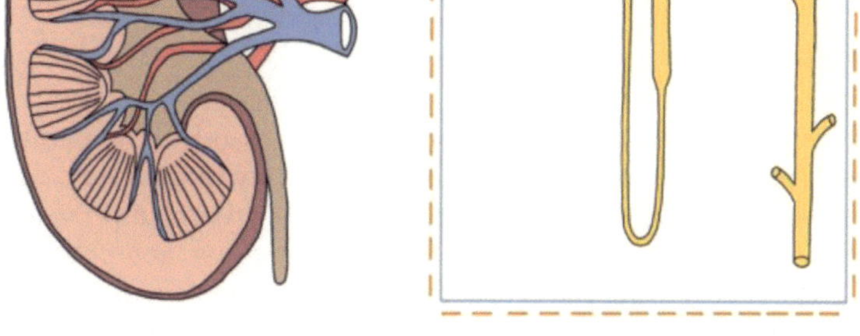

Figure 2.
Shows the site of action of SGLT2i in the nephron.

5.1 Empagliflozin and neuroprotective effects

Since iSGLT2 are lipid-soluble drugs, they can cross the brain–blood barrier and exert interesting neuroprotective effects. Among the ones to be highlighted, empagliflozin states the fact that, when the appropriate brain concentrations are reached (around 0.5 μM), this medicament works as an acetylcholinesterase (AChE) inhibitor. When AChE activity is decreased, acetylcholine M1 receptors face an important increment and thus favor a functional cognitive improvement [25].

T2D patients tend to have low brain-derived neurotrophic factor (BDNF) levels. This becomes relevant when realizing that BDNF plays a crucial role in neuronal growth and plasticity, neurotransmission, memorizing, and learning processes. Hence, cognitive impairment is propitiated, not to mention that it's been associated with inflammation and consequent atherosclerosis risk. When being treated with Empagliflozin, at least in mice, BNDF levels show an important increase [25].

5.2 Empagliflozin and cardioprotective effects

Empagliflozin has been associated, among randomized clinical trials, to lower hospitalization, myocardial infarctions, nonfatal strokes, and death from cardiovascular disease rates. Although these may sound like greater effects, there are other significant ones such as decreases in both systolic and diastolic blood pressures (without compensatory higher heart rates) and reduction in weight, waist circumference, and uric acid level [26].

On the other hand, heart failure is recognized as an important diabetic comorbidity; hence, considering Empagliflozin's diuretic effect, it can be said that its main effect focuses on reducing plasma volume, leading to increased hematocrit and an expected blood pressure drop (3–4 mmHg in 12 weeks), alleviating the heart's workload. Another significant myocardial effect consists of reducing diastolic stiffness and improving diastolic function [27].

5.3 Empagliflozin and nephroprotective effects

T2D patients are susceptible to developing microvascular complications such as kidney disease, which afflicts around 35% of them and magnifies mortality rates. This reason is sufficient to look for innovative therapies, such as SGLT2i's use. In several clinical trials, Empagliflozin has been demonstrated to have renal protective effects, even though the underlying mechanism is not well evidenced. Nevertheless, it is believed to be a summation of the association with blood pressure and body mass reduction, diuresis, and activation of tubuloglomerular feedback [28–30].

5.4 Dapagliflozin and neuroprotective effects

Dapagliflozin exerts no significant improvement in cognitive domains, nor in impaired brain activation, compared to other drugs. However, rat models suggest quite impressive effects. Likewise, it's been associated with the improvement of brain mitochondrial membrane depolarization, function, swelling, and decreased ROS production [31]. Among other numerous benefits, the medicament demonstrated both antioxidant and antiapoptotic properties by alleviating memory and cognition impairment in Streptozotocin (STZ)-induced diabetic rats, probably through its effect on Wnt/β-Catenin and cAMP-response element binding protein (CREB) pathway [32].

5.5 Dapagliflozin and cardioprotective effects

T2D people harbor considerable risk factors, which make them more susceptible to developing atherosclerotic cardiovascular disease and its derivatives. Supporting this idea states the relevance of clinical studies, which show findings such as that prejudicial cardiovascular outcomes in T2D patients treated with Dapagliflozin, according to DECLARE-TIMI 58 clinical trial results, were proven to diminish. This is a fact sustained by an evident lowering of hospitalizations for heart failure and cardiovascular death [33].

5.6 Dapagliflozin and nephroprotective effects

Worrisome renal outcomes in T2D patients, if they have not already progressed into a kidney disease stage, are major events. Therefore, the fact that a sodium-glucose cotransporter-2 inhibitor like Dapagliflozin has been studied and tested in clinical studies represents a scenario leading to new windows of opportunity. Trials such as DAPA-CKD and DECLARE-TIMI 58 found that when administering this medication (compared to placebo), there was a lowering of the declines in the eGFR, meaning a reduction in the progression of kidney disease, a situation that simultaneously translates into less renal-caused deaths [34].

5.7 Others gliflozins

Canagliflozin and Ertugliflozin are also relevant medicaments, belonging to the SGLT2i class. As could be expected, they both have demonstrated their efficacy in lowering hyperglycemia and exerting favorable cardiorenal effects in their principal clinical studies: CREDENCE and VERTIS CV, respectively [35, 36].

6. Glucagon-like peptide 1 receptor agonists

Glucagon-like peptide 1 (GLP-1) is an incretin hormone released from intestinal L-cells of the distal ileum. It is postprandially secreted and binds to a seven-transmembrane G protein-coupled receptor to activate signaling cascades, leading to beneficial downstream effects that include increased insulin secretion in a glucose-dependent manner, somatostatin secretion, lipolysis, decreased glucagon secretion, decreased gastric emptying, and satiety, which leads to a promotion of weight loss (**Figure 3**) [37–39].

The beta-cell mass (responsible for insulin secretion) is reduced in the later stages of T2D, resulting in the requirement of exogenous insulin therapy. Therefore, beta-cell mass preservation and strategies to stimulate beta-cell replication is an important aim in a recent investigation. In this respect, GLP-1 has also shown beta-cell preservation effects (beta-cell proliferation, neogenesis, and prevention of apoptosis) [35, 38]. There are six GLP-1 receptor agonists approved as T2D treatment. Those are dulaglutide, semaglutide (oral and injected), exenatide, albiglutide, liraglutide, and lixisenatide [39].

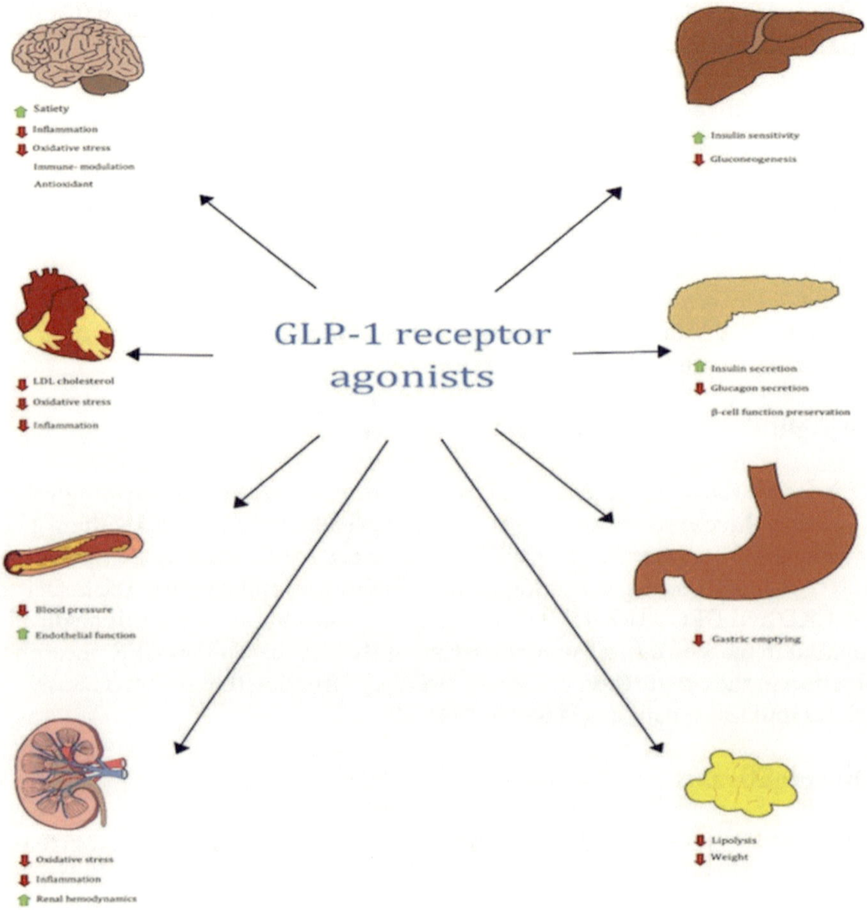

Figure 3.
Shows the different sites of action of GLP-1 receptor agonists.

6.1 Dulaglutide and neuroprotective effects

GLP-1 receptor agonists have demonstrated neuroprotective effects in a range of neurodegenerative conditions. Since GLP-1 receptors are expressed throughout the brain, this type of drug is considered to have neurotrophic and anti-inflammation effects for central nervous system (CNS) diseases. A recent study demonstrated that dulaglutide possessed protective effects on the pathogenesis of experimental autoimmune encephalomyelitis (EAE), which is an established animal model to study human multiple sclerosis [40, 41].

In EAE pathogenesis, the CD4 positive T cells especially Type 1 helper T (Th1) and Type 17 helper T (Th17), which are also interferon (IFN)-y secreting and interleukin (IL)-17 A producing, are inflammatory T cells that mediate the demyelination of neurons in the CNS. In this sense, dulaglutide holds protective effects via immune-modulation of CD4-positive T helper cell lineage in the CNS parenchyma by suppressing the percentage of encephalitogenic Th1/Th17 cells [40].

On the other hand, Parkinson's is one of the most common neurodegenerative diseases that is often linked with diabetes. They both are chronic disorders with pathogenic mechanisms being mitochondrial failure, oxidative stress, and protein aggregation; therefore, patients with T2D are more likely to experience severe Parkinson's disease (PD) symptoms and accelerated neurodegeneration. That being the case, there has been research done to examine the neuroprotective effects of these antidiabetic medications [41–43].

6.2 Dulaglutide and cardioprotective effects

The REWIND trial carried out in 24 countries to assess the cardioprotective effects of dulaglutide in people with cardiovascular risk factors, who were under antihyperglycemic regimens, suggested that dulaglutide reduced cardiovascular events. It also reduced weight, LDL cholesterol, and blood pressure, suggested as the mechanisms by which dulaglutide exerts cardioprotective effects. Moreover, the study also showed dulaglutide's long-term safety effects and durability [44].

6.3 Dulaglutide and nephroprotective effects

In the REWIND trial, renal outcomes were collected as part of the secondary microvascular outcome. It showed that dulaglutide reduced all three components of composite renal outcome (the development of new macroalbuminuria, a sustained ≥30% decline in eGFR, and chronic renal replacement therapy), having a robust effect on the development of macroalbuminuria.

The study suggested that dulaglutide reduced the progression of kidney disease and preserved renal function by reducing HbA1c and systolic blood pressure. However, there is evidence that proposes GLP-1 receptor agonists as agents that directly affect the kidney by reducing inflammation and oxidative stress and improving endothelial function. Therefore, analyses concluded that dulaglutide is an antidiabetic treatment that is likely to confer additional renal benefits [44].

6.4 Semaglutide and neuroprotective effects

Although GLP-1 receptors are expressed in some brain regions, there are some reports suggesting that semaglutide does not cross the blood–brain barrier (BBB). However, it may have access to GLP-1 receptors through leaks in BBB or have an entry into additional regions of the brain. Besides, semaglutide improves insulin resistance and signaling pathways and reduces body mass, which are important factors in the progression of metabolic and neurodegenerative diseases. There have been studies that have demonstrated the neuroprotective efficacy of semaglutide in the rat model and in human neuroblastoma by decreasing inflammation and apoptosis. It has been demonstrated that semaglutide can be safely administered to adults including geriatric patients with renal, hepatic, and cardiovascular disorders [45].

6.5 Semaglutide and cardioprotective effects

Semaglutide is a long-acting GLP-1 analog for T2D with an extended half-life of approximately 1 week that has been shown to inhibit exercise-induced myocardial oxidative stress and inflammation, which are mechanisms that also occur in hyperglycemic states. Semaglutide exerts cardioprotective effects by activating the AMPK pathway and reducing ROS production and inflammation-related proteins. Moreover, this medicament ameliorated myocardial morphological changes and lipid accumulation, which leads to an increase of myocardial oxidative stress response, common in diabetic cardiomyopathy, and decreased the expression of NF-kB, TNF-α, and IL-1β [45, 46].

Both studies (SUSTAIN-6 and PIONEER-6) demonstrated that semaglutide therapy reduces 24% of cardiovascular adverse effects. Moreover, semaglutide-treated patients had a lower risk of nephropathy but a higher risk of diabetic retinopathy complications (vitreous hemorrhage, blindness, or the need for treatment with an intravitreal agent or photocoagulation) in comparison with those receiving placebo. This drug also showed sustained weight loss and a reduction in systolic blood pressure vs. placebo group over 2 years. Given this, semaglutide was the first long-acting GLP-1 receptor agonist to be approved by the United Food and Drug Administration for obesity management [46, 47].

6.6 Semaglutide and nephroprotective effects

Recent evidence supports that GLP-1 receptor agonists improve cardiovascular and renal outcomes in T2D by promoting weight loss, blood pressure, and glycemic control. In this sense, semaglutide has been demonstrated to improve cardiorenal outcomes in patients with T2D. One recent study shows semaglutide's effect on renal outcomes in the db/db UNx-Renin AAV mouse model of hypertension accelerated DKD, which reported a reduced glomerulosclerosis severity and improvements in hyperglycemia, systolic and diastolic blood pressure, and albuminuria. The anti-hypertensive action of GLP-1 receptor agonists may be secondary to their diuretic and natriuretic effects, and there is speculation that the nephroprotective activity of semaglutide could be linked to the improvement in renal hemodynamics. GLP-1 receptors in the kidney are reported to be in the vascular smooth muscle cells; therefore, their activation mediates renal vasorelaxant and blood flow, which translates to the preservation of glomerular function [37, 48].

6.7 Other GLP-1 analogs, dual and triple agonist

Several trials have reported that apart from the improvement in glucose control and the decrease in body mass and blood pressure, liraglutide and albiglutide reported a reduced hazard of the primary cardiovascular outcome (nonfatal myocardial infarction, nonfatal stroke, or death from cardiovascular causes). In addition, liraglutide and lixisenatide reduced the predefined composite renal outcome mainly by a lower incidence of macroalbuminuria [39, 49].

Regarding the neuroprotective effects of the GLP-1 agonists, lixisenatide was found to be a protective treatment of behavioral and neurological functions. It also has a suppressing effect on cerebral oxidative stress and inflammation in diabetic rats. On this subject, liraglutide was reported to suppress neuroinflammation. Lastly, exenatide was also found to have neuroprotective effects in preclinical models of Parkinson's disease [50, 51]. Finally, a novel dual glucose-dependent insulinotropic polypeptide and GLP-1 receptor agonist tirzepatide (**Figure 4**) and a GIP/GLP1/Glucagon triagonist retatrutide are being investigated, both in clinical trials and in experimental studies, respectively, which have shown a benefit in metabolic control through the reduction of HbA1c, and in body mass mainly, with reductions around 20–30% compared with the results observed through bariatric surgery, although currently, they are neither FDA approved nor of routine treatment [52, 53].

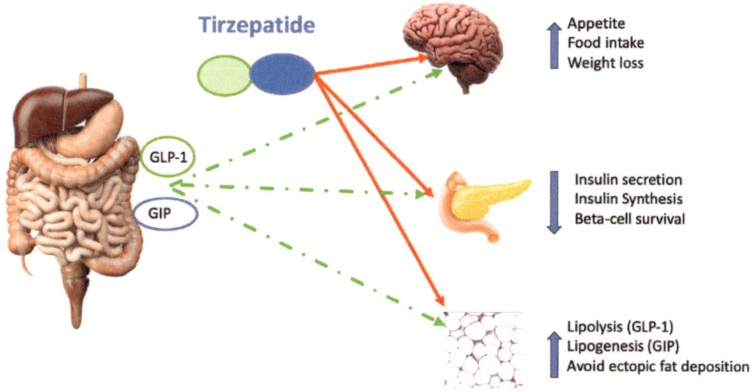

Figure 4.
Shows the different mechanisms of action of Tirzepatide.

7. Conclusion

With all this information and in view of this promising panorama with these new molecules whose outcomes favor a better prognosis regarding, control glucose, weight reduction, microvascular, and macrovascular complications, it is necessary to consider a personalized holistic therapy for each patient to improve their quality of life and reduce their morbidity and mortality.

Author details

Fernando Grover-Páez*, Arantza Maya Gómez, Alejandra Hernández Suárez and Andrea Martínez Echauri
Health Sciences University Center, University of Guadalajara, Mexico

*Address all correspondence to: fgroverp@hotmail.com

References

[1] International Diabetes Federation. IDF Diabetes Atlas 10th edition 202. diabetesatlas.org. 2021. Available from: https://diabetesatlas.org/

[2] Conget I. Diagnóstico, clasificación y patogenia de la diabetes mellitus. Revista Española de Cardiología. 2002;**55**(5):528-535

[3] DeFronzo RA. From the triumvirate to the ominous octet: A new paradigm for the treatment of type 2 diabetes mellitus. Diabetes. 2009;**58**(4):773-795. DOI: 10.2337/db09-9028

[4] Yap-Campos K, Sánchez-Gálvez X, Rivero-López C. El papel de los inhibidores de la DPP4: un enfoque actual en el manejo de la diabetes mellitus tipo 2. Aten Fam. 2017;**24**(3):136-139

[5] Huang D, Refaat M, Mohammedi K, Jayyousi A, Al Suwaidi J, Abi KC. Macrovascular complications in patients with diabetes and prediabetes. BioMed Research International. 2017;**2017**:1-9

[6] Viigimaa M, Sachinidis A, Toumpourleka M, Koutsampasopoulos K, Alliksoo S, Titma T. Macrovascular complications of type 2 diabetes mellitus. Current Vascular Pharmacology. 2019;**18**(2). DOI: 10.2174/1570161117666190405165151

[7] Wilson PWF. Diabetes mellitus and coronary heart disease. Endocrinology and Metabolism Clinics of North America. 2001;**30**(4):857-881. DOI: 10.1016/S0889-8529(05)70219-X

[8] Lehrke M, Marx N. Diabetes mellitus and heart failure. The American Journal of Medicine. 2017;**130**(6S):S40-S50. DOI: 10.1016/j.amjmed.2017.04.010

[9] Lukovits TG, Mazzone T, Gorelick PB. Diabetes mellitus and cerebrovascular disease. Neuroepidemiology. 1999;**18**(1):1-14. DOI: 10.1159/000026190

[10] Huysman E, Mathieu C. Diabetes and peripheral vascular disease. Acta chirurgica Belgica. 2009;**109**(5):587-594. DOI: 10.1080/00015458.2009.11680493

[11] Faselis C, Katsimardou A, Imprialos K, Deligkaris P, Kallistratos M, Dimitriadis K. Microvascular complications of type 2 diabetes mellitus. Current Vascular Pharmacology. 2020;**18**(2):117-124. DOI: 10.2174/1570161117666190502103733

[12] Summary of Revisions. Standards of medical Care in diabetes—2020. Diabetes Care. 2019;**43**(Supplement 1):S4-S6. DOI: 10.2337/dc20-srev

[13] Gerstein HC, Miller ME, Byington RP, et al. Effects of intensive glucose lowering in type 2 diabetes. The New England Journal of Medicine. 2008;**358**(24):2545-2559

[14] Patel A, MacMahon S, Chalmers J, et al. Intensive blood glucose control and vascular outcomes in patients with type 2 diabetes. The New England Journal of Medicine. 2008;**358**(24):2560-2572

[15] Duckworth W, Abraira C, Moritz T, et al. Glucose control and vascular complications in veterans with type 2 diabetes. The New England Journal of Medicine. 2009;**360**(2):129-139

[16] Dluhy RG, McMahon GT. Intensive glycemic control in the ACCORD and ADVANCE trials. The

New England Journal of Medicine. 2008;**358**(24):2630-2633

[17] Group AS, Gerstein HC, Miller ME, et al. Long-term effects of intensive glucose lowering on cardiovascular outcomes. The New England Journal of Medicine. 2011;**364**(9):818-828

[18] Dal Canto E, Ceriello A, Ryden L, et al. Diabetes as a cardiovascular risk factor: An overview of global trends of macro and microvascular complications. European Journal of Preventive Cardiology. 2019;**26**(2S):25-32

[19] Pickup JC, Reznik Y, Sutton AJ. Glycemic control during continuous subcutaneous insulin infusion versus multiple daily insulin injections in type 2 diabetes: Individual patient data meta-analysis and meta-regression of randomized controlled trials. Diabetes Care. 2017;**40**:715-722

[20] Chlup R, Runzis S, Castaneda J, Lee S, Nguyen X, Cohen O. Complex assessment of metabolic effectiveness of insulin pump therapy in patients with type 2 diabetes beyond HbA1c reduction. Diabetes Technology and Therapeutics. 2018;**20**(2):153-159

[21] Gough SC, Bode B, Woo V, Rodbard HW, Linjawi S, Poulsen P, et al. Efficacy and safety of a fixed-ratio combination of insulin degludec and liraglutide (IDegLira) compared with its components given alone: Results of a phase 3, open-label, randomised, 26-week, treat-to-target trial in insulin-naive patients with type 2 diabetes. Lancet Diabetes Endocrinol. 2014;**2**(11):885-893. DOI: 10.1016/S2213-8587(14)70174-3

[22] Davies MJ, D'Alessio DA, Fradkin J, et al. A consensus report by the American Diabetes Association (ADA) and the European Association for the Study of diabetes (EASD). Diabetes Care. 2018;**2018**(41):2669-2701

[23] Buse JB, Wexler DJ, Tsapas A, et al. A consensus report by the American Diabetes Association (ADA) and the European Association for the Study of diabetes (EASD). Diabetes Care. 2018;**2020**(43):487-493

[24] Davies MJ, Aroda VR, Collins BS, et al. A consensus report by the American Diabetes Association (ADA) and the European Association for the Study of diabetes (EASD). Diabetes Care. 2022;**2022**(45):2753-2786

[25] Pawlos A, Broncel M, Woźniak E, Gorzelak-Pabiś P. Neuroprotective effect of SGLT2 inhibitors. Molecules. 2021;**26**(23):7213. DOI: 10.3390/molecules26237213

[26] Zinman B, Wanner C, Lachin JM, Fitchett D, Bluhmki E, Hantel S, et al. EMPA-REG OUTCOME Investigators. Empagliflozin, cardiovascular outcomes, and mortality in type 2 diabetes. The New England Journal of Medicine. 2015;**373**(22):2117-2128. DOI: 10.1056/NEJMoa1504720

[27] Pabel S, Wagner S, Bollenberg H, et al. Empagliflozin directly improves diastolic function in human heart failure. Journal of Cardiac Failure. 2018;**20**(12):1690-1700. DOI: 10.1002/ejhf.1328

[28] Kowalska K, Walczak J, Femlak J, Młynarska E, Franczyk B, Rysz J. Empagliflozin—A new chance for patients with chronic heart failure. Pharmaceuticals (Basel). 2021;**15**(1):47. DOI: 10.3390/ph15010047

[29] Wanner C, Inzucchi SE, Lachin JM, Fitchett D, von Eynatten M, Mattheus M, et al. Empagliflozin and progression

of kidney disease in type 2 diabetes. The New England Journal of Medicine. 2016;**375**(4):323-334. DOI: 10.1056/NEJMoa1515920

[30] Perrone-Filardi P, Avogaro A, Bonora E, Colivicchi F, Fioretto P, Maggioni AP, et al. Mechanisms linking empagliflozin to cardiovascular and renal protection. International Journal of Cardiology. 2017;**241**:450-456. DOI: 10.1016/j.ijcard.2017.03.089

[31] Erdogan MA, Yusuf D, Christy J, Solmaz V, Erdogan A, Taskiran E, et al. Highly selective SGLT2 inhibitor dapagliflozin reduces seizure activity in pentylenetetrazol-induced murine model of epilepsy. BMC Neurology. 2018;**18**(1):81. DOI: 10.1186/s12883-018-1086-4

[32] El-Safty H, Ismail A, Abdelsalam RM, El-Sahar AE, Saad MA. Dapagliflozin diminishes memory and cognition impairment in streptozotocin induced diabetes through its effect on Wnt/β-catenin and CREB pathway. Brain Research Bulletin. 2022;**181**:109-120. DOI: 10.1016/j.brainresbull.2022.01.017

[33] Wiviott SD, Raz I, Bonaca MP, Mosenzon O, Kato ET, Cahn A, et al. DECLARE–TIMI 58 Investigators. Dapagliflozin and cardiovascular outcomes in type 2 diabetes. The New England Journal of Medicine. 2019;**380**(4):347-357. DOI: 10.1056/NEJMoa1812389

[34] Heerspink HJL, Stefánsson BV, Correa-Rotter R, Chertow GM, Greene T, Hou F-F, et al. For the DAPA-CKD trial committees and Investigators. Dapagliflozin in patients with chronic kidney disease. The New England Journal of Medicine. 2020;**383**:1436-1446. DOI: 10.1056/NEJMoa2024816

[35] Jardine MJ, Zhou Z, Mahaffey KW, Oshima M, Agarwal R, Bakris G, et al. Renal, cardiovascular, and safety outcomes of canagliflozin by baseline kidney function: A secondary analysis of the CREDENCE randomized trial. Journal of the American Society of Nephrology. 2020;**31**(5):1128-1139. DOI: 10.1681/ASN.2019111168

[36] Pratley RE, Cannon CP, Cherney DZI, Cosentino F, McGuire DK, Essex MN, et al. Cardiorenal outcomes, kidney function, and other safety outcomes with ertugliflozin in older adults with type 2 diabetes (VERTIS CV): Secondary analyses from a randomised, double-blind trial. Lancet Healthy Longev. 2023;**4**(4):e143-e154. DOI: 10.1016/S2666-7568(23)00032-6

[37] Lee Y-S, Jun H-S. Anti-diabetic actions of glucagon-like peptide-1 on pancreatic beta-cells. Metabolism. 2014;**63**(1):9-19. DOI: 10.1016/j.metabol.2013.09.010

[38] DeFronzo RA, Abdul-Ghani MA. Preservation of β-cell function: The key to diabetes prevention. The Journal of Clinical Endocrinology and Metabolism. 2011;**96**(8):2354k-23566k. DOI: 10.1210/jc.2011-0246

[39] Tommerdahl KL, Kendrick J, Bjornstad P. The role of glucagon-like peptide 1 (GLP-1) receptor agonists in the prevention and treatment of diabetic kidney disease: Insights from the AMPLITUDE-O trial. Clinical Journal of the American Society of Nephrology. 2022;**17**(6):905-907. DOI: 10.2215/CJN.00020122

[40] Kristensen SL, Rørth R, Jhund PS, Docherty KF, Sattar N, Preiss D, et al. Cardiovascular, mortality, and kidney outcomes with GLP-1 receptor agonists

in patients with type 2 diabetes: A systematic review and meta-analysis of cardiovascular outcome trials. The Lancet. 2019;**7**(10):776-785

[41] Madsbad S. Review of head-to-head comparisons of glucagon-like peptide-1 receptor agonists. Diabetes, Obesity and Metabolism. 2016;**18**(4):317-332. DOI: 10.1111/dom.12596

[42] Chiou H-YC, Lin M-W, Hsiao P-J, Chen C-L, Chiao S, Lin T-Y, et al. Dulaglutide modulates the development of tissue-infiltrating TH1/Th17 cells and the pathogenicity of encephalitogenic Th1 cells in the central nervous system. International Journal of Molecular Sciences. 2019;**20**(7):1584. DOI: 10.3390/ijms20071584

[43] Maskery MP, Holscher C, Jones SP, Price CI, Strain WD, Watkins CL, et al. Glucagon-like peptide-1 receptor agonists as neuroprotective agents for ischemic stroke: A systematic scoping review. Journal of Cerebral Blood Flow & Metabolism. 2021;**41**(1):14-30. DOI: 10.1177/0271678X20952011

[44] Gerstein HC, Colhoun HM, Dagenais GR, Diaz R, Lakshmanan M, Pais P, et al. Dulaglutide and cardiovascular outcomes in type 2 diabetes (REWIND): A double-blind, randomised placebo-controlled trial. The Lancet. 2019;**394**(10193):121-130. DOI: 10.1016/S0140-6736(19)31149-3

[45] Mahapatra M, Karuppasamy M, Sahoo BM. Therapeutic potential of semaglutide, a newer GLP-1 receptor agonist, in abating obesity, non-alcoholic steatohepatitis and neurodegenerative diseases: A narrative review. Pharmaceutical Research. 2022;**39**(6):1233-1248. DOI: 10.1007/s11095-022-03302-1

[46] Marso SP, Bain SC, Consoli A, Eliaschewitz FG, Jódar E, Leiter LA, et al. Semaglutide and cardiovascular outcomes in patients with type 2 diabetes. The New England Journal of Medicine. 2016;**375**(19):1834-1844. DOI: 10.1056/NEJMoa1607141

[47] Bain SC, Mosenzon O, Arechavaleta R, et al. Cardiovascular safety of oral semaglutide in patients with type 2 diabetes: Rationale, design and patient baseline characteristics for the PIONEER 6 trial. Diabetes, Obesity & Metabolism. 2019;**21**:499-508. DOI: 10.1111/dom.13553

[48] Dalbøge LS, Christensen M, Madsen MR, Secher T, Endlich N, Drenic V, et al. Nephroprotective effects of semaglutide as mono- and combination treatment with lisinopril in a mouse model of hypertension-accelerated diabetic kidney disease. Biomedicines. 2022;**10**(7):1661. DOI: 10.3390/biomedicines10071661

[49] Mann JFE, Ørsted DD, Brown-Frandsen K, Marso SP, Poulter NR, Rasmussen S, et al. Liraglutide and renal outcomes in type 2 diabetes. The New England Journal of Medicine. 2017;**377**:839-848. DOI: 10.1056/nejmoa1616011

[50] Adel-Latif RG, Heeba GH, Taye A, Khalifa MMA. Lixisenatide, a novel GLP-1 analog, protects against cerebral ischemia/reperfusion injury in diabetic rats. Naunyn-Schmiedeberg's Archives of Pharmacology. 2018;**391**:705-717. DOI: 10.1007/s00210-018-1497-1

[51] You J, Manaenko A, Hakon J, Hansen-Schwartz J, Tang J, Zhang JH. Liraglutide, a long-acting GLP-1 mimetic, and its metabolite attenuate inflammation after intracerebral haemorrhage. Journal of

Cerebral Blood Flow and Metabolism. 2012;**32**:2201-2210. DOI: 10.1038/jcbfm.2012.133

[52] Sattar N, McGuire DK, Pavo I, Govinda J, et al. Tirzepatide cardiovascular event risk assessment: A pre-specified meta-analysis. Nature Medicine. 2022;**28**:591-598. DOI: 10.1038/s41591-022-01707-4

[53] Knerr PJ, Mowery SA, Douros JD, et al. Next generation GLP-1/GIP/glucagon triple agonists normalize body weight in obese mice. Molecular Metabolism. 2022;**63**:101533. DOI: 10.1016/j.molmet.2022.101533

Chapter 6

Dyslipoproteinaemia: Important Concern in Type 2 Diabetes

Mick John Kumwenda

Abstract

Dyslipoproteinaemia, also known as dyslipidaemia, occurs in more than 70% of people with diabetes and is a significant risk factor for atherosclerotic cardiovascular disease (ASCVD) associated with obesity, hypertension, and poor glycaemic control. The prevalence of diabetes worldwide is increasing, and so is the death rate in people with diabetes. The causes of dyslipoproteinaemia are divided into primary (genetic) or secondary, which are diagnosed from history (diabetes, obesity, endocrine disorders, and chronic kidney disease). The pattern of dyslipoproteinaemia in diabetes typically consists of increased levels of fasting and post-prandial triacylglycerols (TAGs), Low Dense Lipoprotein-C (LDL-C), non-HDL-C, small LDL particles and Apo-B and lower levels of non-atherogenic HDL-C and ApoA1. Treating dyslipoproteinaemia includes patients' risk stratification and targeting those at high risk. It consists of lifestyle modification, statins, cholesterol absorption inhibitors (ezetimibe), drugs that increase HDL and reduce LDL (niacin, fibrates), triglycerides (Omega-3) and bile acid sequestrants. Proprotein convertase subtilisin–kexin type 9 inhibitors reduce LDL by 60–80%, ApoB by 50% and Lp (a) by 25% and should be considered in all people with diabetes with other risk factors and with coexisting primary dyslipoproteinaemia before developing ASCVD as well as those with established ASCVD.

Keywords: dyslipidaemia, dyslipoproteinaemia, diabetes, cardiovascular disease, atherosclerosis

1. Introduction

Dyslipoproteinaemia, also known as dyslipidaemia, is a lipid metabolism disorder characterised by increased levels of plasma cholesterol, triacylglycerols (TAGs), or both, and a low high-dense lipoprotein cholesterol (HDL-C) level that is strongly associated with atherosclerotic vascular disease. In addition, the link between increased levels of Apo protein B or lipoprotein (A) and lower levels of Apo lipoprotein A-1 and atherosclerotic vascular disease has led to the broader use of the term dyslipoproteinaemia in preference to dyslipidaemia. Dyslipoproteinaemia in diabetes is common. It can affect up to 70% of people with type 2 diabetes mellitus. Cardiovascular disease is the leading cause of death in people with diabetes, and mortality rates are 40% higher in men and 50% higher in women with diabetes compared to those without diabetes [1]. The prevalence of diabetes continues to rise, affecting 537 million people (1 in 10) worldwide and is predicted to rise to 783.2 by 2045 [2].

Dyslipidaemia in diabetes typically consists of the following lipid abnormalities:

- Increased levels of fasting and postprandial TAGs, Low Dense Lipoprotein-C (LDL-C), non-HDL-C, small LDL particles and Apo-B
- Decreased HDL-C and ApoA1

In this chapter, the importance and scale of dysproteinaemia in diabetes as a vital risk factor for cardiovascular disease is outlined, and there is a focus on pathophysiology, current clinical management, and guidelines of dyslipoproteinaemia for primary and secondary prevention in people at high risk of cardiovascular disease.

2. Epidemiology of dyslipoproteinaemia

By 2019, over 4 million deaths were attributable to high plasma LDL-C levels, more commonly affecting men than women. Although deaths have been reduced since 1990 in middle-income compared to middle-low-income countries, ischaemic heart disease caused 8.54 million deaths, of which 44.3% were due to high plasma LDL-C levels. 2.73 million deaths were due to ischaemic stroke, of which 26.5% were attributable to high plasma LDL-C levels [3]. Estimates from the World Health Organisation in 2008 showed that the prevalence of hypercholesterolemia was 53.7% in Europe, 47.7% in the USA and lower prevalence in South East Asia and Africa [4]. Large-scale RCTs have shown that targeted dyslipidaemia treatment reduced all-cause and coronary mortality. Reducing LDL-C by one mmol/l minimises the risk of stroke, coronary revascularisation, and major cardiovascular events by about 20% [5].

3. Causes of dyslipoproteinaemia

The causes of dyslipoproteinaemia are divided into primary (genetic) or secondary, diagnosed from history and the measurement of abnormally high plasma levels of total cholesterol, TAGs, and individual lipoproteins. The treatment of dyslipoproteinaemia is primarily 2-fold, through lifestyle modifications and lipid-lowering drugs.

Primary dyslipoproteinaemia is due to genetic defects in lipid metabolism, predominantly causing impaired clearance of plasma LDL and a deficiency in LDL receptors. Levels of LDL-C in people with familial hypercholesterolemia are abnormally high at birth and are associated with the deposition of cholesterol in the arteries, skin, tendons, and corneas. Environmental factors and diseases such as diabetes, hypothyroidism, obstructive liver disease and drugs (e.g., thiazide diuretics and anabolic steroids) are often associated with secondary dyslipoproteinaemia. A thorough history and clinical examination are imperative for accurately diagnosing dyslipoproteinaemia.

4. Pathophysiology

4.1 Role of lipids

Lipoproteins are particles that transport lipids to tissues for energy utilisation, steroid hormone production and bile acid formation. Lipoproteins are made of esterified and unsterilised cholesterol, phospholipids, triglycerides, and Apo lipoproteins. Apo lipoproteins are crucial to forming cellular receptor binding, activating, and inhibiting enzyme reactions and the composition of cellular structural components. Lipoproteins are divided into seven different classes: chylomicrons, chylomicron remnants, very low dense lipoprotein (VLDL), intermediate-dense lipoprotein (IDL), intermediate-dense lipoprotein (IDL), HDL and Lp (a) depending on their size, lipid composition and Apo lipoproteins. All lipoproteins are atherogenic except anti-atherogenic HDL. **Table 1** shows lipoprotein characteristics.

Since the publication of the Framingham Heart Study [6], cholesterol has been identified as a critical contributory risk to coronary heart disease. A vast number of epidemiologic studies and randomised clinical trials (RCTs) have demonstrated the causal link of LDL-C to atherosclerotic cardiovascular disease (ASCVD) [7]. Managing serum cholesterol levels is now the cornerstone of primary prevention (in those individuals before developing ASCVD and secondary prevention in individuals where the ASCVD event has occurred) worldwide, focusing on lipoproteins reflected in LDL-C, non-HDL-C and TGs levels. Many studies have shown a log-linear relationship between LDL-C and the risk of ASCVD. Lowering LDL-C lowers the risk of ASCVD, providing solid support for causal and cumulative impact in the development of ASCVD dependent on exposure to high LDL-C. Equally, high levels of TAGs are associated with an increased risk of the development of ASCVD, whereas lower levels of TAGs reduce risk. The inverse association between HDL-C and the risk of ASCVD is well recognised through epidemiology studies. However, the evidence for this association needs to be more strictly and consistently compelling [8]. In a systematic review and meta-analysis of a dose response in prospective cohort studies, high TC and LDL-C serum levels were associated with increased ASCVD mortality. There is a wide ethnicity variation in the prevalence of LP (a), more common in blacks and South Asians than Chinese and whites [8]. High Lp (a) has been linked to calcific with aortic valve disease, and the oxidised phospholipids carried by Lp (a) make it more pro-atherosclerotic and proinflammatory, independently promoting ASCVD [9].

The absorption of dietary lipids occurs via enterocytes through passive diffusion or specific transporters. Within the enterocytes, TAGs, cholesteryl esters and other lipids are associated with Apo lipoprotein (ApoA-IV and ApoA-I) to form chylomicrons. Chylomicrons are then exported into the lymph and the bloodstream. Lipoprotein lipase on the luminal surface is responsible for chylomicron clearance. Lipolysis of chylomicrons produces chylomicron remnants taken up by the liver via the LDL receptor in conjunction with the LDL receptor-related protein that binds ApoE. From the liver, lipids are exported into the bloodstream as VLDLs. Like chylomicrons, TAGs from VLDLs are hydrolysed by LPL lipase in plasma, producing non-esterified fatty acids (NEFA), used as fuel in the heart and skeletal muscle or for storage within adipocytes. As the depletion of VLDLs occurs, the transfer of part of the lipoprotein surface layer closely related to phospholipids, ApoC and ApoE to HDLs occurs and is responsible for forming IDLs. Most of the formed IDLs are converted into LDL through lipolysis by hepatic enzymes, whereas the liver clears the rest through lipid receptor protein and LDL receptors. Cholesterol is transported mainly by LDL as a core of esterified cholesterol wrapped up in a shell of phospholipid, unesterified cholesterol and a single molecule of ApoB-100 bound to the LDL receptor regulated by the binding of the lysosomal enzyme Proportion Convertase Subtilizing/Kevin type 9 (PCSK9) to the LDL-receptor/LDL complex preventing the receptor to enter back to the surface and into the lysosomal catabolic pathway.

	Density (g/mL)	Diameter (nm)	TGs (%)	Cholesterol ester (%)	PLs (%)	Cholesterol (%)	Apolipoprotein major	Others
Chylomicrons	<0.95 1	80–100	90–95	2–4	2–6	1	ApoB-48	ApoA-I, A-II, A-IV, A-V
VLDL	0.951–1.006	30–80	50–65	8–14	12–16	4–7	ApoB8-14 1-100	ApoA-I, C-II, C-III, E, A-V
IDL	1.006–1.019	25–30	25–40	20–35	16–24	7–11	ApoB-100	ApoC-II, C-III, E
LDL	1.019–1.063	20–25	4–6	34–35	22–26	6–15	ApoB-100	
HDL	1.063–1.210	8–13	7	10–20	55	5	ApoA-I	ApoA-II, C-III, E, M
Lp(a)	1.006–1.125	25–30	4–8	35–46	17–24	6–9	Apo(a)	ApoB-100

Apo = apolipoprotein; HDL = high-density lipoprotein; IDL = intermediate-density lipoprotein; LDL = low-density lipoprotein; Lp (a) = lipoprotein (a); PLs = phospholipids; TGs = triglycerides; VLDL = very low-density lipoprotein.

Table 1.
Lipoprotein characteristics.

Produced by the liver and intestine, HDL is involved in reverse cholesterol transport, which protects against atherosclerosis through its anti-apoptotic, anti-thrombotic, anti-inflammatory, and anti-oxidative properties. Soon after secretion, HDLs bind Apo A-I to membrane-associated ATP-binding cassette protein-1 (ABCA-1) transporter responsible for the transport of non-esterified cholesterol and phospholipids from the cytoplasm into HDL and is followed by esterification of non-esterified cholesterol on HDL particle by lecithin–cholesterol acyltransferase which attracts more cholesterol from peripheral tissue and also recruits macrophages within artery walls through ABCA-1 and the ATP-binding cassette G1 transporters. HDL returns cholesterol to the liver through scavenger receptor B1 (SR-B1) or is taken up directly by the liver, which undergoes hydrolysis. Cholesteryl esters are transferred from HDL to VLDL, and TAGs from VLDL to HDL through cholesteryl ester transfer protein (CETP). HDL is further enriched with TAGs and phospholipids by receiving ApoC and ApoE from VLDL in circulation, later degraded by hepatic lipase to smaller HDL particles, which are removed by the liver or form part of reverse cholesterol transport. The formed lipid-poor ApoA-I is filtered from circulation by the renal proximal tubules and degraded by binding to cubilin, a protein on the apical surface of renal tubular cells.

Two hormones significantly affect lipid metabolism: adiponectin and insulin. Adiponectin promotes ApoA-I-mediated cholesterol efflux from macrophages by upregulating ABCA1 expression [10]. Adiponectin may directly reduce HDL metabolism and, therefore, is antiatherogenic. On the other hand, insulin is antilipolytic by inhibiting hormone-sensitive lipase, which then promotes the storage of TAGs in adipose tissue. In addition, insulin directly inhibits hepatic VLDL production by reducing circulating levels of NEFA, substrates for VLDL. Insulin increases LDL-receptor expression and activity, accelerating LDL clearance [11].

In high plasma concentrations, the oxidation of cholesterol promotes intercellular monocyte influx and cytokine generation of tumour necrosis factor-α, interleukin-1 and interleukin-6 (IL-6) by macrophages, lymphocytes, natural killer cells, and vascular smooth muscle cells producing a cascade for further production of cytokines causing the formation of an unstable plaque that is prone to rupture [12]. Themonocytes differentiate into macrophages, which absorb oxidised cholesterol to become foam cells and are deposited on the blood vessels' walls, causing the formation of more atherosclerotic plaques. In parallel, LDL is transported into the extracellular matrix of the sub-endothelial space, undergoes oxidation and recruits monocytes that are transformed into macrophages to increase LDL oxidation, further causing more inflammatory reaction and damage within the vessel wall. A fibrous cap's formation accelerates as the plaque's damage and repair process continues. The size of the plaque can increase to a critical extent, which may become unstable and vulnerable to rupture and cause blood flow obstruction that causes unstable angina, myocardial infarction, and death in some cases. Therapies to maintain plaque stability and inhibit plaque rupture and subsequent coronary thrombosis are critical to preventing cardiovascular events [13]. Lipid-lowering therapies may reduce the increase in the size of the plaque and prevent ASCVD events [14].

The mechanism for diabetic dyslipoproteinaemia is not fully understood. Both glycaemic control and insulin resistance play a role. Insulin decreases levels of VLDL by reducing free fatty acids in circulation, which are substrates of VLDL that directly inhibit VLDL production in the liver. Insulin also inhibits the hepatic secretion of TAG-VLDL and ApoB-100. Insulin resistance in people with type 2 diabetes mellitus causes an increase in microsomal transfer protein expression and lipid bioavailability, which results in the overproduction of TAG-VLDL and VLDL-ApoB.

5. Measurement of lipids

Risk assessment of ASCVD is essential to guide therapies for primary and secondary prevention, and measurements of lipid profile form part of patient evaluation. A clear, detailed history and thorough patient examination are essential to obtain clinical features of coexisting conditions such as diabetes, obesity, thyroid, liver, and kidney disorders. More importantly, medication and other supplements may be responsible for dyslipoproteinaemia, and this can only be diagnosed from a careful history. Other essential elements include any family history of premature ASCKD events. The pattern of plasma sterols may indicate different categories of familiar hyperlipidaemias. For example, raised VLDL-C and LDL-C may indicate familial hypercholesterolemia if sterols levels are normal, familial combined hyperlipidaemia if lathosterol is high, dysbetalipoproteinemia when β-sitosterol is moderately increased, phytosterolemia if β-sitosterol is very high and cerebrotendinous xanthomatosis if very high levels of cholestanol are determined.

Assays of apo A-I provide a characterisation of HDL and its influence. It is beneficial to diagnose conditions with significant HDL deficiencies, such as apoA-I deficiency and variants, Tangier disease, and lecithin/cholesteryl acyltransferase deficiency, whereas measuring apoB may provide evidence to diagnose abetalipoproteinemia or hypobetalipoproteinaemia.

Total cholesterol is distributed among the three major lipoproteins: VDL. LDL and HDL, but some are distributed between IDL and Lp (a). Most laboratories measure total cholesterol, HDL and TAGs from which LDL-C is estimated. Direct measurement of LDL-C is possible. However, cost and inaccuracies in assays limit their availability and reproducibility.

A fasting serum sample is preferred when assessing the lipid profile due to the lower TAG levels in the fasting state, which gives more accurate LDL-C estimations. However, the changes in TAG levels in fasting and non-fasting states are small [15]. If a non-fasting sample is taken, TAG and LDL-C levels should be interpreted cautiously, especially in patients with diabetes, metabolic syndrome, and hypertriglyceridemia. Non-fasting lipid measurements can be used for population screening because of the inconvenience to patients to fast, but also the fact that systematic reviews have shown a small and non-significant difference between fasting and non-fasting lipid parameters in predicting patient prognosis when considering these levels [16].

Other laboratories also measure Lp (a) as part of a routine lipid profile, which is more informative for diagnosis and primary and secondary prevention risk stratification.

LDL-C is usually calculated from the Friedewald equation:
LDL-C 1 divided by four times TC HDL-C (TAGs/2.2) in mmol/L.
The formula is inaccurate when TAG levels are higher than 4.5 mmol/L.

Current guidelines recommend using one of the available risk assessment systems relevant to the patient population's region. The SCORE (Systematic Coronary Risk Estimation) system is country specific. It is calibrated by considering population differences primarily adjusted for prevalence and mortality for ASCVD in those regions [17]. Cardiovascular risk means the likelihood of a person developing an atherosclerotic event over time. Assessing the combined effects of all identifiable risk factors of the individual is critical to estimating the risk of future cardiovascular events to determine treatment strategies for primary or secondary prevention of ASCVD events. Through total risk assessment, the cut-off points identify low, moderate, high, and very high-risk categories [18] on which lipid-lowering treatment is based. Clinicians and their multidisciplinary teams must agree on which guidelines apply to their patient populations and healthcare systems.

Examples of categories from low to high risks:

- Patients at low risk have a calculated SCORE of less than 1% over ten years to develop fatal ASCVD.

- Those at moderate risk are young people with T2DM younger than 50 years old and T1DM less than 35 years old with diabetes duration of less than ten years, without other risk factors have a calculated SCORE of 1% - 5% risk for ten years to develop fatal ASCVD.

- Those at high risk have TC more than eight mmol/L, LDL-C more than 4.9 mmol/L, or BP higher than 180/110 mmHg, people with FH without other major risk factors or with diabetes without target organ damage, with diabetes duration of more than ten years or another additional risk factor or those with moderate CKD (eGFR 30–59 mL/min/1.73 m^2) have a calculated SCORE of at least 5% - 10% risk over ten years to develop fatal ASCVD.

- Those at very high risk are people with any of the following: documented ASCVD or have diabetes with target organ damage, or at least three major risk factors, or early onset of T1DM duration of at least 20 years or CKD stage 4 (eGFR <30 mL/min/1.73 m^2) have a calculated SCORE of at least 10% over a 10-year to develop of fatal ASCVD.

The Task Force for the Management of Dyslipidaemias of the European Society of Cardiology and European Atherosclerosis Society for lipid profile assessment [17] recommends the following:

- TC should be measured routinely to estimate total ASCVD risk using the SCORE system.

- HDL-C analysis should be measured to refine risk estimation using the online SCORE system.

- LDL-C analysis should be used for screening, diagnosis, and management.

- Non-HDL-C is recommended for risk assessment, particularly in people with high TAG levels, obesity, or very low LDL-C.

- ApoB analysis is recommended for risk assessment in people with high TAG levels, diabetes, obesity, metabolic syndrome, or very low LDL-C levels. ApoB can be used as an alternative to LDL-C as the primary measurement for very low LDL-C levels.

- Consider Lp (a) measurement at least once in each adult person's lifetime to identify those with very high risk.

6. Dyslipoproteinaemia in special groups

6.1 Diabetes

Substantial evidence supports the targeting of LDL-C lowering to reduce the risk and mortality of ASCVD. Still, the benefit of treating hypertriglyceridemia in people with has been questioned. However, more recently, a meta-analysis of studies of fibrates in primary prevention of ASCVD in people with type 2 diabetes reported that fibrates significantly reduced the risk of non-fatal MI by 21% but had no effect on the overall mortality risk [18]. All people with diabetes at high risk should be considered for statin therapy and lifestyle modification. Those that do not reach target levels should be offered non-statin therapy. Targeting dyslipoproteinaemia in individuals at risk of developing diabetes is one aspect of managing risk factors before they develop diabetic complications and ASCVD. Specific clinical characteristics may indicate a risk of progressing to diabetes, e.g., metabolic syndrome, obesity, hypertension, fasting glucose >6.0 mmol/l and raised TAGs. More recently, the hypertriglyceridemia waist phenotype (waist circumference over 85 cm in women and over 90 cm in men and raised TGs) has been proposed as a more robust marker of ASCVD risk than metabolic syndrome [19].

6.2 Familial dyslipidaemias

Familial dyslipidaemias can be monogenic when one major gene is responsible for the condition or heterogenic when more than one gene variant affects lipid metabolism. The association of familial dyslipidaemia with ASCVD and premature deaths is well recognised, and early diagnosis is critical for primary and secondary prevention of ASCVD. The treatment requires a combination of statin and non-statin therapies, and in severe cases, lipid apheresis may be necessary.

6.3 Familial hypercholesteraemic (FH)

FH is a monogenic dyslipidaemia with autosomal dominance inheritance occurring in 1/200–250 population, predominantly causing a lifelong increase in LDL-C and premature death if left untreated. This condition is due to the mutation of the gene that encodes for the LDL receptor or Apo gene and can be diagnosed by the presence of characteristic clinical physical findings (tendon xanthomata, arcus senilis and xanthelasma) and the demonstration of the gene mutations. More than 1000 gene mutations for the LDL receptor have been identified. When a single gene mutation is inherited from both parents, the condition is called homozygous FH and heterozygous when inheritance is from one single parent only. Typically, in FH, the TC is higher than 8 mmol/l in patients <40 years old or there is a history of premature CVD under 60 years old and characteristic clinical findings on examination. Both the Dutch Lipid Clinic Network (DLCN) criteria and the Simon Broome Register (SBR) have been adopted worldwide to diagnose FH [20]. These criteria are based on a score generated from a personal and family medical history, clinical characteristics, LDL-C concentration, and DNA testing. The higher the score, the higher the chances of the person having FH.

6.4 Familial dysbetalipoproteinemia (FD)

FD is rare and is inherited as an autosomal recessive disorder with variable penetrance. The characteristics of FD are increased levels of both TC and TGs, tuberoeruptive xanthomas over the elbows and knees, and palmar xanthomata of the hands and wrists. The risk of CVD is very high and includes atherosclerosis of the femoral and tibial arteries; most cases are homozygous for the E2 isoform of ApoE. ApoE promotes the clearance of chylomicron remnants and IDL.

6.5 Familial combined hyperlipidaemia (FCH)

FCH is more common than previously recognised, occurring at a frequency of 1:100–200 in the population, and typically presents with increased levels of LDL-C, TAGs, or both. The diagnosis is frequently missed. High levels of ApoB improve the detection of this condition [20].

6.6 Familial hypertriglyceridemia (FHTG)

FHTG is polygenic due to the involvement of multiple gene mutation defects in the catabolism pathway for chylomicrons and VLDL, causing elevated levels and a high risk for CVD and pancreatitis [21].

7. Management of dyslipoproteinaemia

7.1 Lifestyle modification

European Cardiology and European Atherosclerotic Societies recommended lifestyle modification for primary and secondary prevention of ASCVD based on sufficient evidence from observational studies and RCTs, which have shown a positive effect of cholesterol and other biomarkers on reducing cardiovascular risk. In the INTERHEART study in 52 countries, nearly 50% of risk factors for myocardial infarction were modifiable lifestyle parameters: physical activity and intake of fruit and vegetables reduced risk, whereas alcohol use and smoking increased risk. The cumulative risk of myocardial infarction increased as the number of risk factors (smoking, diabetes, obesity, raised ApoB/ApoA1 ratio, hypertension, lack of fruit and vegetable consumption and exercise) increased too [22].

Other epidemiological studies have also shown that high fruit consumption and non-starchy vegetables, nuts, legumes, fish, vegetable oils, yoghurt, and whole grains, in addition to lower intake of red and processed foods, salt and switching from animal fats to vegetable sources of fats lowered risk of ASCVD. Saturated fatty acids increase LDL-C, whereas unsaturated fat-rich oils from sunflower, flaxseed, corn, olives, or soybeans reduce LDL-C levels. Although weight loss has a negligible impact on LDL-C reduction, its effects on lowering TAGs and increasing HDL-C are significant.

The ACC–AHA Risk Calculator is recommended for adults 40 to 75 years of age who do not have diabetes and whose LDL cholesterol level is 70 mg per decilitre or higher to estimate the risk of ASCVD. Those with low to moderate risk can be managed through lifestyle modification alone, but those with high risk require pharmacological interventions. The presence of multiple risk factors such as a strong family history or premature ASCVD, preeclampsia, South Asian ancestry,

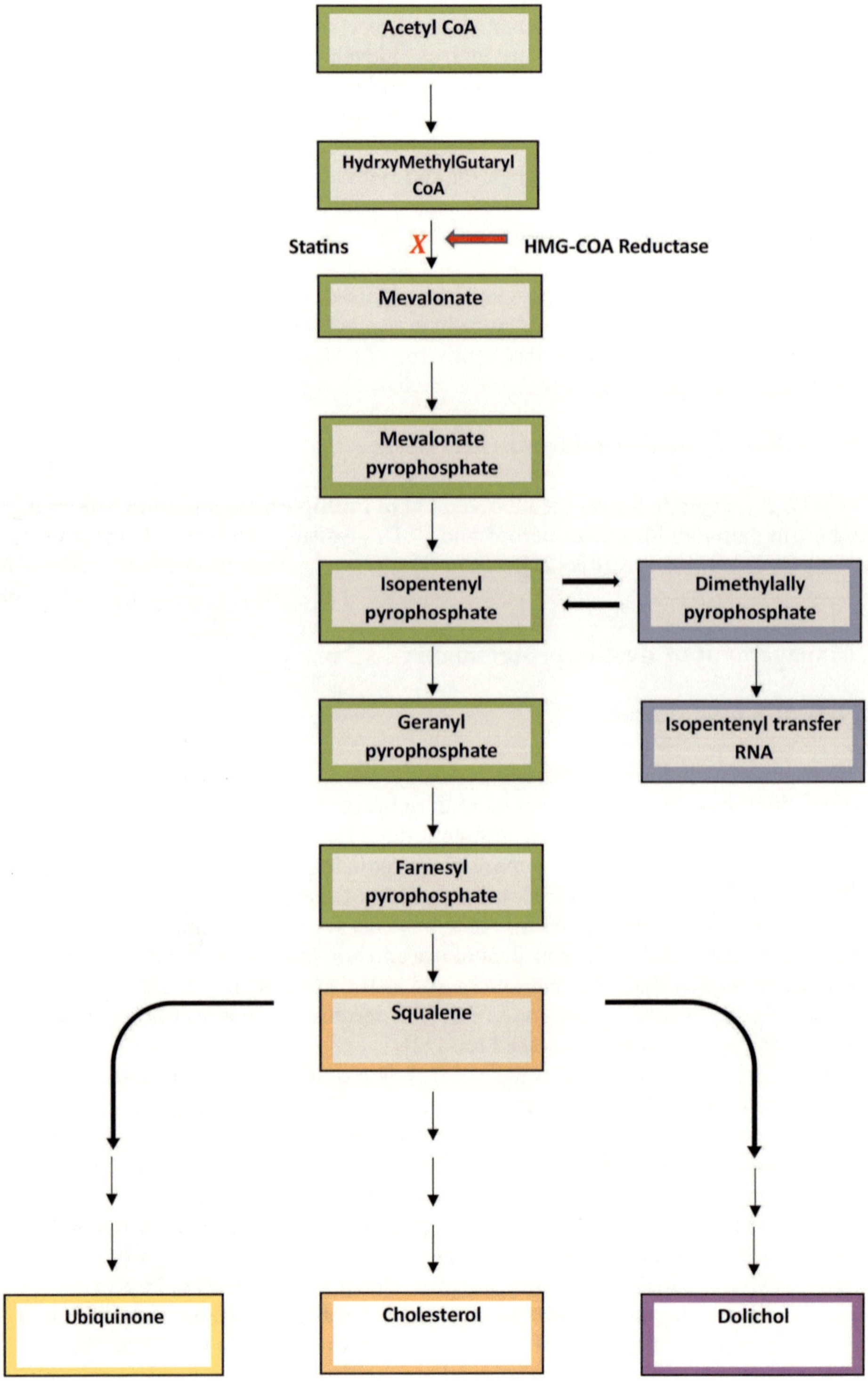

Figure 1.
Cholesterol metabolism.

Characteristic	Atorvastatin	Rosuvastatin	Simvastatin	Pravastatin	Lovastatin
High intensity (Lowers TC by ≥50%)	40–80	20–40			
Moderate intensity (Lowers TC by 30–50%)	10–20	5–10	20–24	40–80	40
Low intensity (Lowers TC by <30%			10	10–20	20
HDL % increase	7–8	11–14	8–12	3–8	6–9
TGs % increase	28–47	29–38	19–32	20	10–23

Table 2.
Common statin drug characteristic.

hypertension, early menopause, chronic kidney disease, HIV, persistently elevated triglyceride levels, and elevated levels of high-sensitivity C-reactive protein and Lp(a) requires pharmacological interventions for primary prevention of ASCVD. The same principle applies to individuals without multiple risk factors who have severe primary hyperlipidaemia when their LDL cholesterol level is≥190 mg per decilitre. People with diabetes and LDL cholesterol levels>70 decilitres do not require risk calculation as they are at high risk of ASCVD anyway and require pharmacological treatment [23].

8. Drug therapy in dyslipoproteinaemia

8.1 Statins

8.1.1 Evolution of statins

3-hydroxy-3-methyl-glutaryl-CoA (HMG-CoA) reductase is the rate-limiting enzyme in the cholesterol biosynthetic pathway (**Figure 1**), which is inhibited by statins resulting in the lowering of LDL-C serum levels. The first statin in the world was mevastatin, a naturally derived statin from fungal species Aspergillum and Penicillium in the 1970s, but it was never marketed. Lovastatin, also a naturally occurring statin, was granted FDA approval for commercial production in 1987 and was later modified semi-synthetically to form simvastatin. Later, pravastatin was modified from mevastatin. Synthetic statins soon followed on the market (**Table 2**). Extensive studies have shown that statins stabilise atherosclerotic plaques to prevent rupture and the development of ASCVD events. Statins are among the most widely used drugs, with atorvastatin as the best-selling statin worldwide. Estimates showed that more than 145 million people were taking statins by 2018 [24] (**Figure 2**).

8.1.2 Adverse effects of statin

- Myopathy is the most common adverse reaction with statin therapy, whereas rhabdomyolysis can be one of the most severe, occurring on average at 13 cases/100,000 patient-years. Rhabdomyolysis typically presents with severe muscular pain, muscle necrosis and myoglobinuria and may progress to severe acute kidney injury, and creatine kinase may rise 10 to >40 fold before death occurs.

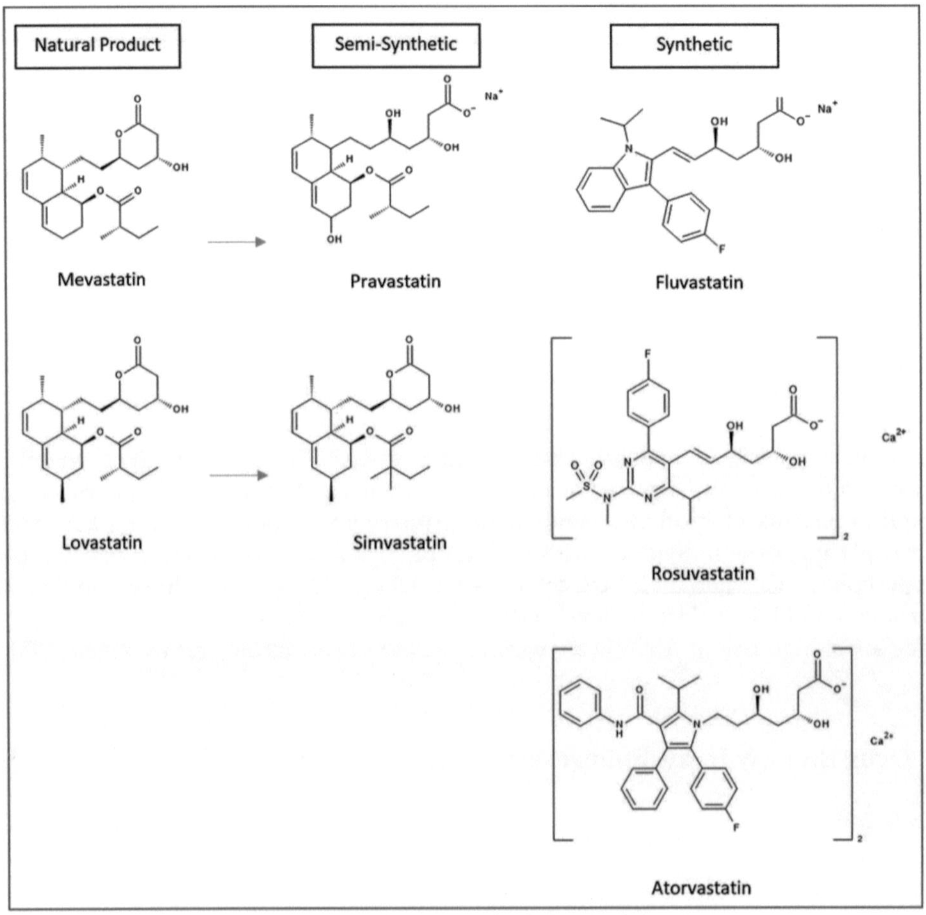

Structures of some popular natural, semi-synthetic and synthetic statins.

Figure 2.
Evolution of statins.

- Statins are contraindicated in acute liver failure or decompensated liver disease.
- The association of statins and cancer has been the subject of exciting debates concerning those studies that involved individuals with LDL-C below two mmol/l. However, many meta-analyses of randomised trials that recruited large numbers of cancers showed that current standard statin regimens do not increase the relative risk of any cancer over five years [25].
- Other important adverse reactions include liver failure, alopecia, memory loss, pancreatitis, paraesthesia, sexual dysfunction, new-onset diabetes, and haemorrhagic stroke.

Follow-up and monitoring of statin therapy:

- Statins are indicated for both primary and secondary prevention.

- Monitor liver function tests at baseline and within three months of starting treatment.
- Avoid statins if transaminase (alanine aminotransferase or aspartate aminotransferase) levels three or more times the upper limit of normal and in pregnancy.

8.1.3 Bile acid sequestrants

- Synthesised in the liver from cholesterol bile sequestrants work by binding bile and depleting bile salts from enterohepatic circulation, forcing the liver to synthesise more, thereby increasing LDLR expression and reducing LDL-C.
- Bile acid sequestrants are polymeric compounds that serve as ion exchange resins.
- Bile acid sequestrants are indicated for hypercholesterolemia without hypertriglyceridemia for individuals intolerant to statins or as an add-on therapy when the statin is insufficient.
- Bile acid sequestrants reduce LDL-C by 15–30% at total doses.
- In addition to a bad taste in the mouth, bile sequestrants may cause constipation, diarrhoea, bloating, and flatulence.

Three commonly used bile acid sequestrants are:

- Cholestyramine – taken at 4 g 1–2 times a day, and the maximum dose is 24 g/day.
- Colestipol – is taken at 2 g 1–2 times a day, and the maximum dose is 20 g, which reduces LDL-C by 20% with very few adverse effects.
- Colesevelam – available at a maximum dose of 3.75 g/day.

8.2 Cholesterol absorption inhibitors

Cholesterol absorption inhibitors prevent intestinal cholesterol absorption but do not affect TGs and bile acid absorption.

8.2.1 Ezetimibe

- Reduces the cholesterol content of triglyceride-rich lipoproteins and the concentrations of atherogenic remnant particles and can be combined with other lipid-lowering medications.
- It inhibits the sterol transporter Neimann-Pick C1 located on the border cells in the small intestine.
- Due to the long half-life, Ezetimibe is administered once daily at 10 mg.

- It lowers LDL-C by 10–15% and has a good safety profile.
- Adverse reactions include asthenia, gastrointestinal symptoms, muscle aches, thrombocytopenia, and hypertension.

8.2.2 Fibrates

Fibrates act on peroxisome proliferator-activated receptor alpha (PPAR-a) to regulate various steps in lipid lipoprotein metabolism, reduce TAGs and TAG lipoprotein-rich remnant particles, and increase HDL-C levels. Outcome studies in lowering ASCVD have been disappointing. However, a subgroup analysis from the ACCORD trial showed that fibrates, in addition to statins, decreased the risk of nonfatal MI, nonfatal stroke, or death from cardiovascular (CV). In this study, despite lowering fasting triglyceride levels by 26% with pemafibrate, there was no significant impact on major cardiovascular events compared to the placebo [26]. Overall, the role of fibrates as monotherapy is limited.

8.2.3 Nicotinic acid

Nicotinic acid inhibits diacylglycerol acyltransferase-2 and decreases VLDL, Lp (a) and LDL particles and increases HDL-C and ApoA1 in the liver, however in a systematic Cochrane Review [27] of 23 RCTs nicotinic acid had no significant positive impact on cardiovascular and non-cardiovascular mortality. At the recommended dose of 500 mg daily, Nicotinic acid-induced flushing is a significant adverse reaction that may contribute to poor patient compliance with this treatment.

8.2.4 Proprotein convertase subtilizing/kevin type 9 inhibitors

PCSK9 down-regulates LDL receptors on hepatocytes. On binding to the LDL receptor, it causes the degradation of the receptor, leading to increased levels of LDL-C. The monoclonal antibodies alirocumab and evolocumab do the opposite and inhibit PCSK9 binding to LDL receptors and upregulate the recycling of LDL receptors, increasing LDL-C uptake and indirectly lowering circulating LDL-C levels. Both alirocumab and evolocumab are injected subcutaneously once every two weeks. In the ODYSSEY OUTCOMES trial, alirocumab reduced circulating LDL-C and prevented CV events [28].

Similarly, in the FOURIER trial, evolocumab decreased CV events by 15% compared to placebo [29]. The trials mentioned above provided important information on the PCSK9 inhibitor safety profile. Apart from reactions at the injection sites and flulike symptoms, both agents have an excellent safety profile. Together with statins, they can reduce LDL-C by 40–73%, depending on dose regimens. In addition, both agents lower TAGs and Lp (a).

Both alirocumab and evolocumab are indicated in primary prevention in high-risk groups or secondary prevention. Despite maximal conventional lipid-lowering therapies, target LDL goals are not achieved, and stain intolerance is an issue. Evolocumab is administered into the thigh, abdomen, or upper arm at 140 mg every two weeks or 42 mg monthly for primary or mixed hyperlipidaemia or atherosclerotic disease. Alirocumab is administered starting at 75 mg every two weeks and increasing to 150 mg every four weeks or 300 mg every four weeks.

8.2.5 Small interfering ribonucleic acid (siRNA) inhibitors

Inclisiran, a siRNA, inhibits the translation of PCSK9 by cleaving messenger RNA, decreasing PCSK9 production and upregulating LDL receptors, lowering LDL-C levels in circulation. The inclisiran administration regime is simple at days 1, day 90, day 180, followed by six monthly. Inclisiran-related adverse effects commonly reported are headache, cough, back pain, acute nasopharyngitis, hiccups, and local reactions. In the ORION trials [30], Inclisiran reduced LDL-C by 52%, and adverse reactions occurred in 11% in the treatment arm compared to 8% in the placebo. Inclisiran is an alternative therapy to PCSK9 inhibitors.

8.2.6 Omega-3 fatty acids (OM3-FA)

Eicosapentaenoic acid and Docosahexaenoic acid can lower TAGs and VLDL levels, but the mechanism for this indication has yet to be well studied. In a meta-analysis of 32 studies involving 15,903 subjects [31], OM3-FA used as monotherapy or in combination confirmed significant reductions in levels of TAGs, VLDL-C, non-HDL-C, Apo-B, and Apo-AI while increasing the levels of HDL-C. OM3-FA compounds can be considered for treating endogenous hypertriglyceridemia when dietary measures are insufficient to produce an adequate response. The dose is one capsule per day.

8.2.7 Bempedoic acid

Bempedoic acid is an ATP citrate lipase inhibitor that reduces LDL-C. Several studies have shown a reduction of LDL-C by 17–28% [32]. The main advantage of Bempedoic acid was the lack of muscular adverse effects compared to statins. A double-blind, randomised, placebo-controlled trial involving patients intolerant to statin treatment Bempedoic acid reduced significant adverse cardiovascular by 13% compared to placebo [32]. Bempedoic acid should be considered in statin intolerance in combination with ezetimibe. The recommended dose is 180 mg orally per day. Adverse effects include anaemia, gout, diarrhoea, and muscle spasms.

9. Case study

- Referred to lipid clinic Jan 2021
- 54-year-old female
- Smoker
- No family history of premature ASCVD
- On atorvastatin on the first visit to a lipid clinic
- Myocardial infarction 2013 4 stents aged 48 and non-STEMI 2021
- BMI 43 BP 156/47 Corneal arcus nil else
- Genetics: PCSK9:c:1120 GOF variant elevated SNP score

Date	TC (mmol/l)	TG (mmol/l)	HDL C (mmol/l	Non-HDL (mmol/l)	Chol: HDL ratio	LDL-C	Other
May 2019	13.9	5.3	1.2	12.7	11.6	—	Atorvastatin 80 mg
Sep 2019	12.5	5.0	1.1	11.4	11.4	—	Atorvastatin 80 mg
Dec 2019	12.8	5.6	1.0	11.8	12.8	—	Atorvastatin 80 mg
Feb 2020	18.7	6.6	0.7	18.0	26.7	15 (estimated)	—
Jan 2021	12.3	4.i	1.1	11.2	11.2	9.3	Atorvastatin 40 mg
March 2021	8.7	5.5	1.2	5.9	5.9	4.1	Atorvastatin 40 mg Evolocumab 140 mg fortnightly Ezetimibe 10 mg
Nov 2022	3.7	2.8	1.7	2.0	2.2	0.7	As above and added Inclisiran 284 mg
March 2023	3.9	2.8	1.7	3.0	2.8	1.7	As above Inclisiran 284 mg 6monthly

Table 3.
Lipid profile – May 2019 to March 2023.

- Diagnosis: Heterozygous FH
- Treatment: In combination, she responded to maximum doses of statin, Ezetimibe, Evolocumab, and Inclisiran. No adverse reaction was observed (**Table 3**).

10. Conclusion

Dyslipoproteinaemia is a common lipid disorder affecting a very high proportion of people with diabetes at a very high risk of developing cardiovascular disease. Early diagnosis through routine screening and treatment to target as recommended by national and international guidelines is vital in the primary and secondary prevention of ASCVD. Substantial evidence supports the targeting of LDL-C lowering to reduce the risk and mortality of ASCVD. The benefit of hypertriglyceridemia treatment in people with diabetes has been questioned. However, more recently, a meta-analysis of studies of fibrates in the primary prevention of ASCVD in people with diabetes reported that fibrates significantly reduced the risk of non-fatal MI by 21% but had no effect on the overall mortality risk [33]. All people with diabetes at high risk should be considered for statin therapy and lifestyle modification. Those who do not reach target levels should be offered non-statin therapy.

There are five stages to incorporate in the management of dyslipoproteinaemia routinely:

1. Clinical history and examination

    - Family history

- ASCVD risk factors: poor diet, excess alcohol, smoking, diabetes, thyroid disorder, liver and CKD, obesity, premature or any past CVD events and autoimmune disorders

- Pancreatitis – high levels of TAGs

- Xanthoma/xanthelasma/corneal arcus

2. Laboratory tests

    - TC

    - LDL-C

    - TAGs

    - HDL-C

    - ApoB

    - Lp(a)

3. Genetic testing

    - Monogenic or polygenic

4. Management

    - Risk charts

    - Address secondary causes

    - Lifestyle modification

    - Treat risk factors to targets.

    - Treat LDL-C to targets

    - Treat TAGs >10 mmol/l to prevent pancreatitis.

5. Lipid Lowering Agents (guidance according to availability)

    - Statins

    - Ezetimibe

    - Fibrates

    - Bempedoic acid

- Bile acid sequestrants
- OM3-FA
- siRNA
- PCSK9 inhibitors

Author details

Mick John Kumwenda
Glan Clwyd Hospital, Bodelwyddan Rhyl, UK

*Address all correspondence to: kumwendamick@yahoo.com

References

[1] Read SH, Kerssens JJ, McAllister DA, Colhoun HM, Fischbacher CM, Lindsay RS, et al. Trends in type 2 diabetes incidence and mortality in Scotland between 2004 and 2013. Diabetologia. 2016;**59**:2106

[2] Jialal I, Singh G. Management of diabetic dyslipidemia: An update. World Journal of Diabetes. 2019;**10**(5):280-290

[3] Management for the prevention of atherosclerotic cardiovascular disease. The New England Journal of Medicine. 2019;**381**(16):1557-1567

[4] Pirillo A, Casula M, Olmastroni E, et al. Global epidemiology of dyslipidaemias. Nature Review Cardiology. 2021;**18**(10):689-700

[5] Krumholz HM. Circulation: Cardiovascular quality and outcomes: Scholarship to improve health and health care for patients and populations. Circulation. 2008;**1**(1):1-3

[6] Kannel WB, Dawber TR, Kagan A, Revotskie N, Stokes J III. Factors of risk in the development of coronary heart disease-six year follow up experience. The Framingham Study. Annals of Internal Medicine. 1961;**55**:33-50

[7] Schwartz GG, Ballantyne CM, Barter PJ, Kallend D, Leiter LA, Leitersdorf E, et al. Association of Lipoprotein(a) with risk of recurrent ischemic events following acute coronary syndrome: Analysis of the dal-outcomes randomized clinical trial. JAMA Cardiology. 2018;**3**(2):164-168

[8] Jung E, Kong SY, Ro YS, Ryu HH, Shin SD. Serum cholesterol levels and risk of cardiovascular death: A systematic review and a dose-response Meta-analysis of prospective cohort studies. International Journal of Environmental Research and Public Health. 2022;**19**(14):8272

[9] Liu Q, Yu Y, Xi R, Li J, Lai R, Wang T, et al. Association between lipoprotein(a) and calcific aortic valve disease: A systematic review and meta-analysis. Frontier in Cardiovascular Medicine. 25 Apr 2022;**9**:877140

[10] Liang B, Wang X, Guo X, Yang Z, Bai R, Liu M, et al. Adiponectin upregulates ABCA1 expression through liver X receptor alpha signalling pathway in RAW 264.7 macrophages. International Journal of Clinical Experimental Pathology. 2015;**8**(1):450-457

[11] Scherer T, Lindtner C, O'Hare J, Hackl M, Zielinski E, Freudenthaler A, et al. Insulin regulates hepatic triglyceride secretion and lipid content via signalling in the brain. Diabetes. 2016;**65**(6):1511-1520

[12] Bennett MR, Sinha S, Owens GK. Vascular smooth muscle cells in atherosclerosis. Circulation Research. 2016;**118**(4):692-702

[13] Pulipati VP, Alenghat FJ. The impact of lipid-lowering medications on coronary artery plaque characteristics. American Journal of Preventive Cardiology. 9 Nov 2021;**8**:100294

[14] Nordestgaard BG, Langsted A, Mora S, Kolovou G, et al. Fasting is not routinely required for determination of a lipid profile: Clinical and laboratory implications including flagging at desirable concentration cut points-a joint consensus statement from the European Atherosclerosis Society and European Federation of Clinical Chemistry and Laboratory Medicine. Clinical Chemistry. 2016;**62**(7):930-946

[15] Tomasik T, Krzysztoń J, Dubas-Jakóbczyk K, Kijowska V, Windak A. The systematic coronary risk evaluation (SCORE) for preventing cardiovascular diseases. Does evidence exist for its effectiveness? A systematic review. Acta Cardiologica. 2017;**72**(4): 370-379

[16] Sun H, Saeedi P, Karuranga S, Pinkepank M, Ogurtsova K, Duncan BB, et al. IDF Diabetes Atlas: Global, regional, and country-level diabetes prevalence estimates for 2021 and projections for 2045. Diabetes Research and Clinical Practice. Jan 2022;**183**:109119

[17] European Association for Cardiovascular Prevention & Rehabilitation, Reiner Z, Catapano AL, De Backer G, et al. ESC Committee for Practice Guidelines (CPG) 2008-2010 and 2010-2012 Committees. ESC/EAS Guidelines for the Management of dyslipidaemias: The Task Force for the Management of dyslipidaemias of the European Society of Cardiology (ESC) and the European Atherosclerosis Society (EAS). European Heart Journal. 2011;**32**(14):1769-1818

[18] DeFilippis AP, Young R, McEvoy JW, Michos ED, Sandfort V, Kronmal RA, et al. Risk score overestimation: The impact of individual cardiovascular risk factors and preventive therapies on the performance of the American Heart Association-American College of Cardiology-Atherosclerotic Cardiovascular Disease risk score in a modern multi-ethnic cohort. European Heart Journal. 2017; **38**(8):598-608

[19] Karasek D, Spurna J, Macakova D, Cibickova L, Krystynik O, Kucerova V, et al. Hypertriglyceridemic waist in patients with type 2 diabetes: Its relationship to selected markers of vascular damage. Metabolic Syndrome and Related Disorders. 2021;**19**(7): 393-400. DOI: 10.1089/met.2021.0019

[20] Gidding SS, Champagne MA, de Ferranti SD, et al. The agenda for familial hypercholesterolemia: A scientific statement from the American Heart Association. Circulation. 1 Dec 2015;**132**(22):2167-2192

[21] Veerkamp MJ, de Graaf J, Bredie SJ, Hendriks JC, Demacker PN, Stalenhoef AF. Diagnosis of familial combined hyperlipidemia based on lipid phenotype expression in 32 families: Results of a 5-year follow-up study. Arteriosclerosis, Thrombosis, and Vascular Biology. 2002;**22**(2):274-282

[22] Cruz-Bautista I, Huerta-Chagoya A, Moreno-Macías H, Rodríguez-Guillén R, Ordóñez-Sánchez ML, Segura-Kato Y, et al. Familial hypertriglyceridemia: An entity with distinguishable features from other causes of hypertriglyceridemia. Lipids in Health and Disease. 2021; **20**(1):14

[23] Beeres SL. INTERHEART - a global study of risk factors for acute myocardial infarction in 52 countries: Munich, 29 August 2004. Netherland Heart Journal. 2004;**12**(Suppl. 2):17-18

[24] Blais JE, Wei Y, Yap KKW, Alwafi H, Ma TT, Brauer R, et al. Trends in lipid-modifying agent use in 83 countries. Atherosclerosis. 2021;**328**: 44-51

[25] Pirillo A, Catapano AL. Inclisiran: How widely and when should we use it? Current Atherosclerosis Reports. 2022; **24**(10):803-811

[26] Simental-Mendía LE, Simental-Mendía M, Sánchez-García A, Banach M, Atkin SL, Gotto AM Jr, et al. Effect of fibrates on glycemic parameters: A

systematic review and meta-analysis of randomised placebo-controlled trials. Pharmacological Research. 2018;**132**: 232-241

[27] Schandelmaier S, Briel M, Saccilotto R, Olu KK, Arpagaus A, Hemkens LG, et al. Niacin for primary and secondary prevention of cardiovascular events. Cochrane Database of Systematic Reviews. 14 Jun 2017;**6**(6):CD009744

[28] Bittner VA, Diaz R, Edelberg JM, Goodman SG, Hanotin C, Harrington RA, et al. ODYSSEY OUTCOMES committees and investigators. Alirocumab and cardiovascular outcomes after acute coronary syndrome. The New England Journal of Medicine. 2018;**379**(22): 2097-2107

[29] Honarpour N, Wiviott SD, Murphy SA, Kuder JF, Wang H, Liu T, et al. FOURIER steering committee and investigators. Evolocumab and clinical outcomes in patients with cardiovascular disease. The New England Journal of Medicine. 2017; **376**(18):1713-1722

[30] Yang Y, Deng W, Wang Y, Li T, Chen Y, Long C, et al. The effect of omega-3 fatty acids and its combination with statins on lipid profile in patients with hypertriglyceridemia: A systematic review and meta-analysis of randomised controlled trials. Frontiers in Nutrition. 2022;**9**:1039056

[31] Hu B, Zhong L, Weng Y, et al. Therapeutic siRNA: State of the art. Signal Transduction Target Therapy. 2020;**5**:101

[32] Nissen SE, Lincoff AM, Brennan D, Ray KK, Mason D, Kastelein JJP, et al. CLEAR outcomes investigators. Bempedoic acid and cardiovascular outcomes in statin-intolerant patients. The New England Journal of Medicine. 2023;**388**(15):1353-1364

[33] Kim NH, Kim SG. Fibrates revisited: Potential role in cardiovascular risk reduction. Diabetes & Metabolism Journal. 2020;**44**(2):213-221

Chapter 7

The Angiosome Concept and Endovascular Techniques for Limb Salvage

Leonardo da Cruz Renó and Angélica Araújo Cortines Laxe Renó

Abstract

The aim of this chapter is to provide an overview of patients with arteriopathy, especially in the infrapatellar segment, which is the most affected in diabetic patients. In this sense, we always try to analyze the degree of disease of the patient and, if limb salvage intervention is necessary, to evaluate the new technologies that promote higher rates of technical success with less tissue aggression. In addition to the TASK classification, which provides an idea of the degree of obstruction and thus facilitates therapeutic decision-making, the use of various classifications has been demonstrated, which aims to promote better communication between physicians about the state of ischemia and the degree of injury. The different techniques used were presented, thanks to the development of new materials, with more and more possibilities for saving limbs.

Keywords: vascular disease, angiosome, endovascular surgery, diabetic foot, peripheral artery disease

1. Introduction

Peripheral obstructive arterial disease (PAD) classically has smoking, systemic arterial hypertension, and diabetes mellitus as major risk factors, with dyslipidemia as an adjuvant factor. The atherosclerotic disease can affect any part of the body, leading to myocardial infarction, stroke, bowel infarction, or distal amputation, depending on the area affected [1]. It is known that the patient with diabetes mellitus has as a major factor of morbidity and mortality, so-called diabetic foot, which can be neuropathic, ischemic, or infectious, usually with two or more of these associated factors. In these patients, it is very common to observe diffuse arterial occlusions at multiple levels, with a predominance of the territory below the knee (BTK), causing distal hypoperfusion and reducing limb viability, with a high risk of amputation [2].

Nearly 50% of patients with diabetes and foot ulcers have peripheral arterial disease (PAD). At the same time, in different stages of the disease with increased risk of adverse events in the limbs and cardiovascular disease, the management of these patients is different concerns in terms of diagnosis, prognosis, and treatment [3]. Critical limb ischemia is the result of many pathological aspects such as hypertension, diabetes mellitus, hyperlipemia, and renal failure. These conditions lead to an atherosclerotic obstructive disease with diffuse, multilevel, and multivessel calcifications, called Monckberg's disease, which causes enormous technical difficulties in the revascularization of the lesions [4].

The angiosome model was pioneered by Jan Taylor in 1987 through his influential anatomical works in the field of plastic reconstructive surgery. The model portrays the human body in three-dimensional tissue blocks that are supplied by precise arterial and venous irrigation sources, referred to as "angiosomes" [5].

Depending on the underlying cause of the process that leads to arterial obstruction, there are different patterns of obstruction in the arterial tree, as well as the characteristics of the obstruction, which can include soft plaques, thrombi, fibrotic or calcified plaques, and of course, a mixture of these types of plaque. It is known that the mortality rate of diabetic patients after amputation is about five times higher than that of the general population. Amputation rates in the diabetic population are approximately 10–20 times higher than in the nondiabetic population. Of all amputations in diabetic patients, 85% are preceded by foot ulceration that progresses to gangrene or severe infection. It is estimated that a lower limb is amputated every 30 seconds because of diabetes. These ulcerated feet are usually compromised primarily by ischemia and neuropathy [6–8].

Thus, the methods of revascularization evolved, from a time when practically only amputations were indicated evolving to sympathectomies and the use of vasodilators and later via bypass until the appearance of endovascular methods, whose technical and material improvement allow for high rates of limb salvage today. The concept of angiosome has accompanied this evolution, and it is only possible to apply this concept in practice through excellent imaging tests, technical capacity of the surgical and multidisciplinary team, and high-quality materials and technology.

2. Epidemiology

In diabetic patients, PAD is one of the leading causes of amputation. Together with neuropathy and infection, it leads to high rates of limb loss. More than 85% of these amputations are caused by a foot ulcer that progresses to deep infection or gangrene. The prevalence of diabetic foot ulcers is estimated to be 3–8% [9]. The age-adjusted prevalence of diabetes has nearly doubled since 1980, from 4.7 to 8.5% of the adult population. Over the past decade, the prevalence of diabetes has increased rapidly in the poorest countries. Myotonic dystrophy type 2 (DM2) has historically been considered a disease in developed countries, but this epidemiologic pattern is changing, and developing countries are experiencing an increasing prevalence of DM2. Currently, the global prevalence of DM2 in people aged 18 years and older has increased from 4.7% in 1980 to 8.5% in 2014, and this increase is greater in developing countries [10]. Diabetes mellitus was once considered a disease that affected the elderly and people of good socioeconomic status, but it is now believed that more than 80% of diabetic deaths occur in developing countries. About 15% of people with diabetes will develop ulcers in their lifetime, and between 14 and 43% of those will require amputation. Considering the complexity of the illness, a multidisciplinary approach is necessary, which includes endocrinologists, general and vascular surgeons, interventional radiologists, neurologists, orthopedists, and specialized nursing teams. Nevertheless, limited access to some specialties and a lack of consensus on the subject hinder the formation of multidisciplinary teams [11]. Based on the 2015 data from the

International Diabetes Federation, an estimated 9.1–26.1 million people worldwide develop diabetic foot ulcers each year. The number of adults with DM quadrupled from 1980 to 2014, mainly due to the increase in obesity and overweight, and the high number of people with diabetes has led to an increase in the incidence of diabetic foot ulcers and peripheral arterial occlusive disease (PAOD) [12]. The risk of death after 5 years is 2.5 times higher for patients with foot ulcers and diabetes than for patients with diabetes without ulcers [13].

3. Pathophysiology

Peripheral artery disease is usually caused by atherosclerosis. In patients with diabetes, we often observe early development of atherosclerotic lesions that are characteristic of poorly controlled and chronic diabetics. PAD is a significant risk factor for impaired wound healing and amputation of the lower extremities. It is imperative to note that foot ulcers often result from a combination of risk factors, therefore, proper examination by a healthcare professional is essential. A small proportion of foot ulcers materialize in patients with severe, purely ischemic PAD; these ulcers are frequently painful and can manifest themselves after minor injuries. Meanwhile, most foot ulcers occur in individuals with pure neuropathic feet who develop infections because of deformities and plantar insensitivity, as well as a combination of neuropathy and arteriopathy. Patients with neuroischemic ulcers may have no symptoms because of neuropathy despite severe ischemic foot disease. Features of peripheral arterial disease in diabetics are as follows:

- lesions with greater calcification of the physician
- worsening in distal collateral circulation
- rapid progression
- multisegmental lesions
- increased risk of amputation

In addition, the presence of moderate or severe infectious conditions greatly increases the likelihood of amputation by placing greater metabolic demands on tissues where the lack of blood supply is easily overwhelmed by the demand, leading to necrosis.

PAD increases the risk of ulcers, infections, and unhealed amputations independently. Mortality rates in patients with diabetes exceed 70% after diabetes-related amputations at 5 years and 74% at 2 years for those on renal replacement therapy [11].

Arterial disease in diabetic foot syndrome (DFS) has specific characteristics that have led to the development of the concept of diabetic distal arterial disease. These concept group's micro- and macroangiopathic changes such as non-occlusive lesions of the microcirculation (resulting from endothelial dysfunction caused by hyperglycemia and hyperinsulinemia), aggressive atherosclerotic changes with multilevel arterial blockages (involving medium and large caliber arteries), reduced collateral circulation, inflammation, and local sepsis with acute septic thrombosis [14].

4. Diagnosis and clinical examination

When confronted with a patient with diabetes mellitus, in addition to a comprehensive laboratory analysis aimed at establishing the degree of metabolic dysfunction, one should observe aspects that may alert about the prognosis of the lower limbs. Observe first the history and associated risk factors such as smoking, alcoholism, and family history of amputations. When performing the physical examination, observe if the patient is overweight or obese. Then, evaluate the skin of the lower limbs, dryness, fissures, and calluses. Finally, observe pulses from the femoral to the pedis and posterior tibial, and one cannot forget the socioeconomic and cultural evaluation. Complementary studies include continuous wave Doppler, which allows the measurement of the ankle-arm index, where values below 0.9 already indicate a reduction in distal perfusion. In diabetic patients, this generates a problem because the calcification of the arterial wall by the classic Monkberg disease leads to falsely high indices. In this case, it is proposed to measure the pressure in the fingers but, in practice today, there is the ease in performing the triplex Doppler ultrasound that can provide a simple diagnosis (**Figures 1** and **2**), which is cheap and without risks of obstructive pattern compared with the other standard, that is, the arteriography. Within the vascular physical examination, we can include the medication of the ankle-arm index, the Semmes-Weinstein monofilament test, and the tuning fork. The monofilament test and the tuning fork evaluate neuropathy; however, for the vascular surgeon, this information is paramount, not only for some types of classification of diabetic foot but also for other types of preventive measures that should be taken. In an obese patient with neuropathy, the degree of stress on the supporting structures of the feet is very high, with a reduction of protective mechanisms, leading to plantar ulcers or pruning in cases of claw or hammer finger, and this requires not only visual examination, special insoles, and shoes but also guidance of the patient and the whole family regarding diet, skincare, and visual inspection. In practice, only the clinical examination can define the picture of peripheral arterial disease, and the request of complementary tests such as Doppler ultrasound, computed tomography angiography, and

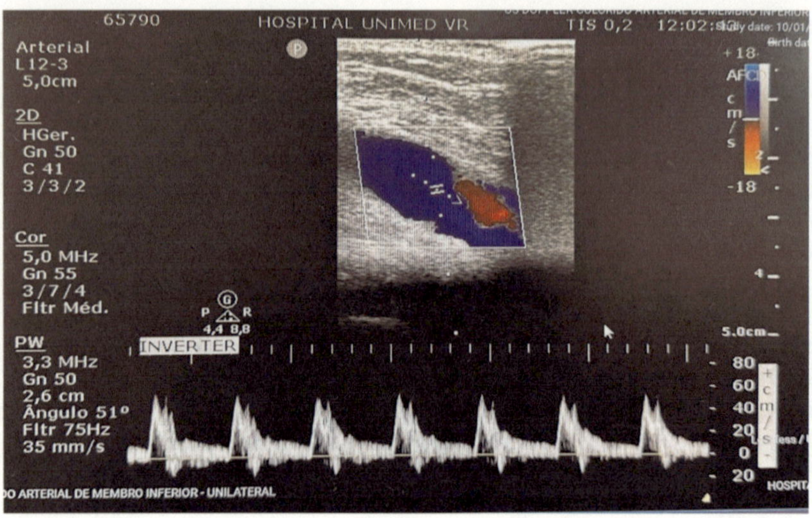

Figure 1.
Popliteal artery with triphasic flow.

DOI: http://dx.doi.org/10.5772/intechopen.1003988

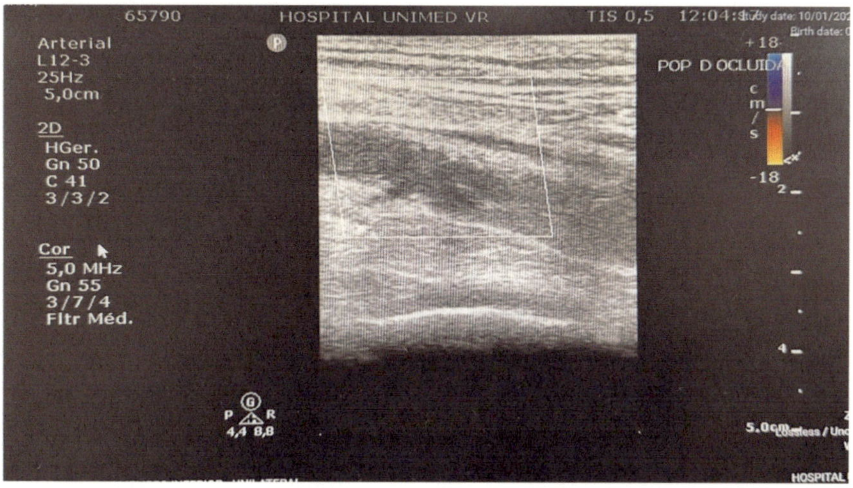

Figure 2.
Popliteal artery occluded.

arteriography would be reserved for patients with prediction of possible renovascular or open approach.

Palpation of the pulses:

1. femoral

2. popliteal

3. tibialis anterior – dorsal of the foot

4. tibialis posterior – retromalleolar.

Because clinical examination does not reliably exclude PAD in most people with diabetes and foot ulcers, it is necessary to evaluate the shapes of the arterial Doppler waves at the wrists of the feet in combination with ankle systolic pressure and ankle-arm index (ABI) or measurement of systolic pressure and finger-arm index (FDI). No single modality has proven to be ideal, and there is no defined threshold above which PAD can be safely excluded. However, the diagnosis of PAD is less likely in the presence of ABI values of 0.9–1.3, BDI $\geq$ 0.75, and three-phase Doppler wave in the wrists of the feet.

5. Classifications used

5.1 Task 2

PAD characteristically presents different patterns according to the fact of associated risk. Thus, in smokers, we observed a greater involvement of the aortoiliac sector. In hypertensive disease, it is the popliteal sector, whereas, in diabetes, it is the infrapatellar pattern with preservation of the fibular artery. From the vascular surgeon's point of view, the TASK2 classification (**Figure 3**) can be used, which provides

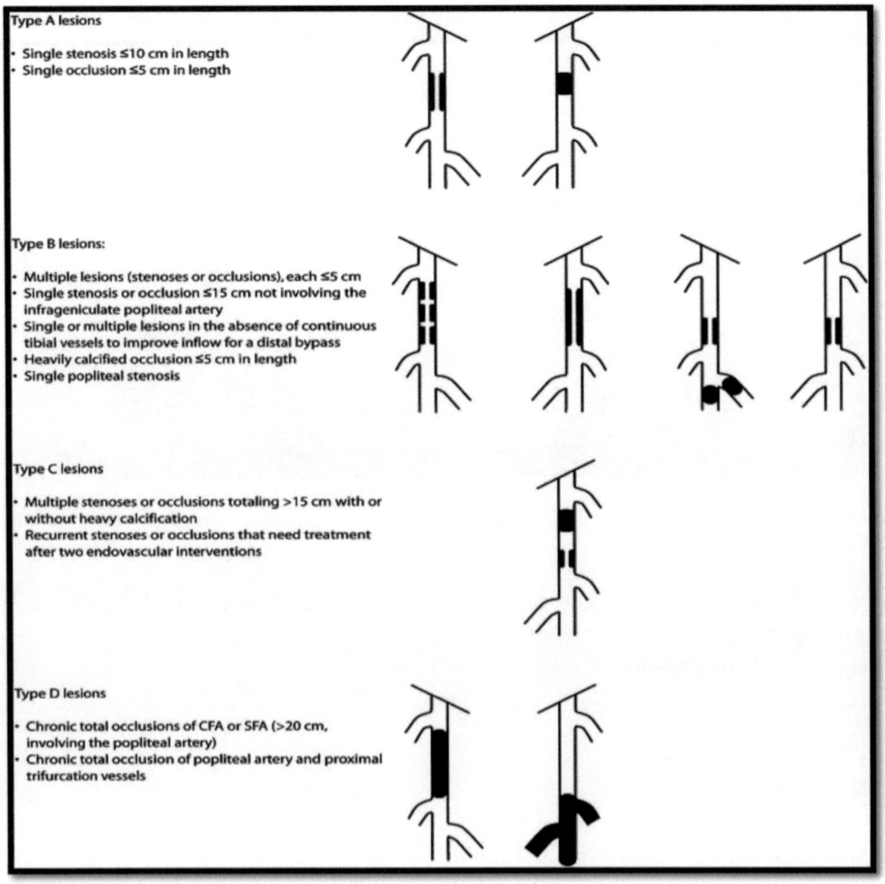

Figure 3.
Task 2 classification.

an anatomical evaluation of the lesion site and its extension and may suggest the best endovascular or conventional treatment. With advances in vascular materials and techniques, we are now treating lesions previously indicated for endovascular treatment.

For the infrapatellar region, the 2015 TASK classification (**Figure 4**) [15] presents the most common types of patterns seen on angiograms and suggests the best approaches for each. In general, in the infrapatellar region, treatment is indicated in cases of critical ischemia, where the ankle-arm index is usually less than 0.3. In patients with high surgical risk and an ankle-arm index greater than 0.5 with a small wound having adequate perfusion as assessed by a clinical examination or other methods such as $TcPO_2$ partial oxygen tension greater than 40 mmHg, we evaluate the use of medications combined with hyperbaric oxygen therapy and appropriate dressings.

5.2 Fontaine and Rutherford's classification

The Fontaine classification (**Table 1**) is used to classify ischemic limbs in general, regardless of etiology. This old classification is well known by vascular surgeons in

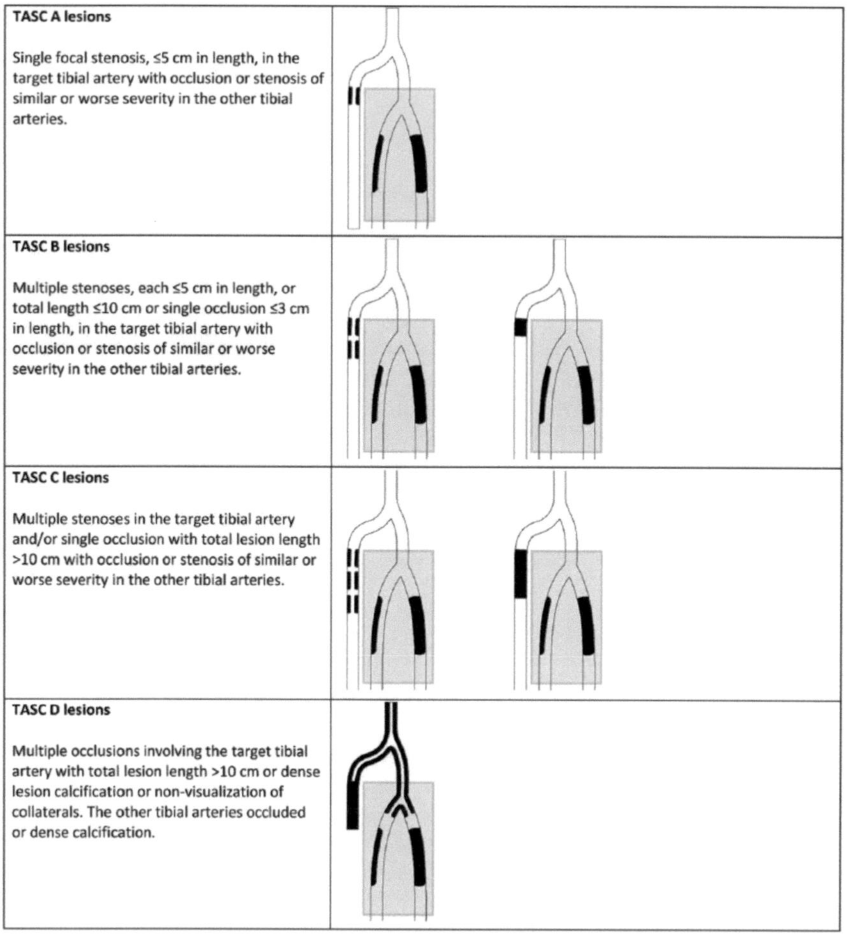

Figure 4.
Task 2 modified for infrapopliteal segment.

Stage	Clinical presentation	Grade	Category	Clinical presentation
I	Asymptomatic	0	0	Asymptomatic
IIa	Mild claudication	I	1	Mild claudication
IIb	Moderate to severe claudication	I	2	Moderate claudication
III	Ischemic pain at rest	I	3	Severe claudication
IV	Gangrene or ulceration	II	4	Ischemic pain at rest
		III	5	Minor tissue lesion
		III	6	Major tissue lesion

Table 1.
Classification of Fontaine and Rutherford's for chronic peripheral arterial disease.

general, is learned early in residency, and is greatly important because of its ease of use. The Rutherford classification provide a 6-category differentiation in ischemic symptoms with 5 and 6 corresponding to grade 4 in Fontaine's classification.

5.3 WIfI classification

From the initial physical examination and anamnesis, we have prioritized the etiologic and anatomic diagnosis to evaluate the best treatment and means of prevention, which are important to classify the patients; now, we have excellent classification systems. Today, the WIfI classification (**Tables 2–4**) is considered one of the best in guiding the best treatment and defining the severity of the ischemic diabetic foot.

When evaluating the optimal revascularization technique for each case, both bypass and endovascular techniques must consider distal outflow as a crucial factor. According to the JVS guideline [16], it is recommended to measure hemodynamic tests, such as hallux pressure. GLASS (Global Limb Anatomic Staging System)

Ulcer graduation	UPD Gangrene
0	No ulcer without gangrene Clinical description: small tissue loss. Recoverable with simple digital amputation (1 or 2 fingers) or coating with the skin.
1	Distal superficial small ulcer(s) without gangrene on the leg or foot; without bone exposure, unless limited to the distal phalanx Clinical description: small tissue loss. Recoverable with simple digital amputation (1 or 2 fingers) or skin coating.
2	Deeper ulcer with bone exposure, gangrene limited to the finger joint or tendon; usually not involving the heel; heel ulcer, without calcaneal involvement Clinical description: large loss of recoverable tissue with multiple finger amputations ≥3 or standard transmetatarsal (TMJ) amputation ± skin lining.
3	Extensive and deep ulcer involving the forefoot. Extensive gangrene involving the forefoot and/or midfoot; deep and/or midfoot heel ulcer; heel necrosis and ± involvement of the calcaneus extensive and ± involvement of the calcaneus Clinical description: extensive loss of tissue recoverable only with a complex reconstruction of the foot or nonstandard TMJ (Chopart or Lisfranc); skin flap or the need for managing complex ulcers for large defects of soft tissues.

Table 2.
WIfI classification. Wound from WIfI system.

Ischemia grade	Ankle-brachial index	Ankle systolic pressure mmHg	Toe pressure, transcutaneous oxygen pressure mmHg
0	≥ 0.80	>100	≥ 60
1	0.6–0.79	70–100	40–59
2	0.4–0.59	50–70	30–39
3	≤ 0.39	<50	<30

Table 3.
WIFI classification. Ischemia from WIfI system.

0	No symptoms or signs of infection Infection present, as defined by the presence of at least two of the following: • local swelling or hardening • erythema >0.5 to ≤2 cm around the ulcer • tenderness or pain at the site • heat on site • purulent exudate (thick, opaque to white or bloody discharge)
1	Local infection involving only the skin and subcutaneous tissue (no involvement of deeper tissues and no systemic signs, as described below).
2	Exclude other causes of the cutaneous inflammatory response (e.g., trauma, gout, Charcot's neuro-osteoarthropathy, fracture, thrombosis, venous stasis). Local infection (as described above) with erythema >2 cm or involving deeper structures of the skin and subcutaneous tissues (e.g., abscess, osteomyelitis, septic arthritis, fasciitis), and No signs of systemic inflammatory response (as described below).
3	Local infection (as described above) with signs of SIRS, manifested by two or more of the following findings: • temperature > 38°C or < 36°C • Heart rate > 90 beats/min • respiratory rate > 20 breaths/min or PaCO2 < 32 mmHg • leukocyte count >12,000 or < 4000 cus/mm or 10% of immature forms (band)

Table 4.
WIFI classification. Foot infection from WIfI system.

evaluates the TAP (Target Artery Path), which is a direct arterial route from the run-off to the area of interest to be revascularized, with the aim of achieving the best possible limb-based patency (LBP). Thus, in addition to the classifications for diabetic foot and degrees of ischemia, there is the GLASS (Global Limb Anatomic Staging System) scheme (**Figures 5** and **6**). This scheme assesses the best direct run-off route to a distal lesion, and in certain cases aims to revascularize a corresponding angiosome. It is important to note that a patent TAP (**Table 5**) is responsible for distributing blood to all the structures of the foot. On the other hand, an incomplete TAP can impede wound healing, even when the corresponding angiosome is used to revascularize the foot [17]. Troisi et al. compared tissue healing, healing time, and survival with PA patency.

GLASS includes the complexity of arterial disease in the distal bed and grades the femoro-popliteal and infra-popliteal segments on a scale of 0–4. This is then plotted on a predetermined matrix based on scientific evidence, resulting in a GLASS combination ranging from 1 to 3. In terms of inflow, GLASS evaluates calcified or non-calcified aortoilic lesions dichotomously.

Aorto-iliac (inflow) disease staging in GLASS.

i. Stenosis of the common and/or external iliac artery, chronic total occlusion of either common or external iliac artery (not both), stenosis of the infrarenal aorta; any combination of these

ii. Chronic total occlusion of the aorta; chronic total occlusion of common and external iliac arteries; severe diffuse disease and/or small-caliber (<6 mm) common and external iliac arteries; concomitant aneurysm disease; severe diffuse in-stent restenosis in the aortoiliac system

FP Grade 0	Mild or no significant (<50%) disease	
FP Grade 1	• Total length SFA disease <1/3 (<10 cm) • May include single focal CTO (< 5 cm) as long as not flush occlusion • Popliteal artery with mild or no significant disease	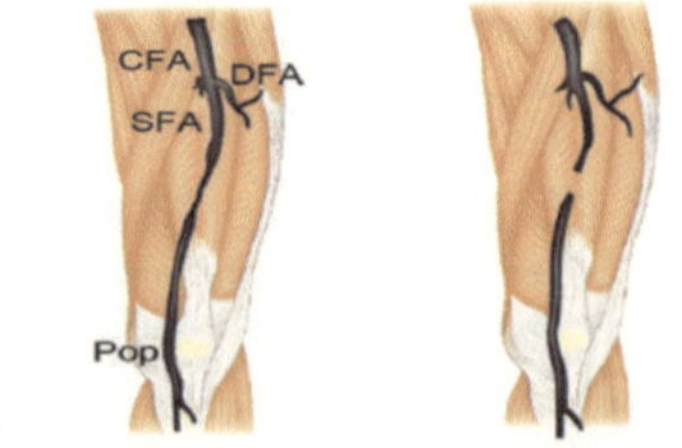
FP Grade 2	• Total length SFA disease 1/3-2/3 (10-20 cm) • May include CTO totaling < 1/3 (10 cm) but not flush occlusion • Focal popliteal artery stenosos <2 cm, not involving trifurcation	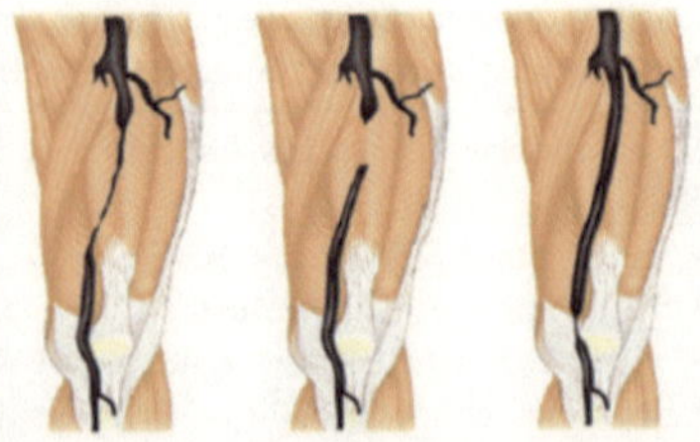
FP Grade 3	• Total length SFA disease >2/3 (>20 cm) length • May include any flush occlusion <20 cm or non-flush CTO 10-20 cm long • Short popliteal stenosis 2-5 cm, not involving trifurcation	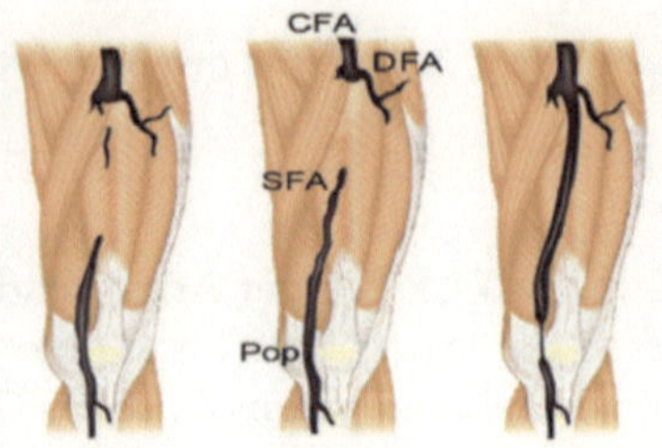
FP Grade 4	• Total length SFA occlusion > 20 cm • Popliteal disease >5 cm or extending into trifurcation • Any popliteal CTO	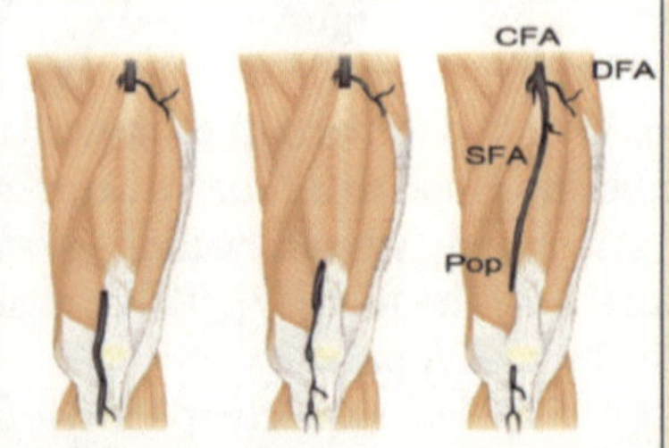

Figure 5.
Femoropopliteal (FP) disease grading in global limb anatomic staging system (GLASS). Trifurcation is defined as the termination of the popliteal artery at the confluence of the anterior tibial (AT) artery and tibioperoneal trunk. CFA ¼ common femoral artery; CTO ¼ chronic total occlusion; DFA ¼ deep femoral artery; pop ¼ popliteal; SFA ¼ superficial femoral artery. (Conte, Bradbury e col., 2019).

The success of revascularization depends on various factors, which differ depending on whether it is a bypass or an endovascular method. In the case of a bypass, a good conduit, inflow and outflow are necessary, and the patient must be in good clinical condition to undergo surgery [18].

For endovascular interventions, it is crucial to assess the degree of atherosclerosis and anticipate any problems with the TAP that could jeopardize the direct arterial line

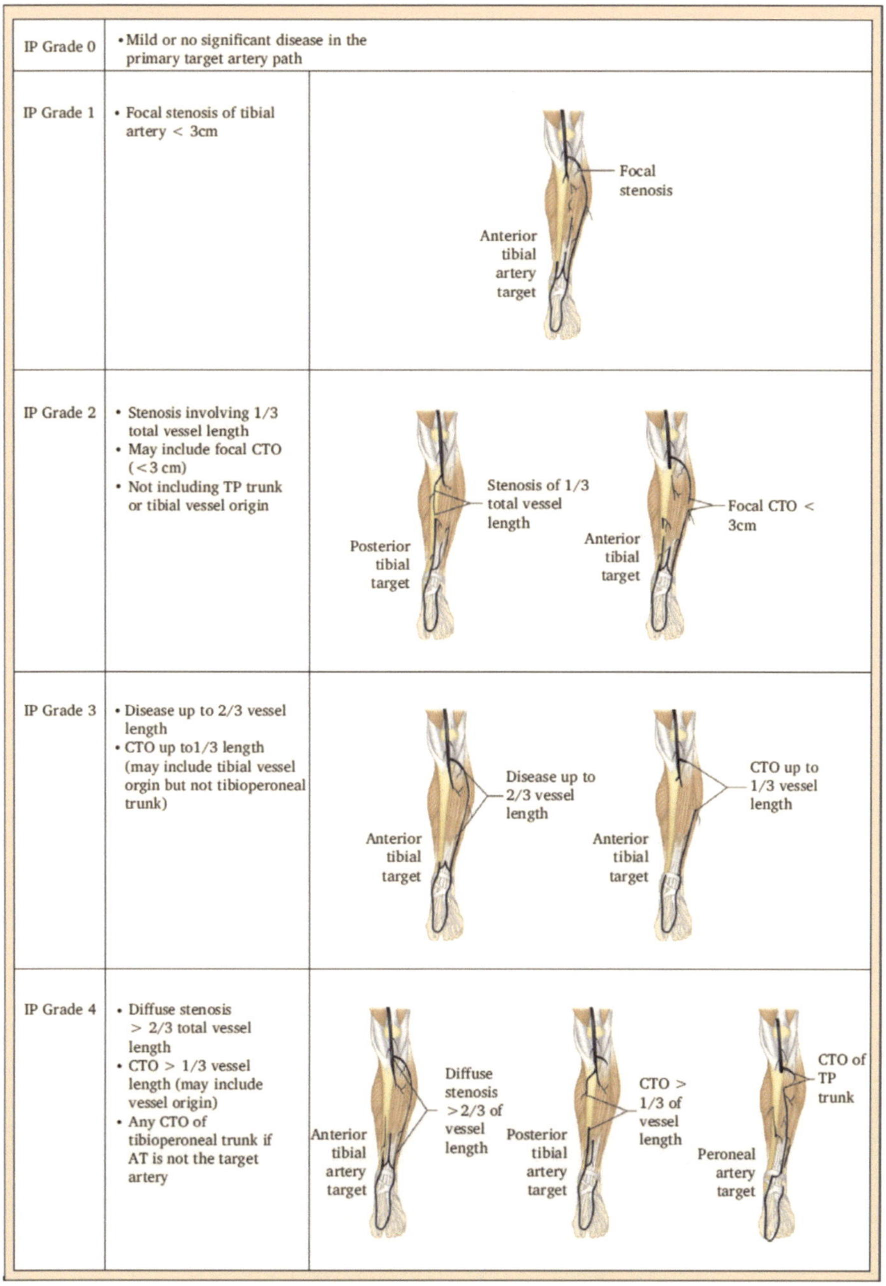

Figure 6.
Infrapopliteal (IP) disease grading in global limb anatomic staging system (GLASS). AT ¼ anterior tibial; CTO ¼ chronic total occlusion; TP ¼ tibioperoneal. (Conte, Bradbury et al., 2019).

to the foot. If the TAP has serial lesions, the success of the procedure will depend on the ability to bypass these lesions.

It is important to note that the artery chosen as the TAP for a bypass may not always be the same for an endovascular intervention (**Figure 7**).

Infra-malleolar/Pedal descriptor	
P0	Target artery crosses ankle into foot, with intact pedal arch
P1	Target artery crosses ankle into foot; absent or severely diseased pedal arch
P2	No target artery crossing ankle into foot

Table 5.
(Conte, Bradbury, et al., 2019).

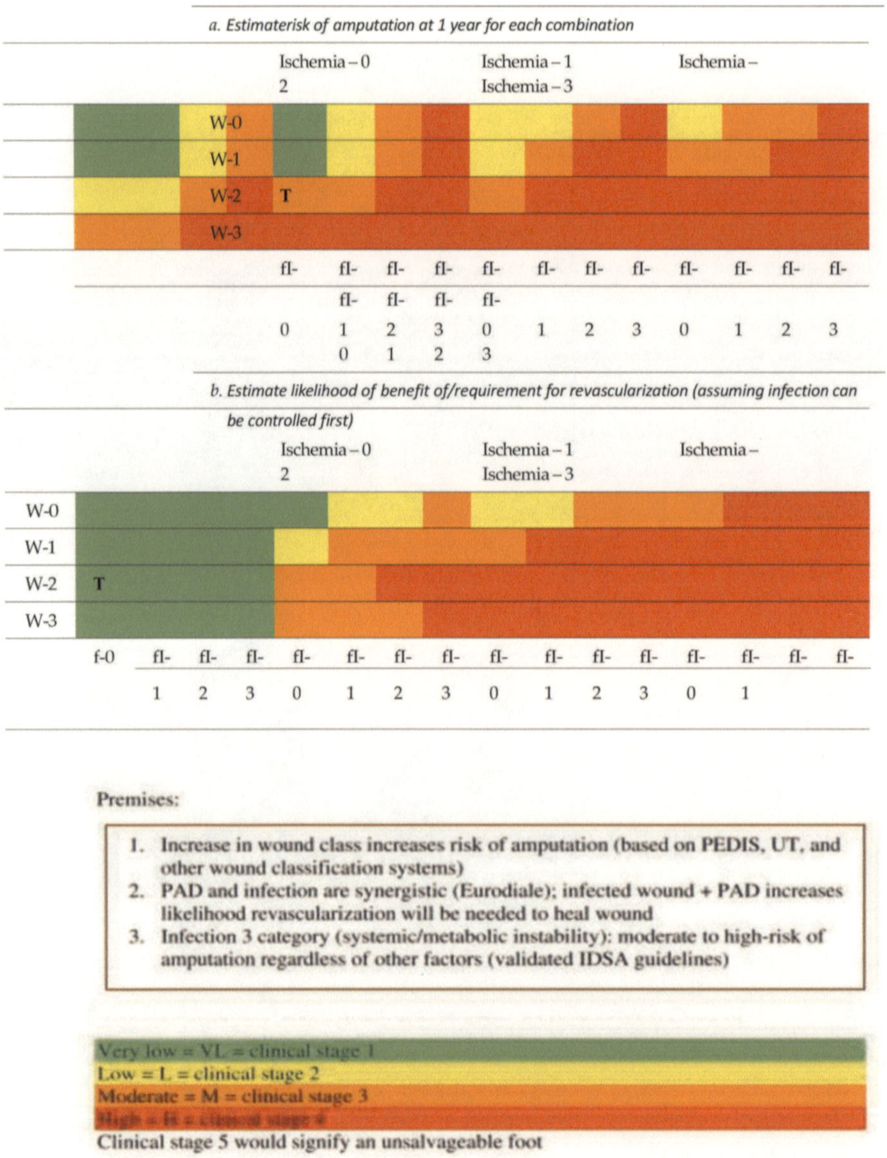

Figure 7.
WIFI classification. WIfI prediction tables. a. Estimaterisk of amputation at 1 year for each combination. b. Estimate likelihood of benefit of/requirement for revascularization (assuming infection can be controlled first).

In the context of malleolar infarction disease, GLASS has three levels to describe the arteries that cross the ankle. GLASS also makes the following assumptions:

- Restoring durable (pulsatile) in-line flow to the affected. Part, particularly in patients with tissue loss, is a primary goal of revascularization in CLTI.
- Using high-quality imaging (Section 3), the vascular specialist chooses and defines a TAP that is most likely to achieve that in-line flow.
- The TAP will usually involve the least diseased IP artery.

The peripheral arteries (PA) can be classified as complete, incomplete, or absent, with only collateral branches present, as proposed by the global limb anatomic staging system (GLASS). A PA is considered complete when a branch of the DP artery (dorsalis pedis) connects with a branch of the plantar arteries via the dorsal and plantar metatarsal arteries [19].

Incomplete peripheral arterial occlusion (PAO) occurs when one of the truncal arteries in the foot is absent, such as the dorsalis pedis artery or the plantar arteries, resulting in incomplete blood flow between the anterior and posterior circulation. Alternatively, incomplete PAO can occur when the plantar arteries and DP artery are present but not connected.

Alternative classifications for foot vascularization have been proposed, such as Hofmann et al.'s [20] classification of the distal pedal bed. It is important to note that these classifications differ from Rutherford's.

This classification includes three types:

1. type 1 – flows into the dorsal artery of the foot or plantar region, without representation of the popliteal artery (PA).
2. type 2 – partial representation of the PA, but no connection between the dorsal and plantar regions.
3. type 3 – complete representation of the PA.

Therefore, it is crucial to conduct a preoperative assessment of the foot's vascularization to determine the appropriate revascularization surgery and predict wound healing [21, 22].

6. Treatment

When faced with a patient with decompensated ischemia who presents with ischemic pain at rest and tissue loss, the possibility of performing invasive procedures to revascularize the limb is evaluated. Conventional infrainguinal revascularization showed higher morbidity and mortality compared to endovascular treatment, according to the BASIL study [23]. In the case of diabetic patients, we often opt for the endovascular technique because these are mostly infrapatellar lesions, for which endovascular treatment is well established as a first-line option. Every year, new materials and more sophisticated techniques appear, allowing extensive and increasingly distal revascularization even in cases previously considered inoperable.

This requires, in addition to a highly trained team, a hospital with an excellent structure and equipment, such as ultrasound in the operating room, high-definition digital fluoroscopy, special guidewires with nitinol bodies, and a heavy weight at the tip to overcome calcified lesions, support catheters, and long and thin balloons to perform the most diverse techniques. The surgeon can choose the anterograde, retrograde, or both approaches, depending on the level of occlusion, the distal artery, and the type of plaque. Another technique widely used in severely calcified arteries where the anterograde route is more difficult to recanalize is the technique of distal micropuncture of the pedal or posterior tibial artery. Today, very thin balloons of up to 1.5 mm are used to dilate the arteries of the foot, in addition to providing support for the guidewire as it advances. Through the concept of angiosome, we should aim to take the pulsatile blood to the most distal regions possible and preferably to the site that directly irrigates the necrotic area, having as a goal the complete revascularization of the plantar arch leaving blood to the toes and perforating branches that irrigate the forefoot, dorsal region of the foot, and calcaneus posteriorly. In terms of techniques used to overcome the lesions anterogradely, we have the technique of using guide wires under a 0.014 catheter to try to slide through the occlusion intraluminal, called the sliding technique. If not effective, we can use guide wires with a thinner, heavier tip and rotate them to perforate the proximal rigid plate (cap), known as the drilling technique. A form of treatment that was once considered only for the supra-patellar area and can now be performed in the infrapatellar area is the subintimal recanalization technique, which requires great technical skill in addition to 0.018 guide wires [24]. According to the 2019 edition of the International Working Group on the Diabetic Foot (IWGDF), patients with ankle pressure < 50 mmHg or ITB <0.5 should undergo vascular imaging for possible revascularization, as well as those with toe pressure < 30 mmHg or $PtcO_2$ < 25 mmHg. Physicians may consider revascularization at higher pressure levels in patients with extensive tissue loss or infection [3]. Classically, the goal of successful revascularization is to deliver pulsatile flow directly to the site of ischemic tissue damage. However, the angiosome approach has recently been proposed as a topic of debate. This theory posits that the foot can be divided into three-dimensional blocks, each with its arterial supply. Direct revascularization results in the restoration of pulsatile blood flow through the supply artery to the area where the ulcer is located. In contrast, indirect revascularization restores flow through collateral vessels derived from nearby angiosomes. Targeting revascularization to the vessel directly supplying the anatomic area (angiosome) where tissue loss has occurred is a more effective method of revascularization than simply targeting the best vessel, which may not supply enough blood to the area where tissue loss has occurred. A recent retrospective analysis of endovascular attempts to salvage limbs in patients with peripheral artery disease revealed that indirect angiosome revascularization was linked to poorer outcomes when compared to direct revascularization.

In cases of arterial obstructions, optimal operative planning should be carried out before proposing treatment. In this case, the access route should be well evaluated based on the obstructive pattern, the patient's physical complexion, and the team's experience. Normally, access to endovascular treatment is via the common femoral artery using the Seldinger technique, either anterograde or retrograde. Today, in some cases, retrograde podal access is used that facilitates the recanalization of distal calcified lesions as the distal region of the obstruction tends to be softer, avoiding the proximal calcium layer. Regarding the material to be used, the ideal is to have a wide range of materials available, including 0.014 guide wires with a high tip weight, such as the Abbott Command® and a support catheter such as the Trailblazer® or Quickcross®. Peripheral artery disease in patients with diabetes has several characteristics that render it more difficult to treat. The atherosclerotic lesions are multilevel and particularly severe in tibial arteries, with a high prevalence of long occlusions. The predilection for multiple crural vessel involvement combined with extensive arterial calcification increases the technical challenges associated with revascularization using either open bypass or endovascular techniques. In the last decades, new techniques and technologies have been introduced for treating PAD, which might be relevant to patients with diabetes and poorly healing ischemic foot ulcers. Encouraging results have been reported on endovascular approaches, and the field is rapidly evolving [25]. Today, the use of ultradistal revascularization techniques at the level of the plantar arch is made possible using thin 1.5-mm balloons under guide wires and combined retrograde and anterograde puncture techniques, as well as auxiliary techniques such as atherectomy and subintimal re-entry catheters. The goal of revascularization is to restore online flow to at least one of the arteries in the foot, preferably the artery supplying the anatomic region of the wound. However, evaluating the benefit of revascularization in patients to whom the risk-benefit ratio for the likelihood of success is unfavorable. Evaluate the distribution of PAD, the availability of an autogenous vein, the patient's comorbidities, and the operator's experience, as well as the available materials and hospital support structure. Lower extremity ischemia affects the healing potential of a foot ulcer. If ischemia is identified during assessment, its treatment should always be considered. Based on the IWGDF/ESVS/SVS intersocial guidelines [26], the following treatment recommendations are made: In a person with ankle pressure < 50 mmHg or ITB < 0.4, consider urgent vascular imaging, always with detailed visualization of the arteries below the knee and foot, and revascularization. In addition, consider urgent evaluation for revascularization if toe pressure is <30 mmHg or $TcpO_2$ is <25 mmHg. However, clinicians may also consider revascularization at higher pressure levels in patients with extensive tissue loss or infection, that is, higher WIfI scores. In terms of treatment, there is a classification called Task 2 that provides a guideline for management. The best course of action for each case depends very much on the service, socioeconomic conditions, and clinical aspects of the patient involved. A Task D patient can successfully undergo an endovascular procedure in a hospital with a dedicated team, using state-of-the-art materials and equipment, and with appropriate intensive care support.

Optimized clinical management to reduce the very high cardiovascular risk associated with PAD in people with diabetes (smoking cessation, control of hypertension and dyslipidemia, use of antiplatelet agents, SGLT2 inhibitors, or GLP1 agonists) [27].

The natural history of patients with diabetes, PAD, and foot ulcers remains poorly defined. However, in two studies that reported outcomes in patients with diabetes and ischemia who did not undergo revascularization, the limb salvage rate was approximately 50% at 1 year. After revascularization, most studies report limb salvage rates of 80–85% and ulcer healing rates of greater than 60% at 12 months [26]. In a different situation, for example in a developing country, we may have to indicate primary amputations without being wrong because, without the conditions to perform revascularization with adequate limb salvage rates, we are putting the patient's life at risk. In this respect, the recent WIfI classification can be considered the most rational, as it assesses the risk of amputation in 1 year, but the good judgment of the medical team is still the determining factor for success. In a recently published meta-analysis combining data from 12 studies (11 prospective and 1 retrospective), the WIfI classification was shown to be a good prognostic method for amputation at 1-year follow-up.

A positive statistical correlation was observed between stage progression (from 1 to 4) and increased incidence of amputation [28].

As the level of heterogeneity was very high because of differences between studies (mainly population characteristics, inclusion criteria, and endpoint), the level of evidence was considered low or very low depending on the stage, and it was not possible to demonstrate the usefulness of using the WIfI classification for clinical practice, that is, for recommending limb revascularization. Specifically for diabetic patients, a very important correlation has been identified, with wound healing proving to be more relevant than direct revascularization (guided by the angiosome) or assessment of the quality of the plantar arch [29].

One of the weaknesses identified in the meta-analysis of the WIfI classification was the inadequate correlation because it does not take into account the anatomical state of the arterial circulation. Thus, nonrevascularization was considered only because it was impossible (clinically or anatomically), and not because it might be necessary. The combination of the WIfI classification with a classification that assesses anatomical impairment would have the role of assessing the patient globally to better support the indication of revascularization [30].

The wide variety of lesion distributions in DM patients requires the use of devices that can be effective in endovascular treatment of tortuous arteries in the aortoiliac of the aortoiliac segment, femoropopliteal arteries and, above all, stenoses of infrapopliteal and inframalleolar arteries. The infrapopliteal vessels are affected in more than 70% of patients [2, 31].

The conventional balloon in long lesions has relatively low patency rates, ranging from 25 to 40% at 1 year. After balloon inflation, they can lead to elastic retraction dissection and therefore dissection, resulting in high rates of stenting after angioplasty (bailout). Still, about angioplasty balloons, new types with different design features have recently been introduced with the aim of improving angioplasty outcomes. These devices appear to reduce the incidence of restenosis and flow-limiting dissection and may increase the ability to fix drugs in pharmacological balloons [32, 33].

Cases such as this may require the use of atherotomes aiming at plaque reduction and better preparation of the lesion for subsequent angioplasty with a drug-eluted balloon.

If endovascular revascularization is indicated, it may be necessary to bypass the lesion via the subintimal (Bolia) or intraluminal route, in which case techniques such as POBBA may be required, requiring materials such as atherotomes, support catheters, high-pressure balloons, and stents. The use of stents in the popliteal artery is problematic because it is an area that is subject to various stresses that can lead to stent fracture. In addition to the use of endoluminal techniques with support catheters and atherotomes, retrograde recanalizations are very useful, and the new stents for this region, such as Supera®, have become indispensable.

In the case of associated infrapatellar occlusion, if the lesions are short, there is usually no great difficulty in bypassing these lesions anterogradely using simple or pharmacologically thin balloons. It is important to keep the balloon inflated for approximately 3 min to ensure good impaction of the plates on the wall. Associated anterograde/retrograde techniques, as well as others such as subintimal techniques, have led to success in situations that were previously virtually impossible to treat endovascularly. In any case, we should evaluate distal bypasses within situ, reverse, or *ex vivo* devolved saphenous veins, which have high patency rates but require a refined technique and the use of autologous grafts in good condition and, of course, a good distal bed to receive the flow.

Patients with diabetes and ischemia represent a subgroup with a worse prognosis, thus, the angiosome model proposed by Jan Taylor in 1987 has reappeared as a target to be achieved in order to obtain favorable results [30].

In the original article by Prof. Jan Taylor [26], he first stated that the angiosome corresponds to a volumetric block of subcutaneous cellular tissue and skin with a single, specific venous and arterial irrigation and with extensive collateral communication between adjacent angiosomes.

This has been adapted to the ischemic diabetic foot in the planning of surgical and endovascular revascularization procedures in patients with Stage III and IV Rutherford classification. The model defines six angiosomes for the foot, divided by the territory of the tibial and peroneal arteries. The medial calcaneal artery and the medial and lateral plantar arteries, which are the branches of the posterior tibial artery, would each irrigate three angiosomes. The pedicle artery, the terminal branch of the anterior tibial artery, would flush another angiosome; and the lateral calcaneal and lateral perimalleolar arteries, which are branches of the peroneal artery, would flush the final two angiosomes in the foot. In the ankle, there are also angiosomes in the territory of the lateral malleolar artery (branch of the anterior tibial artery), which also give off median malleolar branches, and the angiosome of the anterior perforating artery (branch of the peroneal artery (**Table 6** and **Figure 4**).

Several studies have shown that using the angiosome concept, limb salvage rates with direct revascularization techniques are significantly better than with indirect revascularization techniques [34]. An article by Iida et al. showed worse results in limb salvage rates in diabetic patients with elevated CRP, possibly due to increased blood demand. Indirect revascularization without direct pulsatile flow to the angiosome in question was observed. The results of this article would lead to the conclusion that in Rutherford 5 and 6 patients, indirect or direct revascularization would lead to similar results, except in patients with diabetes and wound infection, where direct revascularization in the angiosome leads to significantly better results [35]. Another study by Kahn et al. suggests always try to revascularize as many infrapatellar arteries as possible in patients with diabetes and distal necrotic lesions, regardless of the angiosome of the lesion, to promote overall improvement of foot perfusion pressures at the microcirculatory level leading to better outcomes [36]. The figures below show arteriograms of diabetic patients with infrapatellar artery occlusion. The arteries to be recanalized were indicated (**Figures 8–12**). This is a case of a

Location of the ischemic lesion	Arterial territory to revascularize
Calcanean	median calcaneal artery (branch of the posterior tibial artery) lateral calcaneal artery (branch of the peroneal artery) collaterals between the two anterior territories
Posterolateral side of the ankle and perimalleolar	median perimalleolar network anterior perforating artery (branch of the peroneal artery) anterolateral malleolar branches (branches of the anterior tibial artery)
Plant	median and lateral plantar arteries (branches of the posterior tibial artery) tarsal arteries (branches of the pedicle artery)

Table 6.
Revascularization strategy based on the location of ischemic lesions.

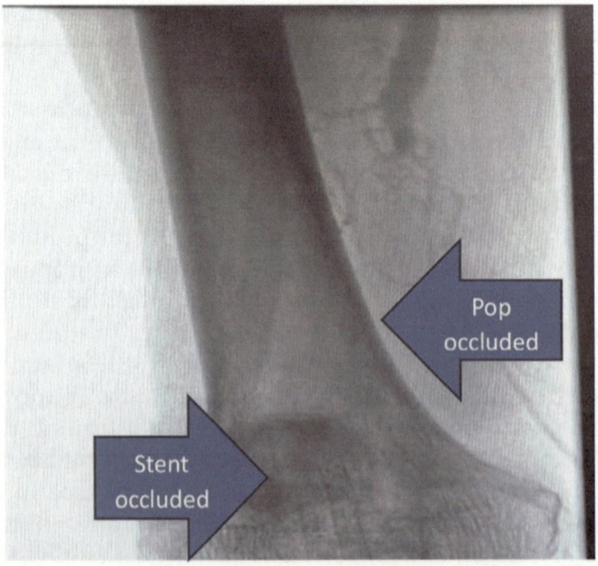

Figure 8.
Example of popliteal occlusion with calcified plaque and occluded stent in popliteal artery.

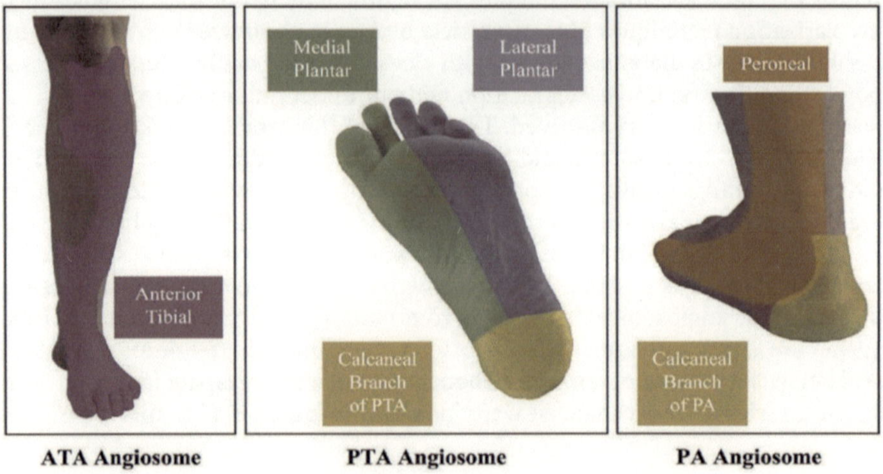

Figure 9.
Angiosome distribution in the foot.

patient with a trophic lesion of the hallux, insulin-dependent diabetes mellitus, and ischemic pain at rest. The arteriography showed a patent fibular and occlusion of the anterior and posterior tibial arteries. In this case, we opted for foot amputation and clinical management because of the presence of extensive collateral circulation, a distal Tcpo2 above 40 mmHg, and the availability of hyperbaric oxygen therapy and a dressing team.

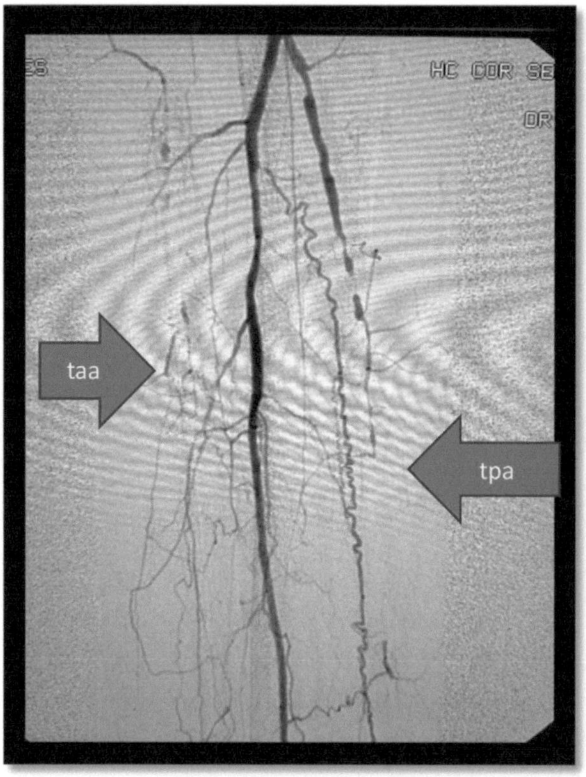

Figure 10.
Image of infra popliteal vessels and distal runnoff, with occlusion of anterior and posterior tibial arteries.

The effectiveness of a revascularization procedure should preferably be assessed with objective perfusion measurements. After revascularization of a limb with an ischemic lesion, it is recommended to wait approximately 2 weeks, if possible, before performing minor amputations or debridements due to the progressive increase in tissue oxygen tension after angioplasty.

7. Conclusions

When we studied the articles on the application of the angiosome concept to the ischemic diabetic foot, we observed a great concern to reduce the MALE and save the limb, and it is necessary to consider not only the anatomical aspects but also the functional aspects of the patient and the institution. The treatment of the diabetic foot will always be multidisciplinary. The vascular surgeon should be responsible for the final treatment strategy aimed at saving the foot in advanced stages. The clinician, physiatrist, physiotherapist, and dietician should be responsible for preventive issues. Finally, the patients themselves and their family members should be trained to recognize early changes that indicate decompensation of the diabetic foot.

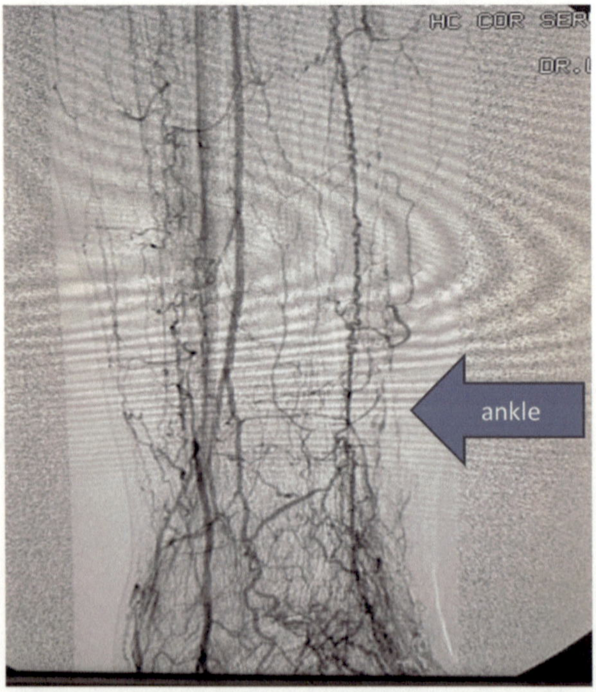

Figure 11.
Image of infra popliteal vessels and distal runnoff, with occlusion of anterior and posterior tibial arteries and and refilling of distal collaterals by the distal branches of the peroneal artery.

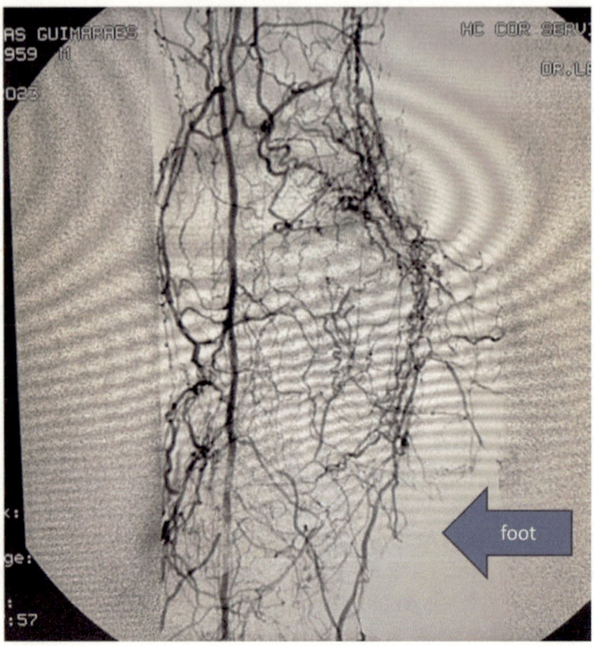

Figure 12.
Image of pedal arteries with dorsal pedis artey and incomplete pedal arch.

Author details

Leonardo da Cruz Renó* and Angélica Araújo Cortines Laxe Renó
Unimed Hospital, Volta Redonda, Rio de Janeiro, Brazil

*Address all correspondence to: c.t.v.r@hotmail.com

References

[1] Bosiers M, Deloose K. New developments in diabetic limb salvage. The Journal of Cardiovascular Surgery. 2012;**53**:1-2

[2] Pinto E, Gomes A, Costa A. Síndrome do pé diabético: A perspectiva do radiologista de intervenção. Revista Clínica do Hospital Professor Doutor Fernando Fonseca. 2014;**1**(2):37-43

[3] Schaper NC, Van Netten JJ, Apelqvist J, Bus SA, Hinchliffe RJ, Lipsky BA. Diretrizes do IWGDF sobre a prevenção e O tratamento de pé diabético. In: Lançamento da Tradução Brasileira das Diretrizes IWGDF. Vol. 2019. Rio de Janeiro. 2019. p. 34. Availbale from: https://iwgdfguidelines.org › uploads › 2020/12

[4] Mustapha JA, Finton SM, Diaz-Sandoval LJ, Saab FA, Miller LE. Percutaneous transluminal angioplasty in patients with infrapopliteal arterial disease: Systematic review and meta-analysis. Circulation: Cardiovascular Interventions. 2016;**9**(5):e003468

[5] Alexandrescu V, Hubermont G. The challenging topic of diabetic foot revascularization: Does the angiosome-guided angioplasty may improve outcome. The Journal of Cardiovascular Surgery. 2012;**53**(1):3-12

[6] Apelqvist J. Diagnostics and treatment of the diabetic foot. Endocrine. 2012;**41**:384-397

[7] Boulton AJ, Vileikyte L, Ragnarson-Tennvall G, et al. The global burden of diabetic foot disease. Lancet. 2005;**366**: 1719-1724

[8] Lep Cantalo M, Apelqvist J, Setacci C, et al. Chapter V: Diabetic foot. European Journal of Vascular and Endovascular Surgery. 2011;**42**:S60-S74

[9] Apelqvist J, Larsson J. What is the most effective way to reduce incidence of amputation in the diabetic foot? Diabetes/Metabolism Research and Reviews. 2000;**16**(S1):S75-S83

[10] Organización Mundial de la Salud. Diabetes. Ginebra: Centro de prensa. OMS; 2016. Available from: http://www.who.int/mediacentre/factsheets/fs312/es/ [Accessed: March 2, 2016]

[11] Mendoza Romo MÁ, Padrón Salas A, Cossío Torres PE, Orozco MS. Prevalencia mundial de la diabetes mellitus tipo 2 y su relación con el índice de desarrollo humano. Revista Panamericana de Salud Pública. 2018;**41**: e103

[12] Armstrong DG, Boulton AJM, Bus SA. Diabetic foot ulcers and their recurrence. New England Journal of Medicine. 2017;**376**:2367-2375

[13] Ref Walsh JW, Hoffstad OJ, Sullivan MO, Margolis DJ. Association of diabetic foot ulcer and death in a population-based cohort from the United Kingdom. Diabetic Medicine. 2016;**33**:1493-1498

[14] Parekh N, Nanjundappa A, Dieter RS. Pharmacological interventions on critical limb ischemia in diabetic patients. The Journal of Cardiovascular Surgery. 2012;**53**(1): 39-43

[15] TASC Steering Committee, Jaff MR, White CJ, Hiatt WR, Fowkes GR, Dormandy J, et al. An update on methods for revascularization and expansion of the TASC lesion classification to include below-the-knee arteries: A supplement to the inter-society consensus for the management of

peripheral arterial disease (TASC II). Vascular Medicine. 2015; **20**(5):465-478

[16] Conte MS, Bradbury AW, Kolh P, White JV, Dick F, Fitridge R, et al. Global vascular guidelines on the management of chronic limb-threatening ischemia. European Journal of Vascular and Endovascular Surgery. 2019;**58**(1):S1-S109

[17] Troisi N, Turini F, Chisci E, Ercolini L, Frosini P, Lombardi R, et al. Pedal arch patency and not direct-angiosome revascularization predicts outcomes of endovascular interventions in diabetic patients with critical limb ischemia. International angiology: A journal of the International Union of Angiology. 2017; **36**(5):438-444

[18] Davies MG, Saad WE, Peden EK, Mohiuddin IT, Naoum JJ, Lumsden AB. Impact of runoff on superficial femoral artery endoluminal interventions for rest pain and tissue loss. Journal of Vascular Surgery. 2008;**48**(3):619-626

[19] Sommerset J, Karmy-Jones R, Dally M, Feliciano B, Vea Y, Teso D. Plantar acceleration time: A novel technique to evaluate arterial flow to the foot. Annals of Vascular Surgery. 2019; **60**:308-314

[20] Hofmann WJ, Walter J, Ugurluoglu A, Czerny M, Forstner R, Magometschnigg H. Preoperative high-frequency duplex scanning of potential pedal target vessels. Journal of Vascular Surgery. 2004;**39**(1):169-175

[21] Cheun TJ, Jayakumar L, Ferrer L, Miserlis D, Mitromaras C, Sideman MJ, et al. Implications of early failure of isolated endovascular tibial interventions. Journal of Vascular Surgery. 2020;**72**(1):233-240

[22] Buril GDO. Comparação entre o índice de resistência e a arteriografia na avaliação pré-operatória da isquemia crítica dos membros inferiores (Master's thesis, Universidade Federal de Pernambuco). Journal of Endovascular Therapy. 2015. 2022;**22**(5):663-677

[23] Adam DJ, Beard JD, Cleveland T. Bypass versus angioplasty in severe ischaemia of the leg (BASIL): Multicentre, randomised, controlled trial. Journal of Vascular Surgery. 2006; **44**(2):430

[24] Carnevale FC. Tratado de Radiologia Intervencionista e Cirurgia Endovascular. Rio de Janeiro-RJ, Brazil: Thieme Revinter Publicações LTDA; 2017

[25] Graziani L, Silvestro A, Bertone V, Manara E, Andreini R, Sigala A, et al. Vascular involvement in diabetic subjects with ischemic foot ulcer: A new morphologic categorization of disease severity. European Journal of Vascular and Endovascular Surgery. 2007;**33**(4): 453-460

[26] Fitridge R, Chuter V, Mills J, Hinchliffe R, Azuma N, Behrendt CA, et al. The intersocietal IWGDF, ESVS, SVS guidelines on peripheral artery disease in people with diabetes mellitus and a foot ulcer. Journal of Vascular Surgery. 2023;**78**(5)

[27] Hinchliffe RJ, Forsythe RO, Apelqvist J, Boyko EJ, Fitridge R, Hong JP, et al. Effectiveness of revascularization of the ulcerated foot in patients with diabetes and peripheral artery disease: A systematic review. Diabetes/Metabolism Research and Reviews. 2016;**32**:136-144

[28] van Reijen NS, Ponchant K, Ubbink DT, Koelemay MJW. Editor's choice – The prognostic value of the

WIfI classification in patients with chronic limb threatening ischaemia: A systematic review and meta-analysis. European Journal of Vascular and Endovascular Surgery. 2019;**58**(3): 362-371

[29] Weaver ML, Hicks CW, Canner JK, et al. The society for vascular surgery wound, ischemia, and foot infection (WIfI) classification system predicts wound healing better than direct angiosome perfusion in diabetic foot wounds. Journal of Vascular Surgery. 2018;**68**(5):1473-1481. Classificação task2

[30] Hingorani A, LaMuraglia GM, Henke P, et al. The management of diabetic foot: A clinical practice guideline by the Society for Vascular Surgery in collaboration with the American podiatric medical association and the Society for Vascular Medicine. Journal of Vascular Surgery. 2016;**63**(2 Suppl):3S-21S

[31] Lowry D, Saeed M, Narendran P, et al. A review of distribution of atherosclerosis in the lower limb arteries of patients with diabetes mellitus and peripheral vascular disease. Vascular and Endovascular Surgery. 2018;**52**(7): 535-542

[32] Neil N. Stent fracture in the superficial femoral and proximal popliteal arteries. Perspectives in Vascular Surgery and Endovascular Therapy. 2013;**25**:20-27

[33] Taylor GI, Palmer JH. The vascular territories (angiosomes) of the body: Experimental study and clinical applications. British Journal of Plastic Surgery. 1987;**40**(2):113-141

[34] Neville RF, Attinger CE, Bulan EJ, Ducic I, Thomassen M, Sidawy AN. Revascularization of a specific angiosome for limb salvage: Does the target artery matter? Annals of Vascular Surgery. 2009;**23**(3):367-373

[35] Iida O, Takahara M, Soga Y, Yamauchi Y, Hirano K, Tazaki J, et al. Worse limb prognosis for indirect versus direct endovascular revascularization only in patients with critical limb ischemia complicated with wound infection and diabetes mellitus. European Journal of Vascular and Endovascular Surgery. 2013;**46**(5): 575-582

[36] Khan SZ, Dosluoglu HH. Should multiple vessels be recanalised for tissue loss irrespective of pedal anatomy and angiosome? European Journal of Vascular and Endovascular Surgery. 2018;**55**(4):528

Chapter 8

Gestational Diabetes Mellitus

Nicolae Gică and Iulia Huluță

Abstract

Formally recognized by O'Sullivan and Mahan in 1964, gestational diabetes mellitus (GDM) is defined as any degree of hyperglycaemia recognized for the first time in the pregnancy, including type 2 diabetes mellitus diagnosed during pregnancy, as well as true GDM which develops in pregnancy. GDM is currently the most prevalent medical complication during gestation, affecting approximately 15% of pregnancies worldwide. Important risk factors for GDM include being obese, advanced maternal age and having a family history of diabetes mellitus. Expectant mothers with GDM face the risk of developing gestational hypertension, pre-eclampsia, and necessitating cesarean section for pregnancy termination. Moreover, GDM amplifies the likelihood of complications such as cardiovascular disease, obesity, and abnormal carbohydrate metabolism, consequently increasing the chances of type 2 diabetes (T2D) development in both the mother and the child. Pregnancy itself places stress on the body's insulin production and utilization, and some women are unable to produce enough insulin to overcome the insulin resistance caused by pregnancy hormones. While gestational diabetes usually resolves after pregnancy, the experience of insulin resistance during pregnancy can unmask an underlying predisposition to insulin resistance, which is a key factor in the development of T2D.

Keywords: gestational diabetes screening, gestational diabetes, pregnancy complication, glycemic control, obstetric management

1. Introduction

Gestational diabetes mellitus, the most common metabolic complication of pregnancy, is a state of hyperglycemia (fasting plasma glucose ≥5.1 mmol/L, 1 h ≥ 10 mmol/L, 2 h ≥ 8.5 mmol/L during a 75 g oral glucose tolerance test according to WHO criteria) diagnosed the first time during pregnancy [1]. The prevalence is increasing consistent with the global increase in obesity and diabetes. GDM affects 14% of pregnancies worldwide, representing approximately 20 million births per year [2].

It is associated with an increased risk of maternal complications like gestational hypertension, pre-eclampsia and termination of pregnancy via cesarean section, as well as neonatal complication as macrosomia, neonatal hypoglycemia, neonatal respiratory distress and birth trauma. In addition, mothers with this condition are at risk of developing cardiovascular disease, obesity and impaired carbohydrate metabolism, leading to the development of T2D in both mother and infant. This relationship between gestational diabetes and the risk of developing type 2 diabetes in the future is thought to be due to shared risk factors, such as genetics, obesity, and insulin resistance. Inadequate control and treatment can lead to major adverse health complications of the mother and child but it is important to note that not all cases of GDM carry the same risk of adverse outcomes. Both clinical and metabolic differences among individuals with GDM may modify the impact of the condition on maternal and fetal health [3].

Historically, screening for GDM consisted of obtaining the patient's medical history and focused primarily on past obstetric outcomes and a family medical history of T2D. The International Association of Diabetes and Pregnancy Study Group (IADPSG) recommend the universal 75 g of glucose, 2 h tolerance test. American College of Gynaecologists and Obstetricians supports the two-step process. At this moment the clinicians can choose to use either the IADPSG's recommendations or ACOG's [4].

The pathogenesis of GDM consists of an intricate mechanism of interaction of many genetic, metabolic and environmental factors. The treatment methods for GDM include an appropriate diet and increased physical activity, and when those are not sufficient, pharmacotherapy, usually insulin is used [5]. Adequate screening, prevention and treatment of GDM are needed to reduce the morbidity complications and economic burden of GDM that affect society.

2. GDM definition and classification

Outside of pregnancy, three distinct forms of diabetes mellitus are described: autoimmune diabetes (type I), diabetes occurring on the background of insulin resistance (type II), and diabetes as a result of other causes, including genetic mutation, diseases of the exocrine pancreas, and drug- or chemical-induced diabetes. While there is evidence that diabetes can occur in all three settings, the vast majority of GDM cases present as β-cell dysfunction on a background of chronic insulin resistance, to which the normal insulin resistance of pregnancy is partially additive [6]. Thus, affected women tend to have an even higher degree of insulin resistance than healthy pregnant women, and therefore have further reductions in glucose utilization and increased glucose production and free fatty acids concentration. It is thought that β-cell deteriorates due to excessive insulin production in response to excess energy consumption and insulin resistance, exhausting the cells over time [7]. Mainly, GDM is defined as a condition in which carbohydrate intolerance develops during pregnancy. Gestational diabetes that is adequately controlled without medication is often termed diet-controlled GDM or class A1GDM. Gestational diabetes that requires medication to achieve euglycemia is often termed class A2GDM. GDM is usually diagnosed in the second and third trimesters. First-trimester hyperglycemia is usually caused by an un-diagnosticated Ty II DM [5].

During a healthy pregnancy, the maternal body goes through a series of physiological transformations to meet the needs of the fetus. These changes encompass various systems such as cardiovascular, renal, hematologic, respiratory, and metabolic. One significant metabolic adaptation involves insulin sensitivity. Throughout gestation, insulin sensitivity fluctuates depending on the demands of pregnancy. In early gestation, insulin sensitivity increases, facilitating the uptake of glucose into adipose stores to prepare for the energy requirements of later pregnancy [8]. Yet, as pregnancy advances, an increase in nearby and placental hormones like estrogen, progesterone, leptin, cortisol, placental lactogen, and placental growth hormone, collaboratively bring about a condition of reduced responsiveness to insulin [8].

Consequently, plasma glucose levels rise slightly. Glucose is readily transported across the placenta to nourish fetal growth. This mild insulin resistance also stimulates endogenous glucose production and the breakdown of fat stores, leading to further elevation of plasma glucose levels and free fatty acids concentrations. Animal studies suggest that pregnant women compensate for these changes by hypertrophy and hyperplasia of pancreatic β-cells, as well as an increase in glucose-stimulated insulin secretion (GSIS), to maintain glucose homeostasis [9]. The involvement of placental hormones in this process is evident from the fact that maternal insulin sensitivity returns to pre-pregnancy levels shortly after delivery [10].

3. Epidemiology

Overweight and obesity represent a growing problem around the world which significantly contributes to the steady increase in the incidence of diabetes, including gestational diabetes of women of reproductive age. According to the 2019 report of the International Diabetes Federation (IDF), more than 20 million women presented with disorders of carbohydrate metabolism, of which approximately 80% were GDM. About 1 in 6 pregnancies is affected by GDM [1]. South-East Asia had the highest prevalence of GDM at 24%, while the lowest prevalence was seen in Africa at 10%. Almost 90% of cases of hyperglycemia in pregnancy occurred in low- and middle-income countries. Even within countries, GDM prevalence varies depending on race/ethnicity and socioeconomic status (**Figure 1**) [11].

4. Risk factors

Inconsistencies in the diagnosis criteria for GDM and measurements of the risk factors make it difficult to compare findings across studies. Despite these, several risk factors emerge consistently. These are obesity, overweight, advanced maternal age, excessive gestational weight gain, ethnicity, genetic polymorphism, family or personal history of GDM and other diseases of insulin resistance such as polycystic ovary syndrome (PCOS) [12–17]. The incidence of hyperglycemia in pregnancy increases with age. IDF data is showing the highest percentage of pregnancies with GDM at ages 45–49, reaching 37%. The delivery of a macrosomic child is another important factor that may increase the risk of both GDM and T2DM by up to 20%. GDM in a

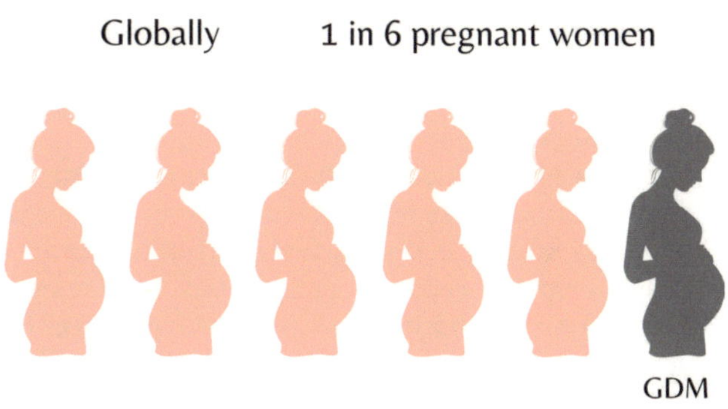

Figure 1.
Global incidence of gestational diabetes.

previous pregnancy increases the risk of reoccurrence by more than six times [18]. In women with a BMI of at least 30 kg/m^2, the frequency of GDM is 12% and in women with first-degree relatives with DM is 11%. The combination of these two factors increases the risk by up to 61%. Women who had prior treatment for PCOS showed an occurrence of gestational diabetes mellitus (GDM) at a rate more than double that of other pregnancies [19].

Gestational diabetes, characterized by a fasting plasma glucose (FPG) level of ≥5.1 mmol/L in the early stages of pregnancy, presents correlations with elevated body weight and BMI at the initiation of pregnancy. Furthermore, it is linked to a heightened propensity for necessitating insulin therapy and is associated with augmented birth weight outcomes. Using IADPSG criteria to diagnose gestational diabetes in the initial phases of pregnancy unveils a subset of pregnant individuals exhibiting discernible contrasts in anthropometric indicators and the trajectory of pregnancy compared to those diagnosed at later stages. Krystynik et al. showed that the early diagnosis of gestational diabetes (indicated by FPG ≥ 5.1 mmol/L) is concomitant with amplified body weight and BMI upon the commencement of pregnancy. Simultaneously, an early diagnosis of gestational diabetes coincides with more frequent utilization of insulin treatment and higher weight at birth [20].

Each of these risk factors is either directly or indirectly linked to the impairment of β-cell function and/or insulin sensitivity. For instance, the association between overweight and obesity with impaired β-cell function and insulin signaling pathways arises from prolonged and excessive calorie intake. This excessive intake overwhelms the capacity of β-cells to produce insulin.

5. Pathophysiology of GDM

As previously discussed GDM is mainly the result of β-cell dysfunction on a background of chronic insulin resistance during pregnancy. Therefore, both β-cell dysfunction and insulin resistance represent critical components of the pathophysiology of GDM. These impairments exist, usually, before the pregnancy and can be progressive. The brain, liver, muscle adipose tissue and placenta contribute to the development of GDM.

5.1 β-Cell dysfunction

The primary function of β-cells is to store and secrete insulin in response to glucose load. β-Cell dysfunction is defined by the impaired ability to adequately sense plasma glucose concentration or release sufficient insulin. The exact mechanisms underlying β-cell dysfunction can be varied and complex, occurring at different stages of the insulin production process [21].

Various susceptibility genes associated with GDM are related to β-cell function. Minor deficiencies in β-cell machinery may only manifest during metabolic stress, such as pregnancy. β-Cell dysfunction is worsened by insulin resistance, as reduced insulin-stimulated glucose uptake leads to hyperglycemia, burdening the β-cells to produce additional insulin. Glucotoxicity, the direct contribution of glucose to β-cell failure, further exacerbates the dysfunction. Thus, once β-cell dysfunction begins, a vicious cycle of hyperglycemia, insulin resistance and further β-cell destruction is set in motion [22]. Animal studies indicate that β-cell number is crucial for glucose homeostasis. Reductions in β-cell mass overload the remaining β-cells, impairing glucose-stimulated insulin secretion and depleting internal insulin stores [23]. Loss of β-cell mass has been linked to epigenetic downregulation of pancreatic transcription factors and inadequate β-cell proliferation [24].

In summary, β-cell dysfunction reduced β-cell mass or number, and impaired β-cell hyperplasia all play a role in the development of GDM, depending on the individual.

5.2 Chronic insulin resistance

Insulin resistance occurs when cells fail to adequately respond to insulin, resulting in impaired insulin signaling and reduced plasma membrane translocation of glucose transporter 4 (GLUT4), the primary glucose transporter in cells. In GDM, insulin-stimulated glucose uptake is significantly reduced compared to normal pregnancy.

Insulin resistance in GDM is often characterized by altered insulin receptor signaling at the molecular level. While insulin receptor abundance is generally unaffected, changes in the phosphorylation of tyrosine or serine/threonine residues on the insulin receptor dampen insulin signaling. Downstream regulators of insulin signaling, including insulin receptor substrate (IRS)-1, phosphatidylinositol 3-kinase (PI3K), and GLUT4, also exhibit altered expression and/or phosphorylation patterns in GDM. These disruptions in insulin signaling and GLUT4 translocation can persist beyond the pregnancy, indicating the long-term effects of GDM [25].

5.3 Neurohormonal dysfunction

The neurohormonal network regulates appetite, active energy expenditure and basal metabolic rate and is highly regulated by the circadian rhythm. The network contributed to GDM by influencing adiposity and glucose utilization. Some of the most important regulators of neurohormonal metabolic control are adipokines-cell signaling proteins that are secreted primarily by the adipose tissue. These include leptin and adiponectin.

Leptin is a hormone produced by the adipocytes in response to sufficient energy stores in the body. Its primary function is to regulate appetite and increase energy expenditure. Leptin acts on specific neurons in the hypothalamus, particularly in the arcuate nucleus, where it suppresses appetite-stimulating substances like neuropeptide Y (NPY) and agouti-related peptide (AgRP), while activating the anorexigenic polypeptide pro-opiomelanocortin (POMC) [26]. Initially, leptin was considered a potential obesity treatment, but it was later discovered that most obese individuals have developed leptin resistance and do not respond to leptin therapy. As a result of leptin resistance, obese individuals tend to have elevated levels of leptin in their blood (hyperleptinemia), and the concentration of leptin is generally proportional to the degree of adiposity. Leptin resistance can occur due to impaired transport of leptin across the blood-brain barrier or through mechanisms similar to insulin resistance within cells. Leptin resistance also occurs to some extent during normal pregnancy, likely to support increased fat storage beyond the non-pregnant state. In GDM, leptin resistance is further heightened, leading to hyperleptinemia [27]. However, it's important to note that pre-pregnancy body mass index (BMI) is a stronger predictor of circulating leptin levels compared to GDM itself. During pregnancy, the placenta also secretes leptin, and it becomes the primary source of circulating leptin. In GDM, placental insulin resistance contributes to increased production of leptin by the placenta, resulting in elevated levels of leptin in the mother's bloodstream. This heightened leptin secretion is believed to enhance the transfer of amino acids across the placenta, potentially contributing to fetal macrosomia.

Adiponectin, like leptin, is a hormone primarily secreted by adipocytes. However, the concentration of adiponectin in the blood is inversely related to adipose tissue mass, with lower levels found in obese individuals [28]. Similarly, GDM is associated with decreased adiponectin levels. Unlike leptin, adiponectin has a stronger association with insulin resistance rather than adiposity, indicating its role in the development of GDM independent of obesity. Adiponectin has several beneficial effects on metabolism. It enhances insulin signaling, promotes fatty acid oxidation, and inhibits gluconeogenesis. These effects are mediated by the activation of AMP-activated protein kinase (AMPK) within insulin-sensitive cells, facilitating insulin receptor substrate-1 (IRS-1) action. Adiponectin also activates the transcription factor peroxisome proliferator-activated receptor alpha (PPAR-alpha) in the liver [29]. Additionally, adiponectin stimulates insulin secretion by increasing the expression of insulin genes and promoting the release of insulin from pancreatic beta cells. In the placenta, adiponectin is expressed at low levels and regulated by cytokines such as tumor necrosis factor-alpha (TNF-alpha), interleukin-6 (IL-6), interferon-gamma (IFN-gamma), and leptin. The role of placental adiponectin in normal and GDM pregnancies is not fully understood. However, emerging evidence suggests that adiponectin may impair insulin signaling and hinder amino acid transport across the placenta, leading to restricted fetal growth. Methylation of the adiponectin gene in the placenta has been associated with maternal glucose intolerance and fetal macrosomia, further emphasizing its potential impact on pregnancy outcomes [30].

5.4 Adipose tissue

Adipose tissue is now recognized as an essential endocrine organ that regulates energy storage and secretes important factors. Adequate storage of excess calories in adipose tissue is crucial for metabolic health. In GDM, reduced adipocyte differentiation and increased adipocyte size hinder the tissue's ability to safely dispose of excess energy, leading to glucose- and lipo-toxicity in other organs. Obesity, T2D, and GDM are associated with increased inflammation in the adipose tissue. Pro-inflammatory cytokines secreted by resident adipose tissue macrophages contribute to insulin resistance by impairing insulin signaling and inhibiting insulin release from pancreatic β-cells [31].

The dysfunction of adipose tissue stands as a well-established factor contributing to heightened levels of insulin resistance. Recent findings have unveiled alterations in the expression of adipokines within women affected by GDM, indicating a pivotal role of malfunctioning adipose tissue and its compromised endocrine function in the progression of hyperglycemia during pregnancy. Among the adipokines, adiponectin and adipocyte fatty acid-binding protein (A-FABP) emerge as prominent members, closely associated with insulin resistance [32].

In a distinct avenue, fibroblast growth factor-19 (FGF-19) assumes the role of a gut hormone, exerting manifold effects. This hormone, predominantly synthesized by the small intestine in response to dietary intake, transcends its involvement in bile acid homeostasis. FGF-19 additionally triggers an insulin-independent endocrine pathway, orchestrating hepatic protein and glycogen metabolism, restraining gluconeogenesis, and fostering glucose uptake within adipocytes. Fibroblast growth factor (FGF)-19 has been shown to improve glycemic homeostasis and lipid metabolism in animal models. In humans, decreased FGF-19 level has been described in diabetes.

Women with GDM had significantly lower mRNA and protein expressions of FGF-19 than control women in the placenta and rectus muscle. FGF-19 expressions are decreased in the placenta and rectus muscle of women with GDM [33].

Women with GDM have significantly lower adiponectin and higher A-FABP levels compared to healthy pregnant, while there are no significant differences in FGF-19 between the groups. Women with GDM showed altered adipokine production even in the first trimester of pregnancy [32].

5.5 Liver

GDM is associated with increased hepatic glucose production (gluconeogenesis), leading to elevated fasting plasma glucose levels. Factors such as insulin signaling pathways and excess gluconeogenesis substrate from increased protein intake and muscle breakdown contribute to this effect. However, the liver is not considered a primary driver of T2D or GDM [5].

5.6 Skeletal and cardiac muscle

Insulin resistance in skeletal muscle is now viewed as a consequence of hyperglycemia rather than a causal factor in diabetes. Skeletal and cardiac muscles develop insulin resistance as a protective measure to divert excess energy to adipose tissue. Treating GDM by targeting skeletal muscle insulin resistance alone, without reducing plasma glucose concentrations, may not be beneficial [34].

5.7 Oxidative stress

Oxidative stress, characterized by an imbalance between pro-oxidants and antioxidants, is implicated in the pathogenesis of GDM. Hyperglycemia and impaired free-radical scavenging mechanisms in GDM women result in increased production of reactive oxygen species (ROS). ROS interfere with insulin signaling and glucose uptake, contributing to insulin resistance. Iron supplementation, homocysteine, and deficiencies of certain micronutrients are associated with oxidative stress in GDM [35, 36].

5.8 Placental transport

The placenta contributes to insulin resistance during GDM by secreting hormones and cytokines. Maternal hyperglycemia affects the placental transport of glucose, amino acids, and lipids. There is strong evidence of changes in the expression of transporters and placental gene expression alterations in lipid pathways in GDM cases (**Figure 2**) [37].

Pregnancy is a phase characterized by heightened metabolic activity in which the maintenance of glucose balance is crucial. When elevated plasma glucose concentrations are detected in pregnant women, it is referred to as GDM, although there is ongoing debate regarding diagnostic criteria. The development of GDM is likely influenced by a combination of genetic, epigenetic, and environmental factors, and the underlying mechanisms are complex and evolve over an extended period. However, in the majority of the cases, the pancreatic β-cells are unable to adequately compensate for prolonged excessive fuel intake, leading to insulin resistance, elevated plasma glucose levels, and increased glucose supply to the developing fetus. Additionally,

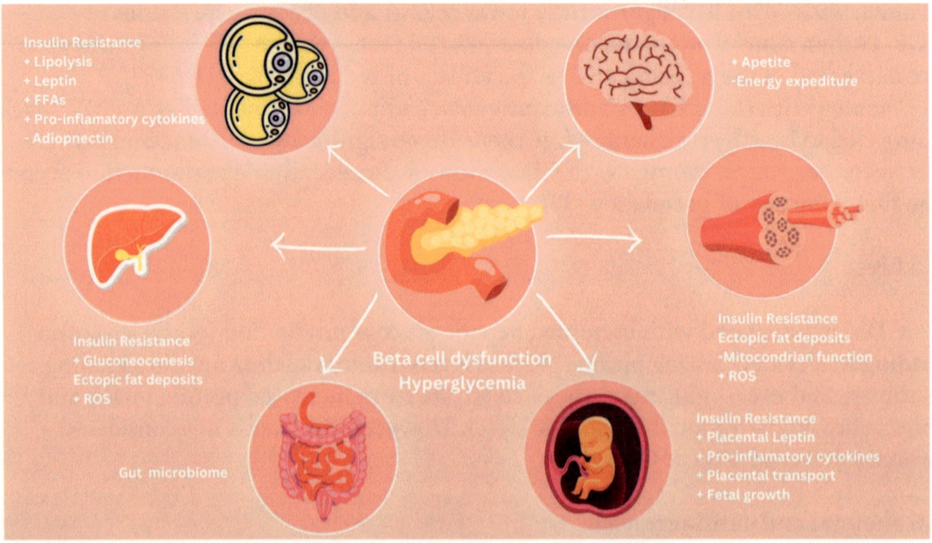

Figure 2.
Organs involved in the pathophysiology of GDM.

adipose tissue expandability, chronic low-grade inflammation, gluconeogenesis, oxidative stress, and placental factors are implicated in the pathology of GDM.

6. Diagnosis

The ongoing debate surrounding the diagnosis of GDM has focused on two key issues: whether to include all pregnant women or only those with risk factors, and whether to use one- or two-stage diagnostic procedures. It is important to note that a GDM diagnosis can only be made after excluding previous diagnoses of diabetes (type I or type II) early in pregnancy. Screening only high-risk groups may result in the underdiagnosis of GDM in as many as 35–47% of pregnant women, which undoubtedly impacts obstetric outcomes [38].

The results of the Hyperglycemia Adverse Pregnancy Outcome (HAPO) study, which involved 23,316 women, provided clear evidence of the relationship between elevated glycemia (below the threshold for overt diabetes mellitus) and maternal and neonatal complications. These complications included large-for-gestational-age (LGA) infants, higher rates of cesarean sections, neonatal hypoglycemia, and increased umbilical C-peptide concentrations [39]. Based on the HAPO study findings, the International Association of Diabetes and Pregnancy Study Groups (IADPSG) introduced current diagnostic criteria for GDM, leading to a threefold increase in GDM diagnoses and suggesting previous underestimation. The aim was to identify screening values that better identify pregnancies at risk of perinatal complications. The study demonstrated a positive linear relationship between screening glucose values and adverse perinatal outcomes, showing that perinatal risks began to increase even in women with glucose values considered "normal" in the past. Consequently, the current basis for GDM diagnosis involves administering 75 g of glucose between 24 and 28 weeks of pregnancy to all pregnant women without previously diagnosed diabetes [40, 41].

	Fasting (mg/dL) mmol/L	1 h (mg/dL) mmol/L	2 h (mg/dL) mmol/L	3 h (mg/dL) mmol/L	Values for diagnosis
ADA/ACOG	95 5.3	180 10	155 8.6	140 7.8	2
ADIPS	92 5.1	180 10	153 8.5	—	1
DIPSI	—	—	140 7.8	—	1
FIGO	92 5.1	180 10	153 8.5	—	1
WHO	92 5.1	180 10	153 8.5	—	1
IADPSG	92 5.1	180 10	153 8.5	—	1
NICE	— 5.6	—	— 7.8	—	—

Table 1.
Criteria for GDM diagnosis according to different societies [4, 38, 43–45].

Treating even mild forms of glucose intolerance in GDM has proven beneficial, as demonstrated by studies such as the Australian Carbohydrate Intolerance Study in Pregnant Women (ACHOIS) and the Maternal-Fetal Medicine Units Network (MFMU) study. These studies showed reduced rates of obstetric complications associated with hyperglycemia and pregnancy weight gain [42]. The ACHOIS study revealed a significant reduction in the composite endpoint (including neonatal death, perinatal injury, hyperbilirubinemia, neonatal hypoglycemia, and hyperinsulinemia) with antihyperglycemic interventions, along with lower weight gain and a decreased incidence of LGA. Most scientific societies have incorporated the recommendations of the IADPSG (2010) and the World Health Organization (WHO) (2013) into their daily practice.

The introduction of IADPSG criteria for GDM screening led to a threefold increase in prevalence without significant improvements in GDM-related events for women without risk factors, except for reduced risks of LGA, neonatal hypoglycemia, and preterm birth [40]. This prompted further research into GDM management. In a large randomized trial involving 23,792 pregnant women, Hillier et al. found that one-step screening, compared to two-step screening, doubled the incidence of GDM diagnosis but did not affect the risks of LGA, adverse perinatal outcomes, primary cesarean section, or gestational hypertension or pre-eclampsia [41]. **Table 1** presents the criteria for the diagnosis of GDM according to different societies.

7. Fetal and maternal effects

Gestational diabetes mellitus raises the likelihood of various short-term and long-term health complications for mothers. Apart from the typical stress associated with pregnancy, GDM is linked to antenatal depression. Furthermore, it increases the chances of additional pregnancy complications such as preterm birth and preeclampsia, often necessitating surgical delivery [46]. Around 60% of women with a history of GDM develop type II diabetes mellitus later in life. Each subsequent pregnancy also amplifies the risk of T2D threefold in women with a GDM history. Additionally, women who previously had GDM face an annual conversion risk of approximately 2–3% to T2D. Recent evidence suggests that women with prior GDM may have permanently altered blood vessels, making them more susceptible to cardiovascular disease (CVD). A recent study revealed a 63% increased risk of CVD in women with a history of GDM, which can only partially be attributed to BMI [13]. This is a significant concern, considering that CVD is the leading cause of death worldwide.

The increased transfer of glucose, amino acids, and fatty acids across the placenta, as mentioned earlier, stimulates the fetus's production of insulin and insulin-like growth factor 1 (IGF-1). This can lead to fetal overgrowth, often resulting in macrosomia or excessive birth weight [47]. Furthermore, the excessive production of fetal insulin can exert stress on the developing pancreatic β-cells, contributing to their dysfunction and insulin resistance, even before birth. Macrosomia also increases the risk of shoulder dystocia, a type of obstructed labour, necessitating cesarean section delivery for babies in GDM pregnancies. Once born, these babies face an increased risk of hypoglycemia due to their dependency on maternal hyperglycemia (fetal hyperinsulinemia), which, if not properly managed, can lead to brain injury [48].

Epidemiological studies have consistently demonstrated that exposure to maternal diabetes in utero increases the risk of cardiovascular disease in the offspring and cardiovascular changes appear from fetal life and extent to adolescence and adulthood [49, 50]. Fetuses of mothers with GDM have more globular hearts with an increase in right and left ventricular sphericity index and subclinical systolic cardiac dysfunction which persists in infancy. These changes are not present at mid-gestation supporting the idea that exposure to glycemia could lead to increased secretion of fetal insulin [51]. Higher systolic and mean arterial blood pressure has also been reported in children and adolescents in association with exposure to maternal diabetes and higher rates of premature cardiovascular heart disease have been shown in offspring of mothers with diabetes in a 40-year follow-up study in Denmark [50].

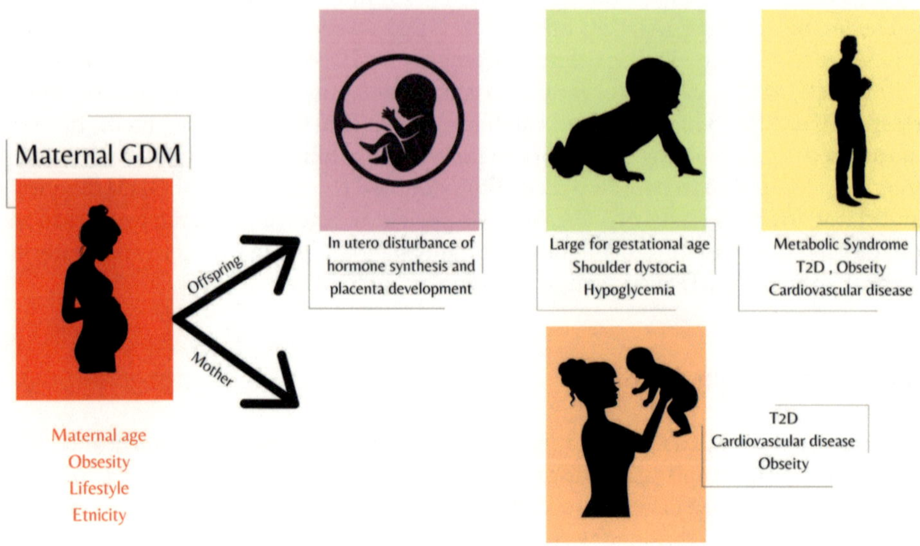

Figure 3.
GDM effects on offspring and mother.

The mechanisms of programming cardiovascular alterations by maternal diabetes remain speculative. It is possible that exposure to glycemia could lead to increased secretion of fetal insulin which can have adverse effects on fetal vascular gene expression and result in vascular and cardiac changes. Inflammatory and oxidative processes may also be involved to modify both gene expression and the vasculature. However, apart from glycemia, offspring of mothers with diabetes tend to be at increased risk of in-utero exposure to many other classical cardiovascular risk factors, such as obesity and higher maternal blood pressure which are commonly prevalent in mothers at risk of GDM and these may also contribute to fetal cardiovascular remodeling (**Figure 3**).

8. Preconception care in women with diabetes

Preconceptional education for women with diabetes is an essential step toward achieving optimal maternal and fetal outcomes. By providing comprehensive information on glycemic control, nutrition, lifestyle, medication management, and psychosocial support, healthcare professionals can empower women to make informed decisions and take proactive steps to ensure a healthy pregnancy.

A cornerstone of preconception care for women with diabetes is achieving and maintaining optimal glycemic control. Insulin therapy, dietary management, or a combination of both are employed to target specific glucose levels. Aiming for fasting plasma glucose levels ≤5.7 mmol/l and postprandial blood glucose levels ≤7.8 mmol/l, along with a glycosylated hemoglobin A (HbA1c) level of less than 53 mmol/mol (<7.0%), helps minimize the risk of complications during pregnancy [52].

Preconception screening for diabetes-related complications, such as retinopathy, nephropathy, and cardiovascular issues, is pivotal. Addressing any identified complications before conception allows for timely intervention and optimization of health. This comprehensive screening approach is vital in reducing the risk of maternal and fetal complications.

Until optimal glycemic control is achieved, the use of contraception is recommended to prevent unplanned pregnancies. This strategy ensures that pregnancy occurs in the most favorable metabolic environment, minimizing potential risks to both mother and fetus [52].

9. Prognosis factors in GDM

It is important to recognize that not all cases of GDM carry the same level of risk for adverse outcomes. While the diagnostic criteria for GDM primarily focus on identifying glucose metabolism dysregulations, GDM is increasingly acknowledged as a heterogeneous disorder affecting all metabolic fuels. Various factors that contribute to metabolic health are considered risk factors for developing GDM, including higher BMI and sociocultural influences. The clinical and metabolic variations among individuals with GDM can modify the impact of the condition on both maternal and fetal well-being. Within the GDM population, individuals with elevated triglyceride levels or markers indicating insulin sensitivity impairment face a greater likelihood of delivering a larger-than-average newborn or a macrosomic one. The simultaneous presence of excess adiposity and GDM is linked to an elevated risk of delivering a larger-than-average newborn or a macrosomic one, as well as complications related to pregnancy [3, 4].

10. Pregnancy management in GDM

10.1 Lifestyle intervention

Gestational diabetes mellitus (GDM) is a condition that requires careful management to achieve normoglycemia, optimal weight gain, and proper fetal development. While pharmacological treatments can be essential, they do not replace the significance of following a tailored diet plan. This chapter explores the importance of individualized nutritional recommendations for women with GDM, taking into account glycemic self-control, pre-pregnancy BMI, energy requirements, macronutrient proportions, and maternal preferences, as well as lifestyle factors such as work, rest, and exercise.

Chao et al. emphasize the effectiveness of personalized dietary recommendations for women with GDM compared to generalized guidelines. A well-designed nutritional plan includes three main meals and 2–3 snacks per day, with a late-night snack around 9:30 pm to safeguard against nocturnal hypoglycemia and morning ketosis [53, 54].

Carbohydrates play a pivotal role in the diet of women with GDM. While excessive consumption may lead to hyperglycemia, glucose remains a vital energy source for the placenta and fetus. The American Thyroid Association (ATA) recommends that saccharides constitute 40–50% of energy intake, with at least 180 g/day, mainly derived from low glycemic index (GI) starchy foods. Adequate dietary fiber intake of 25–28 g per day, primarily from fruits, vegetables, whole grain bread, pasta, and rice, is also recommended [54, 55].

Protein intake should account for about 30% of caloric intake, equivalent to approximately 1.3 g/kg of body weight per day, with a minimum daily intake of 71 g. Favoring plant proteins, lean meat, and fish over red and processed meats can enhance insulin sensitivity and support the treatment of GDM [56].

A high-fat diet is contraindicated for women with GDM, as it may lead to placental dysfunction, infant obesity, and other complications. Recommended fat intake should be 20–30% of the total caloric value, with less than 10% of saturated fat. Instead, emphasis should be placed on consuming polyunsaturated fatty acids (PUFA) n-3 (linolenic acid) and n-6 (linoleic acid) to support fetal growth and development [53].

The recommended weight gain during pregnancy varies depending on the initial body mass index, with an average of 8–12 kg. Excessive weight gain, especially over 18 kg, increases the risk of macrosomia (**Table 2**). Women with GDM may require additional supplementation of vitamins and minerals, particularly folic acid, vitamin D, calcium, and iron, to meet their increased needs during pregnancy [59, 60].

BMI (kg/m^2)	Weight gain in pregnancy (kg)
<18.5	12.5–18
18.5–24.9	11.5–16
25–29.9	7–11.5
>30	5–9

Table 2.
Weight gain in relation to baseline body mass index (BMI) [57, 58].

Personalized nutritional recommendations play a pivotal role in the management of gestational diabetes mellitus. By emphasizing balanced carbohydrate, protein, and fat intake, along with appropriate weight gain and micronutrient supplementation, healthcare providers can help women with GDM achieve optimal health outcomes for both themselves and their unborn children. Further research into emerging therapies and the impact of gut microbiota may shed light on future advancements in GDM management. A comprehensive and individualized approach to nutrition during pregnancy can pave the way for healthier pregnancies and better long-term maternal and fetal health.

The role of exercise and physical activity in improving glycemic control among women with GDM has been a topic of ongoing research. Exercise recommendations for women with GDM have been a subject of ambiguity in terms of their quantitativeness and qualitativeness. It is crucial to consider obstetric indications and contraindications while incorporating physical activity into the management of GDM. Observational studies suggest that physical activity can be safe during pregnancy, but the specific types and intensities need careful evaluation. Certain activities have been deemed safe and beneficial for pregnant women, including walking, cycling, swimming, selected pilates, and low-intensity fitness exercises. Pregnant individuals can continue with activities like yoga, running, tennis, badminton, and strength exercises after consulting with their obstetrician. However, caution is necessary when it comes to contact sports, horse riding, surfing, skiing, and diving [61].

Research indicates that engaging in regular physical activity can significantly reduce the risk of developing GDM. A meta-analysis by Aune et al. revealed a 38% reduction in GDM risk among physically active women. Nasiri-Amiri et al. conducted an intervention study among overweight patients, showing a 24% risk reduction in GDM for women exercising no more than three times a week. Furthermore, in women with normal body weight, increased physical activity was associated with lower weight gain during pregnancy without affecting the child's weight or the frequency of cesarean sections. Ming et al. reported a substantial 42% reduction in GDM risk with increased physical activity [62]. A meta-analysis by Harrison et al. reviewed eight randomized trials, highlighting the positive impact of regular physical activity on fasting and postprandial glucose levels in women with GDM. Engaging in 20–30 min of activity 3–4 times a week showed significant improvements in glycemic control [61, 63, 64].

Exercise and physical activity play a vital role in the management of GDM. Although recommendations may be ambiguous, focusing on safe and beneficial activities tailored to individual needs can yield positive outcomes. Regular physical activity has been associated with a reduced risk of GDM and improved glycemic control in pregnant women. Healthcare providers should encourage and guide pregnant individuals in incorporating suitable exercise routines into their daily lives to promote better maternal and fetal health outcomes. However, caution should be exercised, and obstetric guidance sought to ensure the safety and effectiveness of the chosen physical activities during pregnancy. As more research emerges, a deeper understanding of the link between exercise and GDM can be harnessed to optimize care for expectant mothers and their unborn child.

10.2 Pharmacological treatment

When glycemic targets cannot be achieved through a well-balanced diet and dietary corrections, pharmacological interventions become essential in managing

GDM. This chapter delves into the various pharmacological treatment options available for GDM, with a focus on insulin therapy, oral medications, and emerging agents. The safety and efficacy of these treatments are critically evaluated, along with the importance of evidence-based decisions to optimize maternal and neonatal outcomes.

Numerous studies strongly support insulin therapy as the safest and most effective treatment for GDM. Extensive research has demonstrated the safety of human insulin use during pregnancy, with no passage of insulin analogues across the placenta [62–65]. Oral administration drugs should only be considered when insulin therapy is unsuitable due to patient consent or unavailability [65]. There is no generally accepted treatment plan but we can either use regular insulin, prandial types of insulin or a combination of these [66]. To limit the postprandial spikes, we can either use human insulin or rapid-acting insulin analogues (lispro, aspart, glulisine, and fast-acting aspart) [65]. To control the fasting levels long-lasting analogues (detemir) or human insulin can be used [67]. Plasma glucose levels should be used to adjust insulin dosage.

Metformin and glibenclamide are utilized as oral medications in specific cases of GDM. Although they do cross the placenta, research suggests they are unlikely to be teratogenic. The landmark Metformin in Gestational Diabetes trial, one of the largest randomized controlled trials, provided valuable insights into the safety and efficacy of metformin use in GDM. The results indicated that metformin, with or without supplemental insulin, did not lead to increased perinatal complications. Some studies have indicated potential long-term effects of metformin use on offspring, including higher body mass index, increased visceral and subcutaneous tissue, and elevated blood glucose levels when the offspring reached nine years of age. On the other hand, despite its effectiveness, the use of glibenclamide may lead to a higher percentage of intrauterine deaths and neonatal complications such as hypoglycemia, macrosomia, and fetal growth restriction (FGR) [68, 69]. Therefore, careful consideration of the benefits and potential risks of oral medications is essential [70].

Sodium-glucose cotransporter-2 (SGLT2) inhibitors and glucagon-like peptide-1 (GLP-1) agents are being explored as potential treatments for GDM. While SGLT2 inhibitors have shown promise in reducing plasma glucose concentration, their use during pregnancy is not recommended due to adverse effects noted in animal reproductive studies. GLP-1 agents, including dipeptidyl peptidase-4 (DPP-4) inhibitors and GLP-1 receptor agonists, have demonstrated benefits in treating type 2 diabetes but have not yet become a common choice for GDM [71]. Rigorous clinical trials are needed to establish their safety and efficacy in the context of GDM.

Pharmacological interventions are essential in cases where lifestyle modifications are insufficient to achieve glycemic control in GDM. Insulin therapy remains the preferred and safest option, while oral medications like metformin and glibenclamide require careful consideration of potential long-term effects. Emerging agents like SGLT2 inhibitors and GLP-1 agents hold promise but demand further investigation through well-designed clinical trials. The future of GDM management relies on evidence-based decisions that prioritize the safety and well-being of both mothers and their newborns.

10.3 Maternal care

In the context of GDM, fasting plasma glucose (FPG) measurement and glycated hemoglobin (HbA1c) investigation provide valuable insights into the management and control of blood glucose levels during pregnancy. These tests are crucial tools in diagnosing and monitoring GDM, as well as assessing overall glycemic control.

FPG is a blood test that measures the level of glucose in the blood after an overnight fast, typically of 8–12 h. FPG provides information about how well the body is able to regulate plasma glucose levels after a period of fasting. Elevated fasting glucose levels in GDM can indicate an increased risk of adverse pregnancy outcomes, including macrosomia (large birth weight), preeclampsia, and neonatal hypoglycemia. If FPG levels are consistently elevated, the treatment plan is to be adjusted by modifying the diet, increasing physical activity, or, in some cases, starting insulin therapy.

HbA1c serves as an accepted metric for the preliminary detection of pre-existing diabetes in early pregnancy, the confirmation of glycemic regulation among women employing self-monitoring of blood glucose (SMBG), and the evaluation of glycemic control when SMBG falls short. However, it is noteworthy that HbA1c measurements are influenced by factors affecting the lifespan of red blood cells (RBCs), a category that encompasses pregnancy. The physiological state of pregnancy engenders modified RBC kinetics typified by heightened erythropoiesis, hemodilution, and altered kinetics.

According to The American Diabetes Association (ADA) maintaining HbA1C levels below 6 in the early stages of pregnancy is associated with the lowest incidence of adverse fetal outcomes or maternal complications. Some research posits a connection between elevated HbA1C and adverse outcomes, such as spontaneous abortion and the likelihood of cesarean section. Certain studies suggest that heightened HbA1C in the initial trimester corresponds to severe maternal morbidity (SMM) and mortality risks [72].

The literature suggests a linkage between suboptimal HbA1C control and unfavorable pregnancy outcomes, advocating for improved HbA1C management to mitigate complications. However, challenges persist. Firstly, divergent cutoff values and conclusions arise among various ethnicities and experimental approaches. For instance.

Recognizing the significant influence of maternal blood glucose levels on adverse maternal and infant outcomes in gestational diabetes, meticulous blood glucose management is imperative. Existing studies highlight the association between HbA1C during pregnancy and glycemic levels among pregnant women. Notably, the dynamic values of HbA1C in pregnancy and non-pregnancy states warrant consideration. The ADA recommends utilizing HbA1C for glucose monitoring in gestational diabetes patients, with an optimal target of 42–53 mmol/mol (6–7%) in the initial trimester and below 42 mmol/mol (<6%) in the subsequent trimesters [72].

Glycosylated hemoglobin emerges as a valuable tool for blood glucose management in diabetic patients. The prevailing consensus among researchers affirms the utility of HbA1c for screening and managing gestational diabetes. The International Association of Diabetes and Pregnancy Study Groups (IADPSG) suggests employing HbA1c for gestational diabetes screening, although it should not supplant an oral glucose tolerance test (OGTT) for definitive diagnosis. Current research underscores the feasibility of HbA1c as an indicator for screening and selecting pregnant women warranting further OGTT assessment, especially when used in conjunction with gestational age measurements. In conclusion, the aggregate evidence substantiates the relationship between HbA1c, pregnancy glycemia, and adverse pregnancy outcomes, thereby validating its application in gestational diabetes management to mitigate complications. However, the establishment of precise glycemic control targets demands continued research [72].

It's important to note that while FPG and HbA1c provide valuable information, GDM management often involves multiple tests and considerations, including self-monitoring of blood glucose levels, postprandial glucose measurements, and close collaboration with healthcare providers. The ultimate goal is to achieve and maintain optimal glycemic control to ensure the well-being of both the mother and the developing fetus.

Self-monitoring of blood glucose (SMBG) levels through glucometers has gained increasing recognition as a critical component of diabetes management during pregnancy. Fluctuations in maternal plasma glucose levels can impact fetal development and increase the risk of complications for both mother and child.

SMBG helps pregnant individuals to maintain tight control over their plasma glucose levels, reducing the risk of adverse outcomes such as macrosomia, preterm birth, and preeclampsia and personalize their diabetes management by providing immediate feedback on the effects of food choices, physical activity, and medication regimens.

SMBG aids in the early detection of hypo- and hyperglycemic episodes, allowing timely interventions to prevent complications for both mother and fetus.

Monitoring times during pregnancy include fasting, pre-meal, post-meal, and before bedtime to assess glucose control across different periods of the day. Maintaining a record of SMBG results allows for the tracking of trends and patterns over time. Data from glucometers is used to design tailored treatment plans, ensuring that blood glucose levels are kept within recommended ranges [73].

Self-monitoring of blood glucose levels through glucometers is a pivotal tool for managing diabetes during pregnancy. It empowers pregnant individuals to maintain optimal glycemic control, mitigating risks and enhancing maternal and fetal outcomes.

10.4 Fetal surveillance

The monitoring of fetal well-being in women with gestational diabetes mellitus remains an area with limited evidence and consensus regarding specific antepartum tests and their frequency. Determining the appropriate type and frequency of monitoring depends on one side on the fetal growth and wellbeing but it is also influenced by the presence of other pregnancy complications, such as preeclampsia or fetal growth restriction, as well as the severity of maternal hyperglycemia.

Fetal size and the amniotic fluid are important indicators in GDM management. Large-for-gestational age (LGA) infants can result from inadequately treated GDM, and studies have found that fetal overgrowth is associated with adverse perinatal outcomes including hypoglycemia, respiratory distress syndrome, shoulder dystocia, and Erb's palsy [74]. Ultrasound-guided management may better identify which pregnancies are at risk for fetal overgrowth. In this management framework, fetal ultrasound measurements, specifically fetal abdominal circumference (AC), are used to risk-stratify pregnancies and alter glycemic targets accordingly. Fetal abdominal circumference (AC) measured on ultrasound, equal to or greater than the 75th percentile for gestational age, between 29 + 0- and 33 + 6-weeks' gestation, is associated with evidence of excess fetal growth/adiposity and an increased risk of delivering a large-for-gestational-age (LGA) baby [4, 43]. In such cases, more intensive glucose-lowering therapy may be necessary. However, if fetal ultrasound shows that average growth is maintained, relaxation of glycemic targets may be considered. Longitudinal growth assessment is superior to a single late-pregnancy measurement, especially if abnormalities are detected on the initial scan. Accelerating AC growth, particularly if it exceeds the 95th percentile, holds clinical significance as well and it should not be ignored. Polyhydramnios, defined as the vertical measurement of the deepest pocket of amniotic fluid free of fetal parts more than 8 cm, is considered a consequence of poor glycemic control [43].

For women with unstable diabetes or those requiring pharmacological therapy, or having comorbid risk factors like obesity, hypertension, LGA or SGA, or a previous stillbirth, 2–4 weekly ultrasounds may be considered. Fetal wellbeing monitoring and growth assessment in gestational diabetes demand careful consideration and tailored approaches [4]. Regular ultrasound evaluations, involving fetal abdominal circumference, estimated fetal growth and amniotic fluid index play a crucial role in identifying potential risks and guiding management decisions.

11. Delivery and intrapartum treatment

The timing of delivery and intrapartum treatment in gestational diabetes mellitus (GDM) is a critical aspect of managing maternal and fetal health. Careful consideration of factors such as glycemic control, fetal weight, presence of the polyhydramnios and the need for insulin during labour helps optimize delivery outcomes while minimizing potential risks. This aspect should be discussed in the third trimester.

Timing the delivery in women with GDM is a delicate balance between ensuring adequate fetal lung maturity and reducing the risk of maternal and neonatal complications. Based on current guidelines and evidence, delivery is typically recommended at around 39–40 weeks of gestation. Delivering at around 39–40 weeks helps prevent potential complications associated with prolonged pregnancies, which are common in GDM [4, 43].

Cesarean section may be necessary in cases with an estimated fetal weight equal to or greater than 4500 g (approximately 7.7 pounds) [4, 43]. A cesarean section may be preferred to prevent birth-related complications associated with macrosomia (large birth weight) such as shoulder dystocia. Ultrasound measurements are used to estimate fetal weight and determine if it meets the criteria for considering a cesarean section [4, 43]. This assessment helps healthcare providers make informed decisions regarding the safest delivery method for both the mother and the baby.

During labour, insulin infusion is rarely needed, especially in insulin-depend cases, to maintain stable glycemic control. Monitoring maternal plasma glucose, using capillary plasma glucose every 4 h during labour to determine the appropriate insulin dosage is essential. Frequent checks help avoid fluctuations and ensure a steady balance throughout the delivery process [4].

12. Postpartum management

In the majority of cases GDM will resolve after delivery, but up to one-third of the affected women will have diabetes or impaired glucose metabolism at postpartum screening. The patients should be counseled to stop the insulin treatment if they had it, start breastfeeding, lose weight and have an OGTT at 6–12 weeks postpartum. It is estimated that between 15 and 70% of women with GDM will develop DM later in life. Although the fasting plasma glucose test is easier to perform, it lacks sensitivity for detecting other forms of abnormal glucose metabolism, whereas the results of the OGTT can confirm an impaired fasting glucose level and impaired glucose tolerance.

If the results of the OGGT test are normal (fasting glucose <100 mg/dL, 2 h glucose <140 mg/dL) you should recommend screening for DM at 3 years for the rest of her life. Abnormal results showing impaired fasting glucose, impaired tolerance (fasting glucose 100–125 mg/Dl, 2 h glucose 140–199 mg/dL) or diabetes (fasting glucose >125 mg/dL, 2 h glucose >199 mg/dL) require referral for diabetes management [4]. GDM can increase the risk of postpartum thyroiditis, therefore the assessment of the thyroid function has to be recommended [20].

The recurrence risk for a future pregnancy is estimated at 40–60%. It is recommended to screen for GDM earlier in the pregnancy, providing an opportunity to ensure good glucose control [22].

13. Conclusions

Gestational diabetes is a significant health concern that affects pregnant women worldwide. The prevalence of gestational diabetes has been on the rise in recent years, paralleling the increasing rates of obesity and sedentary lifestyles. Moreover, the condition poses potential risks not only to the mother but also to the unborn child, with adverse effects on fetal development and long-term health outcomes. Identifying the risk factors for gestational diabetes is crucial in early detection and intervention. This includes a family history of diabetes, obesity, previous gestational diabetes, advanced maternal age, and certain ethnic backgrounds. Health professionals should remain vigilant in screening pregnant women for the condition during prenatal care to ensure timely diagnosis and appropriate management.

The management of gestational diabetes typically involves dietary modifications, regular physical activity, and monitoring plasma glucose levels. In some cases, insulin or other medications may be required to maintain optimal plasma glucose levels. Close collaboration between the healthcare team and the expectant mother is essential to achieve successful outcomes for both the mother and the baby. Women diagnosed with gestational diabetes should be educated about the condition and its potential consequences. Empowering them to make informed decisions regarding lifestyle changes and treatment options can significantly improve their ability to manage the condition effectively. Furthermore, long-term follow-up and postpartum care are essential to monitor the mother's health and reduce the risk of developing type 2 diabetes in the future. Encouraging postpartum screenings and lifestyle modifications can help women prevent or delay the onset of diabetes beyond pregnancy.

Prevention is a crucial aspect of combating gestational diabetes. Public health initiatives should focus on promoting healthy lifestyles, emphasizing the importance of balanced nutrition and regular physical activity for all women, especially those planning to conceive or are already pregnant. By addressing modifiable risk factors, we can make significant strides in reducing the burden of gestational diabetes and its associated complications.

In conclusion, gestational diabetes is a complex condition that requires a multifaceted approach from healthcare providers, policymakers, and individuals alike. By raising awareness, facilitating early diagnosis, promoting healthy behaviors, and offering comprehensive care, we can work toward ensuring a healthier future for both mothers and their children. With continued research and collective efforts, we can make a positive impact on the lives of countless women and prevent the potential long-term consequences of gestational diabetes.

Acknowledgements

We would like to express our sincere gratitude to all the individuals who assisted, whether directly or indirectly. Their contributions, no matter how small, have played a significant role in the successful completion of this chapter.

Conflict of interest

The authors declare no conflict of interest.

Author details

Nicolae Gică[1,2]* and Iulia Huluță[1,2]

1 Carol Davila University of Medicine and Pharmacy, Bucharest, Romania

2 Filantropia Clinical Hospital of Obstetrics and Gynaecology, Bucharest, Romania

*Address all correspondence to: gica.nicolae@umfcd.ro

References

[1] Buchanan TA, Xiang AH, Page KA. Gestational diabetes mellitus: Risks and management during and after pregnancy. Nature Reviews. Endocrinology. 2012;**8**(11):639-649

[2] Wang H, Li N, Chivese T, et al. IDF Diabetes Atlas Committee Hyperglycaemia in Pregnancy Special Interest Group. IDF Diabetes Atlas: Estimation of Global and Regional Gestational Diabetes Mellitus Prevalence for 2021 by International Association of Diabetes in Pregnancy Study Group's Criteria. Diabetes Research and Clinical Practice. 2022;**183**:109050

[3] Francis EC, Powe CE, Lowe WL Jr, et al. Refining the diagnosis of gestational diabetes mellitus: A systematic review to inform efforts in precision medicine. medRxiv. 2023.04.19.23288627

[4] ACOG Practice Bulletin No. 190: Gestational diabetes mellitus. Obstetrics and Gynecology. 2018;**131**(2):e49-e64

[5] Plows JF, Stanley JL, Baker PN, et al. The pathophysiology of gestational diabetes mellitus. International Journal of Molecular Sciences. 2018;**19**(11):3342

[6] Buchanan TA, Xiang AH. Gestational diabetes mellitus. Journal of Clinical Investigation. 2005;**115**:485-491

[7] Damm P, Kühl C, Buschard K, JakobsenBK,SvejgaardA,Sodoyez-GoffauxF, et al. Prevalence and predictive value of islet cell antibodies and insulin autoantibodies in women with gestational diabetes. Diabetic Medicine: A Journal of the British Diabetic Association. 1994;**11**:558-563

[8] Di Cianni G, Miccoli R, Volpe L, Lencioni C, Del Prato S. Intermediate metabolism in normal pregnancy and in gestational diabetes. Diabetes/Metabolism Research and Reviews. 2003;**19**(4):259-270

[9] Parsons JA, Brelje TC, Sorenson RL. Adaptation of islets of Langerhans to pregnancy: Increased islet cellproliferation and insulin secretion correlates with the onset of placental lactogen secretion. Endocrinology. 1992;**130**:1459-1466

[10] Ryan EA, O'Sullivan MJ, Skyler JS. Insulin action during pregnancy: Studies with the euglycemic clamp technique. Diabetes. 1985;**34**:380-389

[11] Zhu Y, Zhang C. Prevalence of gestational diabetes and risk of progression to type 2 diabetes: A global perspective. Current Diabetes Reports. 2016;**16**(1):7

[12] Okosun IS, Chandra KMD, Boev A, Boltri JM, Choi ST, Parish DC, et al. Abdominal adiposity in U.S. adults: Prevalence and trends, 1960-2000. Preventive Medicine. 2004;**39**:197-206

[13] Durnwald C. Gestational diabetes: Linking epidemiology, excessive gestational weight gain, adverse pregnancy outcomes, and future metabolic syndrome. Seminars in Perinatology. 2015;**39**:254-258

[14] Zhang C, Tobias DK, Chavarro JE, Bao W, Wang D, Ley SH, et al. Adherence to healthy lifestyle and risk of gestational diabetes mellitus: Prospective cohort study. BMJ. 2014;**349**:g5450. Int. J. Mol. Sci. 2018, 19, 3342 15 of 21

[15] Jenum AK, Mørkrid K, Sletner L, Vange S, Torper JL, Nakstad B, et al. Impact of ethnicity on gestational

diabetes identified with the WHO and the modified International Association of Diabetes and Pregnancy Study Groups criteria: A population-based cohort study. European Journal of Endocrinology. 2012;**166**:317-324

[16] Anghebem-Oliveira MI, Martins BR, Alberton D, de Ramos EAS, Picheth G, de Rego FGM. Type 2 diabetes-associated genetic variants of FTO, LEPR, PPARg, and TCF7L2 in gestational diabetes in a Brazilian population. Archives of Endocrinology and Metabolism. 2017;**61**:238-248

[17] Lao TT, Ho L-F, Chan BCP, Leung W-C. Maternal age and prevalence of gestational diabetes mellitus. Diabetes Care. 2006;**29**:948-949

[18] Song X, Chen L, Zhang S, Liu Y, Wei J, Wang T, et al. Gestational diabetes mellitus and high triglyceride levels mediate the association between pre-pregnancy overweight/obesity and macrosomia: A prospective cohort study in Central China. Nutrients. 2022;**14**(16):3347

[19] Mikola M, Hiilesmaa V, Halttunen M, Suhonen L, Tiitinen A. Obstetric outcome in women with polycystic ovarian syndrome. Human Reproduction. 2001;**16**(2):226-229

[20] Krystynik O, Macakova D, Cibickova L, Karasek D. Fasting plasma glucose and its relationship to anthropometric phenotype in women diagnosed with gestational diabetes according to IADPSG criteria. Life (Basel). 2023;**13**(1):137

[21] Weir GC, Laybutt DR, Kaneto H, Bonner-Weir S, Sharma A. Beta-cell adaptation and decompensation during the progression of diabetes. Diabetes. 2001;**50**(Suppl. 1):S154-S15921

[22] Prentki M, Nolan CJ. Islet beta cell failure in type 2 diabetes. Journal of Clinical Investigation. 2006;**116**:1802-1812

[23] Rahier J, Guiot Y, Goebbels RM, Sempoux C, Henquin JC. Pancreatic beta-cell mass in European subjects with type 2 diabetes. Diabetes, Obesity and Metabolism. 2008;**10**(Suppl. 4):32-42

[24] Van Assche FA, Aerts L, De Prins F. A morphological study of the endocrine pancreas in human pregnancy. British Journal of Obstetrics and Gynaecology. 1978;**85**:818-820

[25] Barbour LA, McCurdy CE, Hernandez TL, Kirwan JP, Catalano PM, Friedman JE. Cellular mechanisms for insulin resistance in normal pregnancy and gestational diabetes. Diabetes Care. 2007;**30**(Suppl. 2):S112-S119

[26] Maple-Brown L, Ye C, Hanley AJ, Connelly PW, Sermer M, Zinman B, et al. Maternal pregravid weight is the primary determinant of serum leptin and its metabolic associations in pregnancy, irrespective of gestational glucose tolerance status. Journal of Clinical Endocrinology and Metabolism. 2012;**97**:4148-4155

[27] Masuzaki H, Ogawa Y, Sagawa N, Hosoda K, Matsumoto T, Mise H, et al. Nonadipose tissue production of leptin: Leptin as a novel placenta-derived hormone in humans. Nature Medicine. 1997;**3**:1029-1033

[28] Williams MA, Qiu C, Muy-Rivera M, Vadachkoria S, Song T, Luthy DA. Plasma adiponectin concentrations in early pregnancy and subsequent risk of gestational diabetes mellitus. The Journal of Clinical Endocrinology and Metabolism. May 2004;**89**(5):2306-2311

[29] Retnakaran R, Hanley AJG, Raif N, Connelly PW, Sermer M, Zinman B.

Reduced adiponectin concentration in women with gestational diabetes: A potential factor in progression to type 2 diabetes. Diabetes Care. 2004;**27**:799-800

[30] Yamauchi T, Kamon J, Minokoshi Y, Ito Y, Waki H, Uchida S, et al. Adiponectin stimulates glucose utilization and fatty-acid oxidation by activating AMP-activated protein kinase. Nature Medicine. 2002;**8**:1288-1295

[31] Rojas-Rodriguez R, Lifshitz LM, Bellve KD, Min SY, Pires J, Leung K, et al. Human adipose tissue expansion in pregnancy is impaired in gestational diabetes mellitus. Diabetologia. 2015;**58**:2106-2114

[32] Karasek D, Krystynik O, Kucerova V, Macakova D, Cibickova L, Schovanek J, et al. Adiponectin, A-FABP and FGF-19 levels in women with early diagnosed gestational diabetes. Journal of Clinical Medicine. 2022;**11**(9):2417

[33] Wang D, Xu S, Ding W, Zhu C, Deng S, Qiu X, et al. Decreased placental and muscular expression of the fibroblast growth factor 19 in gestational diabetes mellitus. Journal of Diabetes Investigation. 2019;**10**(1):171-181

[34] Hoy AJ, Brandon AE, Turner N, Watt MJ, Bruce CR, Cooney GJ, et al. Lipid and insulin infusion-induced skeletal muscle insulin resistance is likely due to metabolic feedback and not changes in IRS-1, Akt, or AS160 phosphorylation. American Journal of Physiology-Endocrinology and Metabolism. 2009;**297**:E67-E75

[35] Patti M-E, Corvera S. The role of mitochondria in the pathogenesis of type 2 diabetes. Endocrine Reviews. 2010;**31**:364-395

[36] Lappas M, Hiden U, Desoye G, Froehlich J, Hauguel-de Mouzon S, Jawerbaum A. The role of oxidative stress in the pathophysiology of gestational diabetes mellitus. Antioxidants & Redox Signaling. 2011;**15**:3061-3100

[37] Hiden U, Maier A, Bilban M, Ghaffari-Tabrizi N, Wadsack C, Lang I, et al. Insulin control of placental gene expression shifts from mother to foetus over the course of pregnancy. Diabetologia. 2006;**49**:123-131

[38] Benhalima K, Hanssens M, Devlieger R, Verhaeghe J, Mathieu C. Analysis of pregnancy outcomes using the new IADPSG recommendation compared with the Carpenter and Coustan criteria in an area with a low prevalence of gestational diabetes. International Journal of Endocrinology. 2013;**2013**:248121

[39] HAPO Study Cooperative Research Group. Hyperglycemia and adverse pregnancy outcome (HAPO) study: Association with maternal body mass index. BJOG. 2010;**117**:575-584

[40] Aubry EM, Raio L, Oelhafen S. Effect of the IADPSG screening strategy for gestational diabetes on perinatal outcomes in Switzerland. Diabetes Research and Clinical Practice. 2021;**175**:108830

[41] Hillier TA, Pedula KL, Ogasawara KK, Vesco KK, Oshiro CES, Lubarsky SL, et al. A pragmatic, randomized clinical trial of gestational diabetes screening. The New England Journal of Medicine. 2021;**384**:895-890

[42] Landon MB, Spong CY, Thom E, Carpenter MW, Ramin SM, Casey B, et al. A multicenter, randomized trial of treatment for mild gestational diabetes. The New England Journal of Medicine. 2009;**361**:1339-1348

[43] Diabetes in pregnancy: Management from preconception to the postnatal

period NICE guideline Published: 25 February 2015 Last updated: 16 December 2020

[44] Zaccara TA, Paganoti CF, Mikami FCF, et al. WHO criteria for diabetes in pregnancy: A retrospective cohort. BMC Pregnancy and Childbirth. 2022;**22**:385

[45] McIntyre HD, Oats JJN, Kihara AB, et al. Update on diagnosis of hyperglycemia in pregnancy and gestational diabetes mellitus from FIGO's Pregnancy & Non-Communicable Diseases Committee. International Journal of Gynecology & Obstetrics. 2021;**154**:189-194

[46] Miller C, Lim E. The risk of diabetes after giving birth to a macrosomic infant: Data from the NHANES cohort. Maternal Health, Neonatology and Perinatology. 2021;**12**:7

[47] Schwartz R, Gruppuso PA, Petzold K, Brambilla D, Hiilesmaa V, Teramo KA. Hyperinsulinemia and macrosomia in the fetus of the diabetic mother. Diabetes Care. 1994;**17**:640-648

[48] Fetita L-S, Sobngwi E, Serradas P, Calvo F, Gautier J-F. Consequences of Fetal exposure to maternal diabetes in offspring. Journal of Clinical Endocrinology and Metabolism. 2006;**91**:3718-3724

[49] Gascho CLL, Leandro DMK, Ribeiro E, Silva T, Silva JC. Predictors of cesarean delivery in pregnant women with gestational diabetes mellitus. Revista Brasileira de Ginecologia e Obstetrícia. 2017;**39**:60-65

[50] Scifres CM, Feghali M, Dumont T, Althouse AD, Speer P, Caritis SN, et al. Large-for-gestational-age ultrasound diagnosis and risk for cesarean delivery in women with gestational diabetes mellitus. Obstetrics and Gynecology. 2015;**126**:978-986

[51] Huluta I, Wright A, Cosma LM, Hamed K, Nicolaides KH, Charakida M. Fetal cardiac function at midgestation in women who subsequently develop gestational diabetes. JAMA Pediatrics. 2023;**177**(7):718-725

[52] Wahabi HA, Alzeidan RA, Bawazeer GA, et al. Preconception care for diabetic women for improving maternal and fetal outcomes: A systematic review and meta-analysis. BMC Pregnancy and Childbirth. 2010;**10**:63

[53] American Diabetes Association. 14. Management of diabetes in pregnancy: Standards of medical care in diabetes—2020. Diabetes Care. 2019;**43**:S183-S192

[54] Chao H, Chen G, Wen X, Liu J, Zhang J. Dietary control plus nutrition guidance for blood glucose and pregnancy outcome in women with gestational diabetes. International Journal of Clinical and Experimental Medicine. 2019;**12**:2773-2778

[55] Morris MA, Hutchinson J, Gianfrancesco C, Alwan NA, Carter MC, Scott EM, et al. Relationship of the frequency, distribution, and content of meals/snacks to glycaemic control in gestational diabetes: The myfood24 GDM pilot study. Nutrients. 2020;**12**:3

[56] Hay WW. Placental-fetal glucose exchange and fetal glucose metabolism. Transactions of the American Climatological and Clinical Association. 2006;**117**:321-340

[57] Kiel D, Dodson E, Artal R, Boehmer T, Leet T. Gestational weight gain and pregnancy outcomes in obese women how much is enough? Obstetrics and Gynecology. 2007;**110**:752-758

[58] Sun Y, Shen Z, Zhan Y. Effects of pre-pregnancy body mass index and gestational weight gain on maternal and infant complications. BMC Pregnancy and Childbirth. 2020;**20**:390

[59] Nordic Nutrition of Ministers. Nordic Nutrition Recommendations 2012. 5th ed. Vol. 2014. Copenhagen, Denmark: Norden. pp. 1-629

[60] Yaktine AL, Rasmussen KM, Youth F, National Research Council; Institute of Medicine; Board on Children; Committee to Reexamine IOM Pregnancy Weight Guidelines. In: Rasmussen KM, Yaktine AL, editors. Weight Gain During Pregnancy: Reexamining the Guidelines (2009). Washington, DC, USA: The National Academies Press; 2009

[61] American College of Obstetricians and Gynecologists. ACOG Committee opinion number 650. Physical activity and exercise during pregnancy and the postpartum period. Obstetrics & Gynecology. December 2015

[62] Aune D, Sen A, Henriksen T, Saugstad OD, Tonstad S. Physical activity and the risk of gestational diabetes mellitus: A systemic review and dose-response meta-analysis of epidemiological studies. European Journal of Epidemiology. 2016;**31**:967-997

[63] Nasiri-Amiri F, Sepidarkish M, Shirvani MA, Habibipour P, Tabari NS. The effect of exercise on the prevention of gestational diabetes in obese and overweight pregnant women: A systemic review and meta-analysis. Diabetology and Metabolic Syndrome. 2019;**11**:72

[64] Ming WK, Ding W, Zhang CJ, Zhong L, Long Y, Li Z, et al. The effect of exercise during pregnancy on gestational diabetes mellitus in normal-weight women: A systemic review and meta-analysis. BMC Pregnancy and Childbirth. 2018;**18**:44

[65] Blum AK. Insulin use in pregnancy: An update. Diabetes Spectrum. 2016;**29**(3):191. Erratum for: Diabetes Spectr. 2016 May;29(2):92-7

[66] Hod M, Mathiesen ER, Jovanovič L, McCance DR, Ivanisevic M, Durán-Garcia S, et al. A randomized trial comparing perinatal outcomes using insulin detemir or neutral protamine Hagedorn in type 1 diabetes. The Journal of Maternal-Fetal & Neonatal Medicine. 2014;**27**(1):7-13

[67] Brown J, Grzeskowiak L, Williamson K, Downie MR, Crowther CA. Insulin for the treatment of women with gestational diabetes. Cochrane Database of Systematic Reviews. 2017;**11**(11):5-11

[68] Gui J, Liu Q, Feng L. Metformin vs insulin in the management of gestational diabetes: A meta-analysis. PLoS One. 2013;**8**(5):e64585

[69] Zeng YC, Li MJ, Chen Y, Jiang L, Wang SM, Mo XL, et al. The use of glyburide in the management of gestational diabetes mellitus: A meta-analysis. Advances in Medical Sciences. 2014;**59**(1):95-101

[70] Yu DQ, Xu GX, Teng XY, Xu JW, Tang LF, Feng C, et al. Glycemic control and neonatal outcomes in women with gestational diabetes mellitus treated using glyburide, metformin, or insulin: A pairwise and network meta-analysis. BMC Endocrine Disorders. 2021;**21**(1):199

[71] Chen C, Huang Y, Dong G, Zeng Y, Zhou Z. The effect of dipeptidyl peptidase-4 inhibitor and glucagon-like peptide-1 receptor agonist in gestational diabetes mellitus: A systematic review. Gynecological Endocrinology. 2020;**36**(5):375-380

[72] Liu X, Wu N, Al-Mureish A. A review on research progress in the application of glycosylated Hemoglobin and glycated albumin in the screening and monitoring of gestational diabetes. International Journal of General Medicine. 2021;**14**:1155-1165

[73] Yeh PT, Kennedy CE, Rhee DK, Zera C, Tunçalp Ö, Lucido B, et al. Self-monitoring of blood glucose levels among pregnant individuals with gestational diabetes: A systematic review and meta-analysis. Frontiers in Global Women's Health. 2023;**4**:1006041

[74] Davidson SJ, de Jersey SJ, Britten FL, Wolski P, Sekar R, Callaway LK. Fetal ultrasound scans to guide management of gestational diabetes: Improved neonatal outcomes in routine clinical practice. Diabetes Research and Clinical Practice. 2021;**173**:108696

Chapter 9

Diabetes in Old Age: Particularities and Specifics

Pavel Weber, Dana Weberová and Hana Meluzinova

Abstract

Diabetes (DM) is a significant risk factor for the onset and development of late diabetic complications at any age. In the elderly, DM often occurs as part of multimorbidity and can contribute to the onset and development of disability. The treatment of DM in old age is based on the same principles as for younger individuals. When choosing therapy for DM, the following should be taken into account: age, life expectancy, the presence of complications, self-sufficiency, economic conditions, eating habits and other handicaps. The authors report their own experience from the outpatient practice of DM type 2 treatment. The authors discuss the growth of the elderly population in relation to organ changes with the ageing process, as well as issues of multimorbidity, the specifics of the clinical picture of diseases in old age and the problem of polypharmacy both from the perspective of ageing and old age and the relationship to diabetes as a comorbidity.

Keywords: aging, diabetes in old age, geriatrization of medicine, multimorbidity, organ specifics and diseases particularities, polypharmacy

1. Introduction

Currently, apart from aging of the population, we are witnessing pandemics of type 2 diabetes (T2DM) and obesity, not only in industrialized countries but literally worldwide [1]. The prevalence of diabetes has doubled since 1980, and similarly, obesity has almost tripled between 1975 and 2020 [2].

Diabetes (DM) represents a significant risk factor for the emergence and development of late diabetic complications, both micro- and macroangiopathic [3]. In the elderly, DM often occurs as part of multimorbidity and can contribute to the onset and development of disability [4]. This can then substantially influence all the other diagnostic and treatment procedures. The treatment of DM in old age is based on the same principles as in younger individuals: diet, physical activity and possible medicines. For these reasons, I will not discuss DM therapy in detail and will leave this to other co-authors. On the contrary, I will focus on some specifics for DM only in old age.

Civilization development increases the hope of reaching old age, and the average life expectancy grows. Until the 1950s, people died prematurely. Over the past 100 years, life expectancy has almost doubled, which is one of the greatest achievements of humanity and science ever. The length of human life is now beginning to approach its biological limit. The probability of living in old age ceases to be an exceptional phenomenon but becomes a normal and mass matter.

The number of old, very old and long-lived people is increasing both absolutely and relatively [5, 6]. This trend will continue and become significantly stronger with aging of the baby boomers (people born after World War II) [6–8]. A basic overview and knowledge of the issues of geriatric medicine will become a necessity. Contemporary geriatric medicine strives to maintain adequate physical and mental activity for as long as possible, to prevent the loss of self-sufficiency and to improve the prognosis of the elderly in case of illness. It, therefore, has an interventional preventive character and supports successful healthy aging [9]. In the chapter, on the contrary, I will try to point out the specifics of organ changes and diseases in old age, which are fully applicable to older diabetics as well. For these reasons, in the text of the chapter, I focus on the issue of the peculiarities of geriatric morbidity and pharmacotherapy in old age (with emphasis on DM).

Demographic forecasts, not only in industrially advanced countries but also in third-world countries, point to a clear trend of global population aging. Understandably, this fact brings a number of new, not yet common and fully identified problems, both in the field of health and social care [10]. The length of life itself ceases to be the main parameter, and the quality of life of an older individual comes to the fore [11].

The senior population as a whole is an extremely heterogeneous group where there are both sick and healthy people [12, 13]. The expected volume of costs in the coming decades is estimated to reach almost twice the current level when it exceeds 40%.

The determination of age bands for old age is a convention and a social construction resulting from the administrative needs of the welfare state. Today, the age of 65 is generally considered to be the beginning of old age, and old age proper (in the narrower sense of the word) is spoken of from 75. At the same time, the most used new age classification of seniors is also derived from this concept:

- 65–74 years: "young old seniors", issues of retirement, free time, activities, self-realization dominate.

- 75–84 years: "old seniors", issues of adaptation, load tolerance, specific moaning, loneliness. Age over 75 years – more significant changes associated with physiological aging develop.

- 85 years and older: "oldest old seniors", usually set aside as a separate category due to the high number of frail seniors and the high risk of the possibility of sudden addiction.

Demographic prognosis clearly indicates the rise of numbers of seniors with limited self-sufficiency or even "fragile" (frailty syndrome) [14–17], who require a specific approach both in the health field (including pharmacotherapy) and in the social sphere [18, 19]. Life expectancy in the middle of the twenty-first century will reach 85–90 years. Seniors at this age will have depleted physiological reserve mechanisms (to a certain extent) such as immunity, adaptability and functional fitness [19].

Similarly, as society is aging, medical science is currently witnessing a phenomenon – the "geriatrization of medicine". This fact is already significantly reflected in all branches of medicine today – starting with the first line (general practitioners) and ending with almost all specialists. The trend of population aging must be understood as a positive phenomenon of the twenty-first century, as it is a consequence of longer life and better health [1]. Future seniors will very soon also have other demands and requirements for health, social and other community services, which will have to adapt more and more to their needs [20].

The current and future challenges of medicine in the care of the elderly will mainly be:

1. Atomization of medicine

2. Absence of a holistic approach

3. Multimorbidity of the elderly, when they seemingly do not belong anywhere or in many different places

4. Excessive socialization of health problems

2. Specificity of diabetes in old age

Diabetes mellitus (DM) affects up to 20% of people in the 7th decade of age, and another 20% have impaired glucose tolerance. In the elderly it is mostly DM type 2 (over 70 years up to 95%). Less frequently, in old age, we can encounter DM type 1, which people bring with them from earlier years. DM1 can, however, also occur in old age, and not only the Latent Autoimmune Diabetes of Adults (LADA) type, where it is an autoimmune insulitis that has been going on for years. Diabetics over 65 years old with DM duration of more than 10 years have more comorbidities and late complications of DM. This fact only proves the huge heterogeneity of the population of older diabetics, where, on the one hand, there will be people with type 1 diabetes with DM duration of several decades and advanced organ complications; on the other hand, a large group of people where T2DM is usually diagnosed in the 7th or 8th decade without corresponding organ complications. Some of them will be fully able to manage their disease, while others will not due to cognitive dysfunction visual or other handicaps. The management of DM in old age must fully respect phenomena such as the duration of diabetes, complications and comorbidities, the chance of survival, the patient's preferences and the functional capacity of a particular senior.

Significant differences in the characteristics of diabetes in the middle and younger ages as compared to the elderly mainly are:

- Worse social-economic situation

- Greater social isolation and loneliness

- Greater need for help and dependence on family, caregivers, etc.

- Polypharmacy

- Frequent occurrence of senile frailty syndrome and limited life expectancy

- Significant comorbidities that limit the senior's independence

- Lower ability to recognize hypoglycaemia and perform self-monitoring

Correct screening is the key to avoiding diabetic complications, morbidity and mortality.

Early diagnosis of DM of seniors in institutional care (nursing homes, etc.) can be of fundamental importance for their care [21].

- Improvement of metabolic control can improve cognitive functions and reduce the risk of hypoglycaemia on the one hand and hyperosmolar coma on the other.

- Early treatment can slow down the development of vascular complications and disability.

- Properly managed dietary and regimen measures can also delay the need for medical treatment.

- Treatment can relieve symptoms of DM and can improve quality of life.

3. Targets of DM treatment in old age

The objectives of DM compensation will be fundamentally different for the elderly without other serious handicaps and for the frail ones [22]. Achieving euglycaemia in elderly diabetics can often be unrealistic and sometimes even dangerous.

Pharmacologic treatment of DM and effective glycaemic control using appropriate and effective procedures can greatly alter the impact of the disease on comorbidities associated with micro- and macrovascular complications of the disease [23]. **Figure 1** depicts the updated approach to DM2T therapy by the Professional Practice Committee (from European Association for the Study of Diabetes (EASD) and American Diabetes Association (ADA) recommendations) in relation to the degree of motivation, cooperation and self-sufficiency. It lists individual groups of antidiabetic drugs in relation to atherosclerosis-related cardiovascular (CVD) diseases (ASCVD); chronic kidney diseases (CKD) and heart failure (HF); further hypoglycaemia; possible weight gain or loss, and from a price point of view.

In 2021, in our diabetological outpatient clinic Ltd.- outpatient departement (DIASTOP) of people with DM2T (2500 persons) we used: diabetic diet only 12%; oral antidiabetics (OAD) 53%; monotherapy with insulin or insulin analogues 17% and a combination of insulin and OAD (18%) – **Figure 2** [24].

Figure 3 shows changes in the use of the diabetic diet itself, sulfonylureas – SU (decrease in both) and metformin (MET) in 2008–2019 [25].

New Antidiabetic Drugs (NAD) (gliptins, gliflozins and incretin mimetics) were used either within monotherapy or in combination in persons with DM2T in 2021 in a total of 35%. Our retrospective data analysis showed a steady trend in increasing NAD (most gliptins) use – shown in **Figures 4-6** [24].

It is not well known whether effective management of DM can improve the diverse impairments, i.e., functional, physical, cognitive, nutritional status and social exclusion, that are often associated with the presence of DM in old age. Therapeutic goals of the treatment of elderly people with DM have been summarized in the guidelines of the European Union Geriatric Medicine Society and the International Diabetes Foundation and must be consistently applied individually

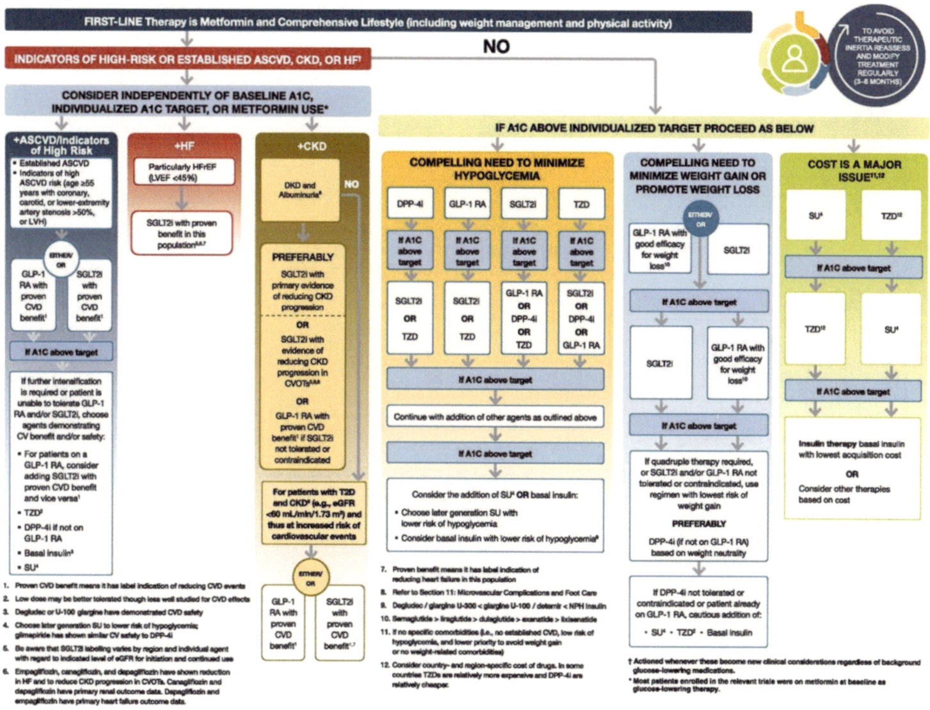

Figure 1.
Updated approach to DM2T therapy by the "professional practice committee (PPC)" of the American Diabetes Association -ADA considering complications, risk of hypoglycaemia, weight changes and cost.

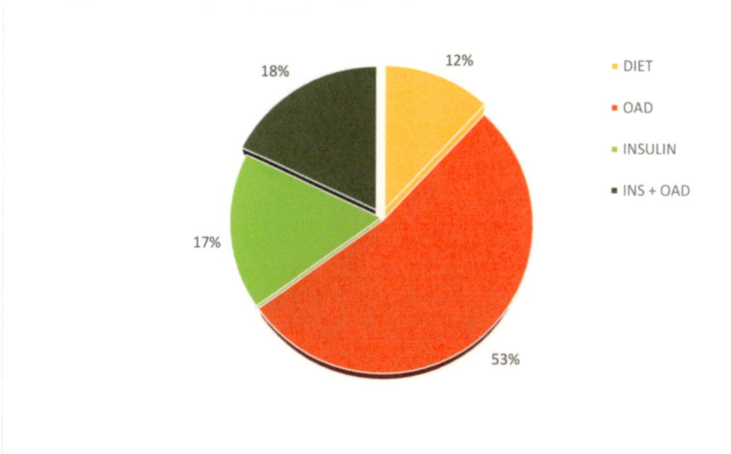

Figure 2.
Basic overview of DM2T treatment used – in 2021: Only diabetic diet; OAD = oral antidiabetic drug; INS insulin (CIT = classic insulin therapy and IIT = intensified insulin therapy); insulin + OAD.

based on the functional status and the presence of comorbidities in elderly persons [26]. It is generally accepted that:

- elderly persons without physical or cognitive disabilities should be treated in a similar way as the adult population.

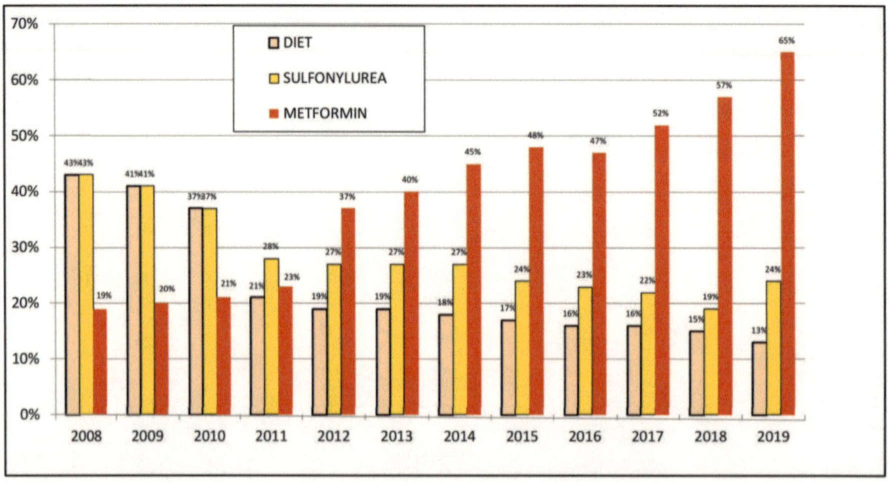

Figure 3.
Changes in the use of diabetic diet alone, sulfonylurea (SU) and metformin (MET) in 2008–2019.

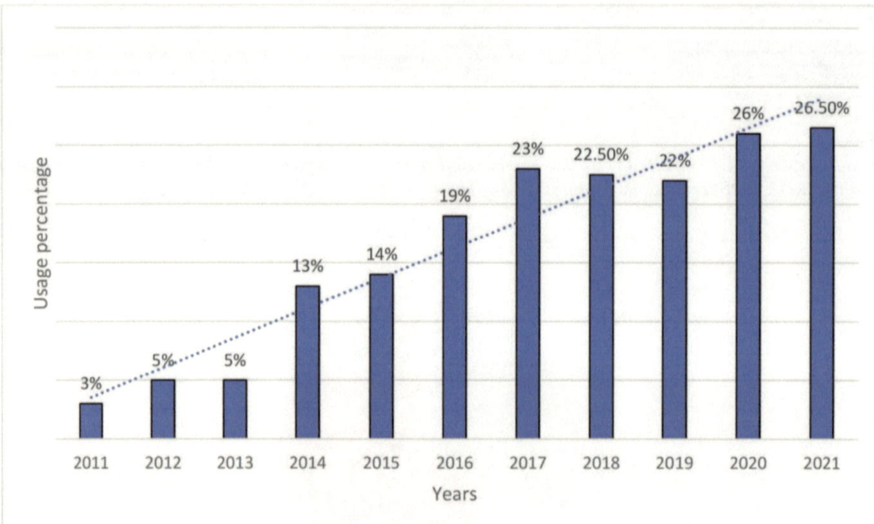

Figure 4.
Changes in the use of DPP4-inhibitors in 2011–2021.

- glycaemic control in elderly persons with physical or cognitive disabilities or with a low life expectancy should be aimed at preventing symptomatic hyperglycaemia and the risk of hypoglycaemia [27]. Considerations when initiating DM therapy must include consideration of hypoglycaemia risk, comorbidities, current drug therapy, body mass and DM compensation options [28–31]. Therapeutic options for T2DM in the elderly are diet, physical activity, various antidiabetic drugs, insulin and education [32–34]. When choosing an appropriate treatment, it is always necessary to take into account the age of the diabetic (including the chance of survival), macro and microangiopathic complications, the level of self-sufficiency, a family environment and economic situation,

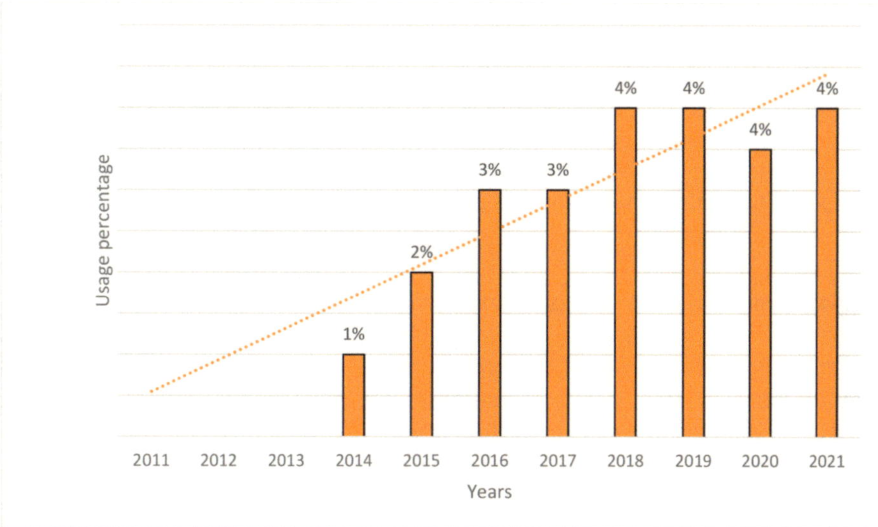

Figure 5.
Changes in the use of SGLT2-inhibitors in 2011–2021.

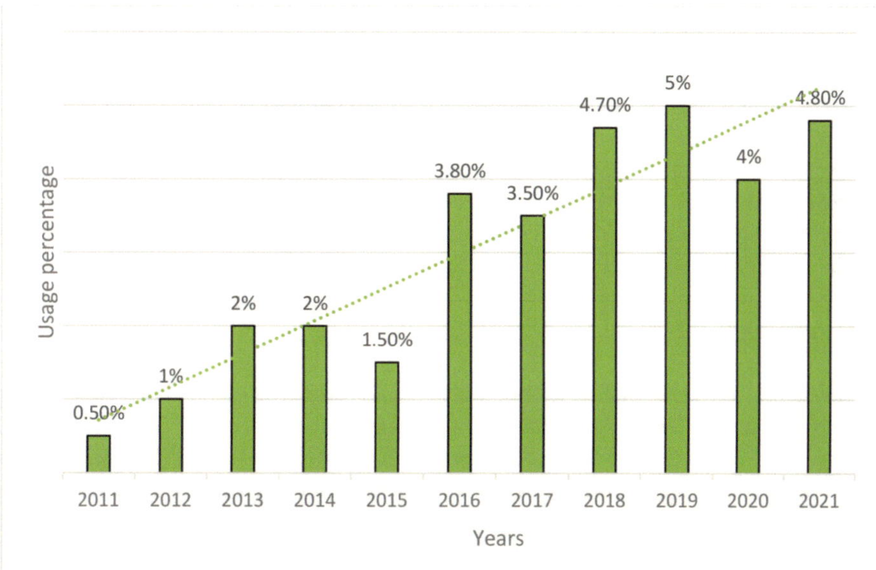

Figure 6.
Changes in the use of GLP1-agonists in 2011–2021.

catering habits (including the state of the teeth) and other handicaps such as disabilities – mental, motor, sight and hearing deficits.

The European Diabetes Working Party for Older, in the published guidelines for the treatment of people with diabetes aged 70+ [26], recommends modifying the HbA1c target values with regard to age and comorbidities. The range HbA1c of 54–59 mmol/mol IFCC (7–7.5% DCCT) is recommended for elderly people with type 2 diabetes without major comorbidities and 60–70 mmol/mol IFCC (7.6–8.5% DCCT) for frail seniors = frail (not self-sufficient, multimorbid, with dementia), where the risk of developing hypoglycaemia is high and the benefit of medical intervention is relatively low. One of the main principles is to reduce the risk of hypoglycaemia, no diabetic should have fasting blood glucose <6.0 mmol/l during treatment. It should never be started if fasting blood glucose is consistently around 7.0 mmol/l. Low glycaemia (glucose levels <5.0 mmol/l) should never be treated with medication, and similarly, random blood glucose levels >11.0 mmol/l as well.

4. Geriatric syndromes: Coexistence with diabetes

Apart from typical acute and late specific and non-specific complications, which I will not discuss here, the emergence and development of typical geriatric syndromes come to the fore in the senior population [3, 4].

DM increases the risk of developing geriatric syndromes – such as dementia, depression, urinary incontinence, falls and a general decline in functional capacity [3, 6, 9].

4.1 Cognitive disorders

DM increases the risk of Alzheimer's dementia by 50 to 100% and vascular dementia by 100 to 200%. Although, on the one hand, some works point to the fact that hyperglycaemia and poor DM control increase the risk of dementia, there are also studies showing that hypoglycaemia as a consequence of tight DM compensation similarly increases the risk of developing mental deterioration. Taking into account that the focus of effective DM treatment is self-monitoring, this will be a limiting factor even in persons with mild cognitive impairment, who will have a problem with adherence to regimen measures, diets and medication and will be unable to recognize potential hypoglycaemia.

4.2 Depression

Depression, as such, itself is associated with adverse side effects, including poorer quality of life, a decline of functional capacity and increased risk of death. Diabetes and depression coexist in 30% of individuals with DM. In 5–10% of diabetics, it can be a severe form of depression. Depression will worsen compliance and adherence to treatment, possibly even self-monitoring as well.

4.3 Urinary incontinence

MI is a problem for 50% of older women with DM. Urgent incontinence is three times higher, and stress incontinence is twice as high. Similar data are not available for men. A higher degree of obesity is also a risk factor for MI; conversely, reducing excess weight reduces the incidence of MI.

4.4 Falls and fractures

In general, individuals with a higher weight have DM more frequently but also a higher bone density, which is associated with a lower risk of fractures. Yu Yang [35] describes a greater risk of falls in older diabetics, and this association is more pronounced in insulin-treated diabetics compared to non-diabetics. The use of insulin, possibly hypoglycaemic insulin secretagogues, poorer eyesight and peripheral neuropathy, belong to the causes of a higher prevalence of falls in older people with DM [36].

5. Changes of organ systems in the elderly

The following paragraphs summarize examples of more serious physiological changes observed in older age people according to individual organ systems [37–39]. These will significantly influence morbidity in old age – including diabetes [8].

Body composition and homeostasis. Changes in body composition include a decrease in lean body mass (primarily the result of muscle loss – sarcopenia is a typical accompanying phenomenon of aging) associated with a proportional increase in fat (especially visceral) [40, 41]. These fundamental changes are important determinants of physiological function and possibilities of therapeutic intervention in the elderly [42]. The reduced volume of striated muscles (e.g. at the age of 90, it can be more than one-third) fundamentally affects insulin sensitivity, and in fact, it only increases insulin resistance [43–45]. This makes the elderly more susceptible to glycoregulation disorders under any load from internal or external causes (illnesses, injuries, surgery, drugs, etc.) [46]. Similarly, reduced muscle mass is largely responsible for the decline in maximal oxygen consumption during exercises (VO2max) which is demonstrable with increasing age. In addition, an increase in body fat can increase the volume of distribution of lipophilic drugs and prolong their pharmacological action. Changes in body composition in the elderly are probably caused not only by the aging process itself but also by such external factors as physical inactivity and changes in the way of catering [47]. Age-related changes include the homeostatic control of impaired baro-reflex sensitivity, which itself may predispose the elderly to orthostatic hypotension, and impaired thermoregulation, which increases the propensity for hypothermia and stroke [6, 7, 9].

Cardiovascular system. Many studies have been conducted to evaluate the functional changes of the cardiovascular system in old age. A well-documented observation is a pattern of left ventricular filling changing with age. In old age, early diastolic filling is reduced, so atrial contractions are increased to maintain adequate left ventricular filling. With age, the content of connective tissue increases in the same way as ventricular hypertrophy presence. As a result of increased left ventricular rigidity, symptoms of pulmonary congestion (murmurs, exertional dyspnoea) may gradually develop in the elderly with the absence of systolic dysfunction. Diastolic dysfunction is of fundamental importance in the elderly. During intense exercises, the heart rate rises less than in younger people. This age-related change is attributed to a weakening beta-adrenergic modulation of heart rate during exercises. Although hypertension cannot, in any case, be considered a physiological manifestation of aging, its incidence increases significantly with age, and higher blood pressure (BP) accelerates the aging process and associated organ changes. More than half of seniors are hypertensive and can benefit to varying degrees from appropriate lifestyle changes or pharmacotherapy. Arterial stiffness, which is of multifactorial origin, also increases with age. Hypertension, increased deposition of collagen in arterial walls, calcification and ongoing atherosclerosis contribute to its development. On the other hand, age modifies the clinical picture, treatment procedure and prognosis in older hypertensive persons. Treatment of hypertension in the elderly leads primarily to a reduction in the number of strokes and, to a lesser extent, to a decrease in cardiovascular events.

Respiratory system. The most typical change in the aged chest wall is rigidity. Lung functions decline with increasing age. During aging, the elastic fraction in the lungs decreases, and there comes a loss of pulmonary alveoli tightly connected with elastic fibers. Reduced lung elasticity contributes to the age-related increase of functional residual capacity (resting expiration) and residual volume. The loss of elasticity leads to early collapse of the peripheral airways during forced expiration and may also partially result in an age-related decline of maximal vital capacity (forced expiratory flow after full inspiration) and forcefully expired volume in 1 second (FEV1). In addition, the decreasing elasticity progressively increases the closing pressure of the airways to such an extent that in some elderly individuals, their closure may occur even during normal respiration.

Loss of maximum breathing capacity decreases by about 40%. At the level of the alveoli, the exchange of oxygen and carbon dioxide decreases by about 50% between the ages of 30 and 65. Although these changes are not observable at rest, older individuals experience fatigue or shortness of breath during increased exertion (exercises or serious illness). Pulmonary reflexes such as cough (ciliary function) decrease with age and thus predispose older people to an accumulation of secretions and development of aspiration pneumonia.

Arterial pressure of oxygen (PaO2) decreases with age over a fairly wide range as a result of ventilation and perfusion imbalance. The reduced ventilatory response to hypoxia and hypercapnia is demonstrable in the elderly and is thought to be a decline in chemoreceptor function. All these changes do not lead to fundamental changes in resting oxygen saturation, but there is a decrease in arterial PaO2. The arterial PaO2 of many people over 80 is around 70-75 mmHg. These changes in blood gases are of minimal importance under resting conditions but dramatically affect survival during severe respiratory disease.

Gastrointestinal tract (GIT). During the aging process, GIT function changes relatively little compared to other organ systems. This is probably due, among other things, to an increase in the secretion of GIT hormones and the relative structural excess of this system. In old age, there is a slight decrease in motility, secretion of digestive juices and absorption of food. A number of dyspeptic problems have a more or less functional character and are rather related to the overall multimorbidity of a specific individual. Even so, the GIT is more vulnerable in old age, and the incidence of GIT diseases increases with age. At the same time, the symptoms of many GIT diseases in old age have a complex character, are discrete and can be difficult to diagnose. In older age, the differential diagnosis of various problems is also very important and difficult, such as pains in the chest (angina or gastroesophageal reflux – up to 30%) and in the abdominal area in general. With the development of atherosclerosis (AS) affection of abdominal vessels, there is also an increase in the occurrence of various angiodysplasias, bleeding lesions of the GIT, complications from vascular ischaemia (ischaemic colitis and vascular ileus), which generally do not occur in younger people.

Uropoetic system. After the age of 40, renal functions gradually decline by about 1 ml/min/year. At the same time, the glomerular filtration evaluated using creatinine clearance can decrease by up to one-third of the original value. This decrease, however, does not occur at all in about one-third of people, so it cannot be unequivocally attributed to involution. Apart from the decrease in glomerular function, renal perfusion, tubular resorption (e.g. glucose, sodium), concentrating and diluting capacity of the kidneys decrease with age as well. Due to the decrease in total muscle mass, serum creatinine may be less informative than it is in younger people. Renal insufficiency – even the chronic one, generally tends to grow with age due to glomerular damage (that is, among other things, diabetic nephropathy) and ischaemic nephropathy (hypertension, atherosclerosis).

The internal environment is usually referred to as all the extracellular fluid consisting of both interstitial and intravascular fluid (i.e. blood plasma). It forms a dynamic system that permanently maintains homeostasis in the body. The older age is not associated with changes in electrolytes or acid-base balance (ABB) in healthy seniors. The changes in the main ions in the serum, sodium, potassium, and chlorides do not take place. The CO_2 does not change either. Only the pH drops very slightly. Unlike creatinine, urea has an upward trend with age (correlation with advanced glomerular sclerosis). Under stress, such as illness, serum urea and creatinine levels rise in the elderly. The occurrence of ion disturbances and ABB also increases with age because the kidneys cannot respond effectively to electrolytes and ABB deviations in the elderly. The occurrence of complications arising from the inability to maintain stable ion homeostasis increases in the presence of intercurrent diseases (DM). In accordance with the decline of glomeru¬lar function, tubular dysfunction also occurs (impaired glucose reabsorption and parathormon excretion). Compared to younger people, the activity of renal ATP-ase also decreases, the decrease in tubule sodium reabsorption, the increase in sodium and water losses, and the decrease in sodium-hydrogen and sodium-phosphate exchange. The acid-base balance is maintained even in old age in a narrow stable pH band of 7.35–7.45.

The age will limit the ability to respond correctly to the load with the compensatory mechanisms of the lungs and kidneys. For example, the ability of the lungs to respond by hyperventilating to acute metabolic acidosis is weakened and only leads to a further drop in pH. Aging kidneys also respond more slowly to acid load, and blood pH recovers more slowly. Many diseases that are frequent in older age (such as heart failure, anaemia, sepsis, diabetes mellitus, kidney and lung diseases) can overload regulatory systems and contribute to the development of acid-base disorders. Similarly, numerous drugs often used in senium (nonsteroidal antiinflammatory drugs, diuretics, laxatives) can contribute to AB-imbalances. The combination of mildly disturbed homeostasis and multimorbidity together with polypharmacy at an advanced age means that disturbances of AB-equilibrium are common. Despite the increase in vasopressin clearance, renal reactivity to it decreases with age, which in turn leads to reduced renal concentrating ability after water deprivation. In addition, in the elderly, the feeling of thirst is reduced, and thus, the drinking regime is affected by water deficit. The impaired concentration capacity of the kidneys and reduced thirst in old age can significantly increase the risk of dehydration during any serious illness.

Endocrine system. Particular attention is paid to changes in glucose metabolism associated with aging. Glucose tolerance decreases with increasing age. In healthy seniors, plasma glucose measured 2 h after a glucose challenge in an oral glucose tolerance test increases by about 0.33–0.72 mmol/l per decade since the age of 50, while fasting blood glucose rises by only 0.05–0.06 mmol/l (= 1 mg%) per decade. This deterioration of glucose tolerance in advanced age tends to be independent of obesity and physical inactivity, which are common accompaniments of the aging process and may themselves contribute to the development of glucose intolerance. The primary cause of the decline in glucose tolerance during aging is insulin resistance in peripheral tissues, especially muscles. A number of studies have demonstrated that there is no age-associated change in the binding of insulin to cell receptors; therefore, the post-receptor abnormality of insulin action (i.e. intracellular defect) is considered to be the cause of age-related glucose intolerance.

Although insulin secretion may be impaired in old age, circulating insulin levels do not decrease, probably due to an age-related decrease in insulin clearance. The impaired glucose tolerance during old age is not generally the same as glycaemia in diabetics. According to the theory of aging, however, emphasizing protein glycation, even moderate long-term increases in glycaemia could influence the development of physiological deteriorations or diseases typically occurring in old age. In this regard, fasting blood glucose and glycated haemoglobin show a high degree of correlation in non-diabetics of older age in the broadest sense of the word. Some epidemiological studies indicate that increases in glycaemia can, therefore, accentuate the development of cardiovascular diseases even in non-diabetics. According to Sinclair, optimal fasting glycaemia in diabetics should be in the range of 7–9 mmol/l but should not exceed 10–13 mmol/l, even in very old and disabled diabetics. Even these disabled elderly diabetics should not be at risk of acute hypoglycaemia. DM affects up to 20% of people in the 7th decade, and another 20% suffer from impaired glucose tolerance. It is the most clinically significant metabolic disease of older age. In the case of seniors, it is mainly DM2T (up to 95% over 70 years).

Another endocrine variable of potential importance during aging is a growth hormone (insulin-like growth factor 1 – IGF 1). Pituitary secretion of the growth hormone decreases with age. Many of the anabolic effects of Growth Hormone (GH) are mediated just by IGF 1, which is produced in the liver and other tissues in response to GH. Similarly to how GH declines in old age, IGF 1 secretion declines with age as well. Changes in body composition in the elderly (i.e. muscle reduction and fat gain) are strikingly similar to findings in younger individuals with growth hormone deficiency. These findings led to a hypothesis that typical changes in body composition in old age are due to a decrease in growth hormone secretion.

During aging, the thyroid gland undergoes mild atrophy, fibrosis, ascent of colloid nodules and lymphocytic infiltration. In the senium, thyropathies will be detected in up to a tenth of individuals, more often in women. During the laboratory examination, there will often be asymptomatic forms, the so-called subclinical hypothyroidism and hyperthyroidism, with TSH deviation without an accompanying change in thyroxine (T_4). Considering the initiation of potential therapy for both subclinical hypothyroidism and hyperthyroidism is a very controversial issue: the overall clinical picture and the degree of possible controllable symptoms from hypofunction or hyperfunction of the thyroid gland will be decisive. The prevalence of hypothyroidism increases significantly in old age. Its clinical symptomatology, however, is less noticeable than in younger individuals. Thyroxine (T_4) secretion decreases by about 30% compared to young adults, while serum T_4 levels remain unchanged. This decrease in T_4 secretion is considered to be a physiological compensation for reduced tissue utilization and not a manifestation of primary thyropathy. The decrease in T_4 utilization correlates with a decrease in the body's active muscle mass. The Thyroid-Stimulating Hormone (TSH) level also increases slightly with age, which can probably explain the higher incidence of Hashimoto's thyroiditis in old age. Autoimmune thyroiditis occurs in up to 1–2% of the elderly population, especially in women. A slight decrease in deiodination in the periphery is also compensatory in old age.

Ovaries show a dramatic decline in oestrogen and progesterone secretion as well as fibrosis and scarring as they get older. Menopause represents the most significant age-related endocrine syndrome. Menopause occurs on average around the age of 50 with accompanying hot flushes; the loss of bone mass and oestrogen-sensitive tissues is accentuated.

Andropause in men with a decrease in testosterone levels begins after the age of 50 (without affecting potency). Sexual functions are relatively well protected, although there is an increase in the refractory period and an increase in the time required for sexual arousal and loss of tissue turgor.

Immune system. A decline in immune functions predisposes the elderly to a higher incidence of infectious diseases and malignancies. For older age, a typical decrease in cellular immunity is characterized by a decrease of T-lymphocytes in response to mitogenic stimulation. The impaired T-cell proliferation in old age may be responsible for defective intracellular transduction of mitogenic signals. In addition, interleukin-2 (IL2) synthesis and IL2 receptor expression, essential for T-cell proliferation, are reduced in late age. The involution of the thymus and the loss of its hormones play a fundamental role in the decline of T-cell functionality in the senium. The age-related changes in humoral immunity include an increased production of autoantibodies and a decrease of the antibody response to foreign stimuli. These changes reflect age-related variations in the functions of T-cells and B-cells.

Musculoskeletal system. Bone mass and density decline with age after reaching the age of 20. In women, this loss is about 1% per year until menopause; afterwards, it can rise to 2–3% per year. After 5–10 years after menopause, the bone loss returns to 1% per year but may accelerate again around the age of 80. Men have primarily more bone mass than women; their loss is similar (approx. 1% per year), but the clinical effect is not apparent until advanced age. The tendons and ligaments become less elastic in old age, which can contribute to a higher incidence of ruptures (especially of the Achilles tendon). The cartilage of the ribs and spine is less elastic and more calcified. At the age of 70, muscle mass decreases by about 25%, both in men and women. At the age of 80, muscle size and strength in people with a predominantly sedentary lifestyle decrease by 30–40%.

Sight disorders affect 1 in 6 people aged 75–84 and every fourth one over 85. 1% of people over 65 are affected by almost complete blindness. Among significant causes of visual impairment in old age, we include age-related macular degeneration, cataracts, diabetic retinopathy and glaucoma. Lens accommodation disorders, which can be corrected with glasses or contact lenses, also increase in old age. Loss of sight is always associated with loss of independence, decreased physical activity and depression. The risk of falls and injuries also increases.

Hearing disorders. Clinically significant hearing impairment occurs in up to one-third of individuals over 65 years of age and in half of people over 75 years of age. The most common disorder is presbycusis, with loss of high-frequency tones, which can be improved by using hearing aids.

6. Multimorbidity: Characteristics

Multimorbidity (usually ≥3 diseases) represents the simultaneous presence of several diseases in one individual either without any causal relationship or with mutually causal conditioning. It brings along several risks not only for the sick seniors but also for their physicians. In essence, it belongs to the characteristics of the geriatric medicine [38].

Among the causes of morbidity in old age, diseases of the cardiovascular system conditioned by atherosclerosis (AS) occupy a leading place, such as coronary heart disease (CHD), heart- attack, angina pectoris, cerebrovascular events (stroke, TIA), ischaemic disease of the lower extremities – IDLE (apparent atherosclerosis – AS is present as an aetiology in up to 90% of people over 75 years of age) [48, 49]. The diseases of the locomotion system, sensory organs, tumours, injuries, diseases of the respiratory (chronic obstructive pulmonary disease – COPD), gastrointestinal (biliary and other problems) and urogenital system (prostate in men, gynaecological organs in women) are also common in old age [43]. Diabetes, and mental and nervous diseases are also frequent. The care for elderly people with multiple, mutually influencing diseases requires a great deal of diagnostic, analytical and synthetic skills and abilities of the physician, including his or her ability to deal with people [50]. Their current, often independent coexistence is exactly typical for senile multimorbidity. After the age of 60, diseases of the cardiovascular system (CHD, stroke, hypertension) show a steady rise, and the prevalence of DM also increases with age. The presence of the disease itself (or several diseases) is not decisive for the quality of life of a senior, but the degree of disability, i.e. functional impairment, to which it leads as a result. Full self-sufficiency can be maintained even in the presence of many diseases at the same time.

The interaction of different independent diseases in the elderly is a problem closely related to multimorbidity [5, 6, 9].

The objective effort to evaluate multimorbidity led to the creation of many internationally recognized scales (Kaplan-Feinstein Index; Charlson index); CIRS-G = Cumulative Illness Rating Scale – Geriatric Version; health-related quality of life (HRQOL); Disease Burden Morbidity Assessment (DBMA); Index of Co-Existent Disease (ICED); Geriatric Index of Comorbidity (GI); Functional Comorbidity Index (FCI); Total Illness Burden Index (TIBI).

The diseases often tend to accumulate and potentiate each other. Multidimensionality is typical in geriatric medicine. The seniors as a bio-psycho-social unit need to be understood much more significantly in old age than in younger age periods, both in the etiopathogenesis of diseases and in clinical practice. In geriatric medicine, psychological and social problems always appear simultaneously with somatic problems; both need to be solved just as urgently. This applies in the full sense of the word to completely typical primary somatic diseases characteristic of old age (strokes, degenerative diseases, tumours and immobilization). The same is fully true for diabetics in old age. Similarly, it is valid for the so-called "primarily" mental disorders (dementia, depression, delirium) or the so-called geriatric social syndromes (geriatric maladaptation syndrome, mistreatment, neglect and abuse).

Most clinicians tend to perceive multimorbidity as an unpleasant phenomenon associated with a decrease in functional capacities, cognitive impairment and, in addition to those, the risk of interactions between the diseases themselves and their possible pharmacotherapy. In the elderly (especially the advanced ones) multimorbidity is more the rule than the exception. The growth of the group of multimorbid seniors goes hand in hand with aging of the population in general. It has apparently increased in the last decade (by 22%). More than 75% of people aged ≥85 years are multimorbid.

6.1 Functional capacities: Multimorbidity and vice versa

Functional loss is the final state of most clinical problems in old age (especially late, i.e. over 80 years). This may be the only symptom of a serious ongoing disease, when the typical symptoms of the given disease are absent [33]. In practice, such functional damage means a decrease in the individual's functional ability and can be easily assessed, for example, with the activities of daily living test (ADL score

– assessment of these tasks: transfer, bed mobility, toileting and eating) and the instrumental test of daily activities (IADL – a tool used to determine the amount of help a person may need). In addition, it is also appropriate to assess cognition, nutritional, behavioural and social status in relation to the health status [51].

Older people, unlike younger people, react non-specifically to deterioration or illness, which actually means a decrease in some function. He or she stops eating and drinking, or new falls, confusion, lethargy, dizziness or incontinence occur. These symptoms may be the first or even the only manifestation of the disease, which in younger people has typical symptoms (such as pneumonia, heart attack, pulmonary embolism, myxedema, etc.). These functional deficits constitute geriatric syndromes (GS) [52]. These then significantly affect self-sufficiency without the presence of obvious or typical symptoms of any disease. In this regard, GS can be defined as a loss of functional capacities typically caused by multimorbidity, in which several organ systems are affected simultaneously.

Thanks to the rich range of medicines and progress in the pharmaceutical form technology, the physician can choose a medicinal product practically "tailored" to a specific men or women. On the other hand, however, this option brings along some negatives. This therapeutic effort can initially lead to a completely justified and purposeful pharmacotherapy, from which it is already very close to polypharmacy with possible health risks for the old people [53].

The vulnerability of the elderly through diseases in general is higher, and the balance of their organ homeostasis is quite fragile [54]. This is true for non-diabetic seniors and even more so for those being treated for diabetes and other related comorbidities. Similarly, it is true for the so-called primarily mental disorders (dementia, depression, delirium) or the so-called geriatric social syndromes (loneliness). Clinical picture of adaptation failure based on chronic stress in old age is a geriatric maladaptation syndrome, which can have a worse course in an elderly diabetic. The stressor is usually in the psychosocial area and its clinical manifestation occurs most frequently in the cardio – an cerebrovascular area (heart attack and stroke) or in the deterioration of immunity (bronchopneumonia), etc., with a higher risk of occurrence of complications in diabetics.

The mentioned somatic, psychological and social problems interact with each other and are characterized by difficult treatability, a chronic course with progression and a relatively unfavourable prognosis. They bring many difficult-to-manage situations and problems to the old people and their surroundings. In very old individuals (the so-called old-old, i.e. people over 80 years of age), diseases progress in a way that is usually significantly different from the course of diseases in middle age, and they also require a different approach, enabling the improvement of health status or at least the maintenance of existing self-sufficiency and accentuating the return to the home environment [55].

Pitfalls and negatives of multimorbidity represent:

- Accelerated decline of the functional capacity
- The higher incidence of symptoms and subjective complaints
- The decline in quality of life
- Increased mortality

- Increased risk of hospitalization
- Increased risk of institutionalization (nursing or residential home, etc.)
- Rising health care costs

6.2 Atypical presentation of diseases in old age

Most biological functions (maximal respiratory capacity, glomerular filtration and cardiac index) reach their peak before the age of 30. Some of them then gradually decrease linearly [40, 44]. This decrease is practically insignificant for everyday normal activity, but it can become serious during periods of greater stress or under a load [56]. Physiological events that decrease with age are blood flow through the kidneys, creatinine clearance, maximum heart rate and, subsequently, stroke volume during exercises, glucose tolerance, vital lung capacity, body mass and cellular immunity [40, 44]. On the contrary, total lung capacity and liver function do not change relatively with age; ADH secretion even increases with age. Many of the above-mentioned declines, previously considered a natural consequence of aging, are significantly influenced by lifestyle, behaviour, diet and the environment in which the person has been living. The most important physiological change in old age is a predisposition to a higher incidence of serious diseases. The respiratory function of a healthy 70-year-old is about 50% of that of a 30-year-old one. Pneumonia is a common and severe disease in older people. In this group of men and women, pneumonia is among the four most frequent diseases leading to death. The diagnosis can often be difficult due to an atypical clinical presentation. Therefore, pneumonia should always be considered as the cause of any deterioration in an older person [57]. Geriatric problems, such as frailty, and physical and psychological limitations, should be recorded as well as the social situation [51]. Renal functions commonly decline by 50% or more after the 70th year of age. This decrease in physiological reserve capacity does not affect normal daily life but can complicate the ability to recover from a serious illness. At the same time, some physiological changes mimic a disease, even though they are a normal part of aging [6, 13]. An essential prognostic element in sepsis is the timeliness of acute treatment in elderly individuals with reduced immune defenses and physiological reserves [58]. Early control of comorbidities is the main plus value of the geriatrician in the acute and post-acute treatment of elderly people with sepsis [58]. In van Son study [59], men and women with an atypical presentation of COVID-19 were more frail compared to persons with a typical presentation. Contrary to our expectations, an atypical presentation was not associated with worse outcomes.

Diabetes mellitus (DM) can occur but also disappear in old age. The ability of insulin to stimulate glucose uptake declines with age and usually manifests itself as postprandial hyperglycaemia with constant normal fasting insulin and glucose levels. In stressful situations, diabetes can be detected in the elderly, but when the stressful situation is over, the chemical symptoms of DM also disappear. This loss of physiological reserves understandably contributes to the increasing prevalence of DM with increasing age. The age-related changes that make older people more vulnerable in everyday life tend to be subtle [60]. In the elderly, both hypothermia and hyperthermia can develop more easily during exposure to extreme environmental influences, as there are several changes in the management of thermoregulation, including those in the field of neurology. The loss of brainstem neurotransmitters can not only cause the typical old-age gait but also predisposes genetically determined individuals to the development of, e.g. Parkinson's disease. Some age-related changes cause specific consequences. Menopause is a physiological event associated with normal aging, but it leads to symptoms that predispose the body to a bone loss and atherosclerosis.

Apart from clinically manifest forms of diseases, a subclinical form of diseases is common in the elderly. Among 6000 individuals over the age of 65 participating in the Cardiovascular Health Study, 31% had clinically manifest cardiovascular disease, while another 37% had a subclinical form of the disease detected by non-invasive examinations.

Atypical or symptom-poor symptomatology of diseases is even higher in elderly diabetics than in the general population. This makes them very risky both in terms of diagnosis and possible therapy. The whole problem is greatly complicated by the decline of physiological functions and changes in organ systems in old age, which can often (and in diabetics) border on pathology more significantly.

- Commonly present symptoms typical of a certain diagnosis are missing

- On the contrary, changes in behaviour and functional abilities are present

- Failure to make a correct diagnosis with atypical symptomatology can lead to wrong conclusions, wrong diagnosis and wrong treatment

Seniors come to central admissions for chest pains lasting more than 6 hours, although they were cardiac people with proven CHD. Among the elderly (70–80 years) and very old (>80 years) subjects who had an acute myocardial infarction, in-hospital mortality was two to three times higher than in younger subjects (<70 years). It emphasizes the need to improve education among older people in relation to some symptoms. Some symptoms such as a loss of consciousness or paralysis of the limbs are understandably never considered normal. Although some symptoms of psychiatric illnesses were not considered normal, they were rarely attributed to serious illnesses (e.g. dementia, etc.).

Although the oldest people had the best prospects for good health, they were also the least able to respond to symptoms of illness. The very old seniors most frequently attributed the symptoms to aging itself and reacted to them by: (1) waiting and watching; (2) by accepting; (3) by denying the danger; (4) postponement or refused medical care. Although the underestimation of disease symptoms in old age with dangerous associations is well-known, many clinicians have in mind the image of the elderly with endless longings, whose investigation, in the end, leads nowhere. The risk of underestimation of symptoms in old age is obvious. Late recognition of the disease leads to delayed initiation of therapy, usually after a more severe course of the disease, which leads to serious consequences and causes deeper functional impairment. Rehabilitation to independence tends to be difficult in these cases, and sometimes, despite "successful treatment," permanent addiction can result. Therefore, the message to clinicians is clear: early detection and therapy of sick people and early detection of at-risk seniors must be the priority.

The pitfalls and negatives of multimorbidity are:

- Accelerated decline of functional capacities

- Higher occurrence of symptoms and subjective problems

- Decline of life quality
- Higher mortality
- Higher risk of hospitalization
- Higher risk of placement in institutional care (home for the elderly, etc.)
- Rising health care costs

According to the data published by Medicare [61], the rise in the costs of care per person and year is quite obvious: from $211 for people without a chronic diagnosis (chr. dg.); to those with ≥2 chr. dg. – $1870; ≥ 5 chr. dg. – $8159 and ≥ 7 chr. dg. – $23,000.

Gathering basic information requires the physician's patience, time and information from the family and care providers.

The first symptoms of an impending infection or serious illness across the disease spectrum can be completely inconspicuous in the elderly. They can present themselves as:

- Change of function: new incontinence; new disturbances in standing or walking;
- Behavioural changes: agitation; delirium;
- Other indicators of change in functional potential: falls, anorexia, fatigue, and weakness.

Due to homeostenosis and a decrease in functional reserves, clinical manifestations may appear in some cases, even at an early stage. Here, even a small improvement of specific symptoms can significantly improve the overall condition of the senior (self-sufficiency). E.g., heart failure can be precipitated by mild hyperthyroidism, a urinary retention by beginning benign prostatic hyperplasia, and hyperosmolar non-ketoacidotic coma in mild glucose intolerance. Paradoxically, the underlying disease can be treated at this stage easily because it is not advanced. Unfortunately, in old age, the development of clinical symptoms (including the ability to describe them) may be limited by reduced mobility and cognitive impairment. For these very reasons, CHD or aortic stenosis can be asymptomatic for a certain period of time.

7. Polypharmacy and old age in combination with multimorbidity

There is a lack of evidence for the specific treatment of multimorbid seniors, as they are usually excluded from large randomized clinical trials (RCT). Exclusion from trials of older people and people with comorbidity and co-prescribing is increasingly untenable given the population ageing and increasing multimorbidity [62]. In a retrospective analysis of five general medical periodicals with the highest IF (impact factor) – out of 284 RCTs from 1995 to 2010, 65% of seniors were excluded due to multimorbidity. In an evaluation of 11 Cochrane Review RCTs according to the presence of four typical chronic diseases (diabetes, heart failure, COPD and stroke), less than half of the participants in these studies had some of the listed chronic diagnoses when they met the entry criteria. Multimorbid seniors usually are not included in

RCTs at all. Clinical guidelines usually do not consider multimorbidity at all (or minimally) and often do not even provide any recommendations that would take into account other comorbidities occurring at the same time, which fully can be applied to older diabetics as well. Despite the great individual and societal burden associated with multimorbidity, little is known about how to effectively manage it [63].

A complex health and social situation is common in multimorbidity. It can often lead to complicated treatment regimens that are difficult for seniors to understand and demanding for physicians to explain. The attending physician requires the ability to coordinate the therapy of various organ systems with other physicians (specialists of various medical branches, including subfields of internal medicine) and the skill of communication with elderly people and their families, so that therapeutic efforts are not only correctly understood, but also carried out. In geriatrics, the primary problem is precisely the lack of studies that would include precisely these multimorbid seniors. This deficit is generally known.

Evidence-based medicines (EBMs) are based on RCTs conducted on defined populations where inclusion and exclusion criteria are applied. Physicians must apply them in the specific situations of individual people. The situation is relatively simple if your men or women belong to the group of fit seniors who meet the guidelines' criteria. It becomes very difficult if they belong to typical geriatric multimorbid persons who are frail and multimorbid and have polypharmacy, cognitive impairment or other functional deficits [64]. Physicians acting strictly according to the guidelines can run into certain risks. Regimens can be either too general or demanding and expensive. An individual approach to the elderly is necessary for choosing a treatment strategy and interventions in general. It is crucial to strictly follow the START/STOP recommendations [65]. A hypothetical patient with hypertension, COPD, DM2, osteoporosis and osteoarthritis should take up to 12 different medications per day according to the guidelines.

Physicians in general are led to use EBM as the gold standard in daily clinical practice. Unfortunately, most RCTs work only with ideal persons, where seniors with a greater risk of developing adverse drug reactions (ADRs), advanced disease and a possible risk of not completing the study are excluded. These non-ideal multimorbid persons, often subject to exclusion criteria, are precisely the typical elderly people of our geriatric practice.

The question the physician should ask before applying any standards and templates is whether and how our men or women are different from the RCT one. It is important to note that the guidelines can usually be applied to relatively healthy seniors. ADRs can exacerbate some of the comorbidities. In patients with functional limitations and disorders, there will be justified fears of falls (antihypertensive therapy, etc.) [66]. The use of warfarin and similar new anticoagulants (dabigatran, rivaroxaban, apixaban, etc.) requires the cooperation of the patient (or a caregiver). Their effective use can be limited in the elderly by possible cognitive impairment (close control of blood clotting - International Normalized Ratio (INR). RCTs focus on outcomes such as mortality or organ-specific outcomes (e.g. cardiovascular endpoints). Other outputs that are often essential in geriatrics for seniors such as maintaining self-sufficiency, mobility and fall prevention or quality of life are often not included in the studies.

7.1 Is there any effective polypharmacy in multimorbid seniors?

Nowadays, thanks to a very wide range of medicines and progress in the field of pharmaceutical form technology, a physician can choose a medicine practically "tailored" to a specific senior [67]. On the other hand, this option brings some pitfalls [68].

Above all, it puts high demands on the professional competence of the physician, on his or her orientation in available medicines and on detailed knowledge of their possibilities and potential risks. For physicians in ambulatory practice, the results of recent studies are sometimes problematically available. This therapeutic effort can initially lead to a completely justified and expedient pharmacotherapy, from which it is already very close to polypharmacy with possible health risks for multimorbid seniors, regardless of the decreasing compliance and increasing costs of therapy [68]. The elderly people living in institutional care consume three times more drugs compared to the same number of individuals in the entire population, and women twice as many as compared to men.

Problems accompanying pharmacotherapy in old age are:

- High economic costs of care and the need to consider the benefit of therapy for the patient's prognosis.
- High degree of polypharmacotherapy and multimorbidity with frequent medication complications.
- Inadequate diagnosis, treatment of some diseases and, more than once, underestimation of some symptoms (pain in old age, depression, etc.)
- Low compliance. In old age, non-compliance is present in 30–50%.

7.2 A basic requirement for pharmacotherapy in old age

Simplicity, expediency and efficiency are essential. Polypragmasy in older age can often be risky and ineffective, many times even harmful. In geriatric medicine, symptomatic treatment generally prevails over the causal treatment. Its adverse effects can fundamentally alter the clinical picture of diseases.

The elderly are generally more vulnerable, the therapeutic range becomes narrow, the compliance decreases, interindividual variability of the effect increases, and the risk of drug interactions increases [69]. In old age, there is a rise in gastric pH, a decrease in gastric and intestinal motility and a decrease in GIT blood flow. Despite these changes, the absorption of most drugs is not significantly affected in old age. Among the most frequent and clinically significant drug interactions are those at the biotransformation level. Inducers and inhibitors of metabolism through the modulation of hepatocyte microsomal enzymes (first pass effect cytochrome CYP 450) substantially affect the levels of other drugs biotransformed by these enzymes. The bioavailability of a drug is determined by the amount of drug that enters the systemic circulation. Thus, it is significantly dependent on gastrointestinal absorption and first pass through the liver.

In older age, most people experience significant changes in the effects of many medications [70]. The spectrum of drugs used changes with age and generally has an upward trend towards polypharmacotherapy. Multimorbidity, nutritional problems and an increased risk of non-compliance are typical. These facts, combined with changes in pharmacokinetics and pharmacodynamics, can lead to serious adverse side effects and drug interactions. With age, the interindividual variability of the doses required to achieve a therapeutic effect increases in general. Pharmacotherapy in geriatric medicine can have significant potential not only therapeutic but also toxic.

Reducing excessive polypharmacy means benefiting the patient's health, improving adherence to treatment and reducing drug costs. Scott [66] directly states that no study has shown that changes (reductions) in polypharmacy could reduce morbidity or mortality in the elderly but lead to a decrease in ADRs (by 35%), a decrease in costs and an improvement in compliance with the remaining medication. De-prescribing is an important concept in older people, given the harm associated with polypharmacy in this age group [71, 72]. Holmes [69] emphasizes geriatric prescription on defining health care goals, individual therapeutic goals, expected average life expectancy and chance of survival, and the need to start with a smaller dose and slowly increase it to the effect. The health care goals in general for the elderly can vary from curative to purely palliative care. Similarly, therapeutic goals may range from preventive to immediate curative [73].

8. Conclusion

As an interdisciplinary field, geriatric medicine emphasizes a holistic approach and the need to perceive older individuals from the point of view of bio-psycho-social integrity, while emphasizing maintaining or improving self-sufficiency and independence for as long as possible. In the broadest sense of the word, successful aging in good physical and mental condition with an acceptable degree of independence and possible active engagement is the de facto goal of modern clinical gerontology.

The increase in average life expectancy (LE) brings along a whole range of health and social problems, not only for the seniors themselves but also for their families and society. The aging of the population, as a typical phenomenon of modern society, requires a change of thinking and attitudes in many areas, starting with the conservatism of doctors and ending with the inattention of politicians. Life expectancy comparisons (see **Figure** 7) is significantly influenced by the composition of the

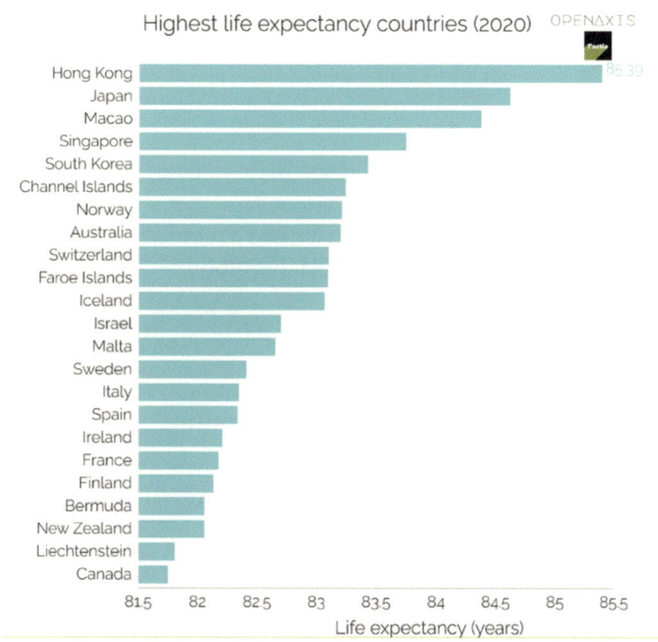

Figure 7.
Highest life expectancy country in 2020 (according Openaxis).

population and will be applied even more significantly in the coming decades (in the Czech Republic is LE 77.2 y., for men 74.1 and women 80.5 in 2020).

When choosing DM therapy, the following should be taken into account: the age of the diabetic, including expected life expectancy; the presence of macro- and microangiopathic complications; degree of self-sufficiency, family environment and economic conditions; catering habits (including state of teeth); other handicaps – mental and motor, sight and hearing.

Therefore, the main goal of DM treatment in old age is to improve the quality of life. It can be summarized in the following few points:

- optimal metabolic compensation
- prevention of the following symptoms: fatigue, weight loss, polyuria, infectious complications
- definition of lifestyle requirements, especially dietary habits
- limitation of drugs used – especially with the risks of hypo- and hyperglycaemia

If insulin therapy is initiated by the clinician, the following questions should always be answered:

- who will administer the insulin?
- what are the checking options (including glycaemia)?
- who will help the diabetic during contingent hypoglycaemia if he lives alone, and how?

Author details

Pavel Weber[1,2]*, Dana Weberová[1,2,3] and Hana Meluzinova[2]

1 Department of Internal Medicine, Geriatrics and Practical Medicine, University Hospital and Masaryk University, Brno, Czech Republic

2 Department of Outpatient for Diabetes, DIASTOP, Ltd., Brno, Czech Republic

3 Department of Gastroenterology and Internal Medicine, University Hospital and Masaryk University, Brno, Czech Republic

*Address all correspondence to: weberpavell@seznam.cz

References

[1] Comer A, Fettig L, Torke AM. Identifying goals of care. The Medical Clinics of North America. 2020;**104**(5):767-775

[2] Hariharan R, Odjidja EN, Scott D, et al. The dietary inflammatory index, obesity, type 2 diabetes, and cardiovascular risk factors and diseases. Obesity Reviews. 2022;**23**(1):e13349

[3] Edelman SV, Henry RR. Diagnosis and Management of Type 2 Diabetes. 13th ed. New York: Professional Communications Inc.; 2017. p. 528

[4] Sinclair AJ, Dunning T, Manas LR, Munshi M. Diabetes in Old Age. 4th ed, Kindle ed. Hoboken, New Jersey: Wiley-Blackwell; 2017. p. 557

[5] Halter J, Ouslander J, Studenski S, High K, Asthana S, Supiano M, et al. Hazzard's Geriatric Medicine and Gerontology. 8th ed. NY: McGraw Hill/Medical; 2022. p. 1824

[6] Morley JE, Vellas B, Sinclair AJ, Cesari M, Munshi M. Pathy's Principles and Practice of Geriatric Medicine. 6th ed. Hoboken, New Jersey: Wiley-Blackwell; 2022. p. 1856

[7] Smailhodzic E, Hooijsma W, Boonstra A, Langley DJ. Social media use in healthcare: A systematic review of effects on patients and on their relationship with healthcare professionals. BMC Health Services Research. 2016;**16**:442. Article number: 442. DOI: 10.1186/s12913-016-1691-0

[8] Lesley KB, James DP, Kunal S, et al. Oxford Handbook of Geriatric Medicine. Third ed. UK: Oxford University Press; 2019

[9] Fillit HM, Rockwood K, Young JB. Brocklehurst's Textbook of Geriatric Medicine and Gerontology. Philadelphia: Elsevier Health Sciences; 2016. p. 1168

[10] Balsa A, Diáz C. Social interactions in health behaviors and conditions. Published online: 26 March 2019. DOI: 10.1093/acrefore/9780190625979.013.17

[11] Hoogendijk EO, Afilalo J, Ensrud KE, et al. Frailty: Implications for clinical practice and public health. Lancet. 2019;**394**(10206):1365-1375

[12] Weber P. Ageing of old community (seniorization) and geriatrization of medicine (in Czech). Geri a Gero. 2018;**7**(4):152-155

[13] Krajčík Š, a kol. (Ed. in Slovac and Czech): Geriatria, 2. vydání, doplněné a přepracované. Bratislava: Herba; 2022. p. 584

[14] Ritt M, Ritt JI, Sieber CC, Gaßmann KG. Comparing the predictive accuracy of frailty, comorbidity, and disability for mortality: A 1-year follow-up in patients hospitalized in geriatric wards. Clinical Interventions in Aging. 2017;**12**:293-304

[15] Romero-Ortuno R, Wallis SJ, Biram RW, Keevil V. Clinical frailty adds to acute illness severity in predicting mortality in hospitalized older adults: An observational study. European Journal of Internal Medicine. 2016;**35**:24-34

[16] Weber P. Elderly Patients with Multi-Morbidity, Frailty and Geriatric Syndromes: Therapeutic Problem of Contemporary and Incoming Medicine at Intensive Care Unit (ICU) from the

Geriatricians Viewpoint. New York: Nova Science Publishers; 2011. p. 82

[17] Fried LP, Cohen AA, Xue QL, et al. The physical frailty syndrome as a transition from homeostatic symphony to cacophony. Nature Aging. 2021;**1**(1):36-46

[18] Kastner M, Cardoso R, Lai Y, Treister V, Hamid JS, Hayden L, et al. Effectiveness of interventions for managing multiple high-burden chronic diseases in older adults: A systematic review and meta-analysis. CMAJ. 2018;**190**(34):E1004-E1012

[19] Ghachem A, Fried LP, Legault V, Bandeen-Roche K, Presse N, Gaudreau P, et al. Evidence from two cohorts for the frailty syndrome as an emergent state of parallel dysregulation in multiple physiological systems. Biogerontology. 2021;**22**(1):63-79

[20] Laurindo LF, Barbalho SM, Guiguer EL, et al. GLP-1a: Going beyond traditional use. International Journal of Molecular Sciences. 2022;**23**(2):739

[21] Saito T, Watanabe M, Nishida J, et al. Zensharen study for prevention of lifestyle diseases group. Lifestyle modification and prevention of type 2 diabetes in overweight Japanese with impaired fasting glucose levels: A randomized controlled trial. Archives of Internal Medicine. 2011;**171**(15):1352-1360

[22] Billings LK, Parkin CG, Price D. Baseline glycated Hemoglobin values predict the magnitude of Glycemic improvement in patients with type 1 and type 2 diabetes: Subgroup analyses from the DIAMOND study program. Diabetes Technology & Therapeutics. 2018;**20**(8):561-565

[23] American Diabetes Association. 9. Pharmacologic approaches to Glycemic treatment: Standards of medical Care in Diabetes-2021. Diabetes Care. 2021;**44**(Suppl.1):S111-S124

[24] Weber P, Meluzínová H, Weberová D. New trends in the approach to the treatment of type 2 diabetes – Observations and benefits in the outpatient practice of a diabetologist (in Czech). Klinická Farmakologie a Farmacie. 2021;**35**(4):3-8

[25] Weber P, Meluzínová H, Weberová D. Trajectories of changes I – in the approach to oral hypoglycemic therapy of type 2 diabetes in post-productive age during the past 12 years – Our own experience (in Czech). Geri a Gero. 2020;**9**(3):61-65

[26] Sinclair AJ, Paolisso G, Castro M, et al. European diabetes working party for older people. European diabetes working party for older people 2011 clinical guidelines for type 2 diabetes mellitus. Executive summary. Diabetes & Metabolism. 2011;**37**(Suppl. 3):S27-S38

[27] Bramlage P, Gitt AK, Binz C, Krekler M, et al. Oral antidiabetic treatment in type-2 diabetes in the elderly: Balancing the need for glucose control and the risk of hypoglycemia. Cardiovascular Diabetology. 2012;**6**(10):111-122

[28] Fayfman M, Galindo RJ, Rubin DJ, et al. A randomized controlled trial on the safety and efficacy of exenatide therapy for the inpatient management of general medicine and surgery patients with type 2 diabetes. Diabetes Care. 2019;**42**(3):450-456

[29] Chon S, Rhee SY, Ahn KJ, et al. KIIT study investigators. Long-term effects on glycaemic control and β-cell preservation of early intensive treatment in patients with newly diagnosed type 2 diabetes: A multicentre randomized

trial. Diabetes, Obesity & Metabolism. 2018;**20**(5):1121-1130

[30] Mahaffey KW, Neal B, Perkovic V, et al. CANVAS program collaborative group. Canagliflozin for primary and secondary prevention of cardiovascular events: Results from the CANVAS program (Canagliflozin cardiovascular assessment study). Circulation. 2018;**137**(4):323-334

[31] Zelniker TA, Wiviott SD, Raz I, et al. Comparison of the effects of glucagon-like peptide receptor agonists and sodium-glucose cotransporter 2 inhibitors for prevention of major adverse cardiovascular and renal outcomes in type 2 diabetes mellitus. Circulation. 2019;**139**(17):2022-2031

[32] Charytan DM, Solomon SD, Ivanovich P, et al. Metformin use and cardiovascular events in patients with type 2 diabetes and chronic kidney disease. Diabetes, Obesity & Metabolism. 2019;**21**(5):1199-1208

[33] Mendes R, Sousa N, Themudo-Barata JL, Reis VM. High-intensity interval training versus moderate-intensity continuous training in middle-aged and older patients with type 2 diabetes: A randomized controlled crossover trial of the acute effects of treadmill walking on Glycemic control. International Journal of Environmental Research and Public Health. 2019;**16**(21):4163

[34] Rossello X, Ferreira JP, McMurray JJ, et al. Editor's choice-impact of insulin-treated diabetes on cardiovascular outcomes following high-risk myocardial infarction. European Heart Journal Acute Cardiovascular Care. 2019;**8**(3):231-241

[35] Yang Y, Xinhua H, Zhang Q, Zou R. Diabetes mellitus and risk of falls in older adults: A systematic review and meta-analysis. Age and Ageing. 2016;**45**(6):761-767

[36] Weber P, Weberová D, Matějovská Kubešová H, Meluzínová H, Jarkovský J, Bieláková K, et al. Falls in anaemic hospitalized elderly patients in 2012-2016–Mutual relationships. Advances in Gerontology. 2019;**32**(5):787-794

[37] Nooijen CFJ, Blom V, Ekblom O, et al. The effectiveness of multi-component interventions targeting physical activity or sedentary behaviour amongst office workers: A three-arm cluster randomised controlled trial. BMC Public Health. 2020;**20**(1):1329

[38] Zulman DM, Sussman JB, Chen X, Cigolle CT, Blaum CS, Hayward RA. Examining the evidence: A systematic review of the inclusion and analysis of older adults in randomized controlled trials. Journal of General Internal Medicine. 2011;**26**(7):783-790

[39] Loscalzo J, Fauci A, Kasper D, Hauser S, Longo D, Jameson JL. Harrison's Principles of Internal Medicine, Twenty-First Edition. 21st ed. Vol. 1 & 2. NY Chicago San Francisco Lisbon London Madrid Mexico City Milan New Delhi San Juan Seoul Singapore Sydney Toronto: McGraw Hill/ Medical; 2022. p. 4384

[40] Barrett K, Barman S, Yuan J, Brooks H. Ganong's Review of Medical Physiology. 26th ed. NY: McGraw Hill/ Medical; 2019. p. 752

[41] Nascimento CM, Ingles M, Salvador-Pascual A, et al. Sarcopenia, frailty and their prevention by exercise. Free Radical Biology & Medicine. 2019;**132**:42-49

[42] Cederholm T, Morley JE. Sarcopenia: The new definitions. Current Opinion in Clinical Nutrition and Metabolic Care. 2015;**18**(1):1-4

[43] Boyd CM, Darer J, Boult C, Fried LP, Boult L, Wu AW. Clinical practice guidelines and quality of care for older patients with multiple comorbid diseases: Implications for pay for performance. Journal of the American Medical Association. 2005;**294**(6):716-724

[44] Dansereau G, Wey TW, Legault V, et al. Conservation of physiological dysregulation signatures of aging across primates. Aging Cell. 2019;**18**(2):e12925

[45] Motta M, Bennati E, Ferlito L, Malaguarnera M. Diabetes mellitus in the elderly: Diagnostic features. Archives of Gerontology and Geriatrics. 2006;**42**:101-106

[46] Huang ES, Laiteerapong N, Liu JY, et al. Rates of complications and mortality in older patients with diabetes mellitus: The diabetes and aging study. JAMA Internal Medicine. 2014;**174**(2):251-258

[47] Ni Lochlainn M, Cox NJ, Wilson T. Nutrition and frailty: Opportunities for prevention and treatment. Nutrients. 2021;**13**(7):2349

[48] Azad N, Molnar F, Byszewski A. Lessons learned from a multidisciplinary heart failure clinic for older women: A randomised controlled trial. Age and Ageing. 2008;**37**(3):282-287

[49] Senni M, Tribouilloy CM, Rodeheffer RJ, et al. Congestive heart failure in the community: A study of all incident cases in Olmsted County, Minnesota, in 1991. Circulation. 1998;**98**(21):2282-2289

[50] American Geriatrics Society expert panel on the Care of Older Adults with multimorbidity. Guiding principles for the care of older adults with multimorbidity: An approach for clinicians. Journal of the American Geriatrics Society. 2012;**60**(10):E1-E25

[51] Rodríguez-Romero R, Herranz-Rodríguez C, Kostov B, et al. Intervention to reduce perceived loneliness in community-dwelling older people. Scandinavian Journal of Caring Sciences. 2021;**35**(2):366-374

[52] Inouye SK. Geriatric syndromes: Clinical, research, and policy implications of a Core geriatric concept. Journal of the American Geriatrics Society. 2007;**55**(5):780-791

[53] Expert Panel. American Geriatrics Society updated beers criteria for potentially inappropriate medication use in older adults. American Geriatrics Society 2012 beers criteria update. Journal of the American Geriatrics Society. 2012;**60**(4):616-631

[54] Jadad AR, Matthew JT, Emara M, Jones J. Consideration of multiple chronic diseases in randomized controlled trials. Journal of the American Medical Association. 2011;**306**(24):2670-2672

[55] Wein B, Seleznova Z, Mueller D, Naumann M, Loeser S, Artmann J, et al. Evaluation of the guideline-adherence of coronary angiography in patients with suspected chronic coronary syndrome - results from the German prospective multicentre ENLIGHT-KHK project. International Journal of Cardiology. Heart & Vasculature. 2023;**46**:101203. DOI: 10.1016/j.ijcha.2023.101203 eCollection 2023 Jun

[56] Emmett KR. Nonspecific and atypical presentation of disease in the older patient. Geriatrics. 1998;**53**(2):50-52

[57] Frohnhofen H, Stieglitz S. Lungenentzündung im Alter. Pneumologe (Berl). 2021;**18**(3):174-181

[58] Putot A, Prendki V. New horizons in sepsis management in older patients. Age and Ageing. 2023;**52**(2):afad016. DOI: 10.1093/ageing/afad016

[59] van Son JE, Kahn ECP, van der Bol JM, Barten DG, Blomaard LC, van Dam C, et al. Atypical presentation of COVID-19 in older patients is associated with frailty but not with adverse outcomes. European Geriatric Medicine. 2023;**14**(2):333-343

[60] Zhao Q, Yin K, Zhou N, Wu Q, Xiao Y, Zheng J, et al. The characteristics of thoracic aortic dissection in autopsy-diagnosed individuals: An autopsy study. Frontiers in Cardiovascular Medicine. 2022;**9**:973530. DOI: 10.3389/fcvm.2022.973530 eCollection 2022

[61] Boult C, Wieland GD. Comprehensive primary care for older patients with multiple chronic conditions: "Nobody rushes you through". Journal of the American Medical Association. 2010;**304**(17):1936-1943

[62] He J, Morales DR, Guthrie B. Exclusion rates in randomized controlled trials of treatments for physical conditions: A systematic review. 2020;**21**(1):228

[63] Skou ST, Nyberg M, Dideriksen M, Overgaard JA, Bodilsen C, Soja AM, et al. Study protocol for a multicenter randomized controlled trial of personalized exercise therapy and self-management support for people with multimorbidity: The MOBILIZE study. Journal of Multimorbidity & Comorbidity. 2023;**13**:26335565231154447. DOI: 0.1177/26335565231154447 eCollection 2023 Jan-Dec

[64] Eidam A, Roth A, Lacroix A, Goisser S, Seidling HM, Haefeli WE, et al. Methods to assess patient preferences in old age pharmacotherapy - a systematic review. Patient Preference and Adherence. 2020;**14**:467-497

[65] Gallagher P, O'Mahony D. STOPP (screening tool of older Persons' potentially inappropriate prescriptions): Application to acutely ill elderly patients and comparison with Beers' criteria. Age and Ageing. 2008;**37**(6):673-679

[66] Cott IA, Gray LC, Martin JH, Mitchell CA. Minimizing inappropriate medications in older populations: A 10-step conceptual framework. The American Journal of Medicine. 2012;**125**(6):529-537

[67] Gurwitz JH. Polypharmacy: A new paradigm for quality drug therapy in the elderly? Archives of Internal Medicine. 2004;**164**(18):1957-1959

[68] Steinman MA, Handler SM, Gurwitz JH, Schiff GD, Covinsky KE. Beyond the prescription: Medication monitoring and adverse drug events in older adults. Journal of the American Geriatrics Society. 2011;**59**(8):1513-1520

[69] Holmes HM, Hayley DC, Alexander GC, Sachs GA. Reconsidering medication appropriateness for patients late in life. Archives of Internal Medicine. 2006;**166**(6):605-609

[70] Aubert CE, Blum MR, Gastens V, Dalleur O, Vaillant F, Jennings E, et al. Prescribing, deprescribing and potential adverse effects of proton pump inhibitors in older patients with multimorbidity: An observational study. CMAJ Open. 2023;**11**(1):E170-E178. DOI: 10.9778/cmajo.20210240. Print 2023 Jan-Feb

[71] Reeve J, Maden M, Hill R, Turk A, Mahtani K, Wong G, et al. Deprescribing medicines in older people living with multimorbidity and polypharmacy: The TAILOR evidence synthesis. Health

Technology Assessment. 2022;**26**(32):1-148. DOI: 10.3310/AAFO2475

[72] Seewoodharry M, Khunti K, Davies MJ, Gillies C, Seidu S. Attitudes of older adults and their carers towards de-prescribing: A systematic review. Diabetic Medicine. 2022;**39**(7):e14801. DOI: 10.1111/dme.14801 Epub 2022 Feb 15

[73] Reeve E, Low L-F, Hilmer SN. Attitudes of older adults and caregivers in Australia toward deprescribing. Journal of the American Geriatrics Society. 2019;**67**(6):1204-1210

Section 3

Paradigm of Type 2 Diabetes Management

Chapter 10

Management of Type 2 Diabetes Mellitus

Leslie Bahn Kawa

Abstract

Type 2 diabetes mellitus is a complex metabolic disease with complex derangements of metabolic pathways that are involved in the glucose metabolism in different organs: the liver, muscles, pancreas, the gut, kidneys, fat cells and the brain. The objectives of the treatment of Type 2 diabetes mellitus are to reverse the underlying eight pathophysiologies called the 'ominous octet', achieve glycaemic control, control comorbidities and prevent or reduce the chronic complications. Lifestyle management and pharmacotherapy remain the mainstay of treatment of Type 2 diabetes mellitus. The development of the newer oral hypoglycaemic agents such as the sodium-glucose transporters 2 receptor inhibitors, the dipeptidyl peptidase 4 inhibitors and the injectables such as the glucagon-like peptide 1 receptor agonists and the analogue insulin in the last decades has provided broad and extended treatment options to achieve the treatment objectives. The recent announcement of the novel combinational peptides, Tirzapatide and Rezatrutide, promises a new era of pharmacotherapy for T2DM.

Keywords: type 2 diabetes mellitus, pharmacological management, drug treatment, oral hypoglycaemic agents, insulin therapy of type 2 diabetes

1. Introduction

Diabetes is a metabolic condition associated with elevated blood sugar levels because of either a relative or an absolute insulin deficiency [1]. Type 2 diabetes mellitus (T2DM) is now known to develop from disturbances in the glucose metabolic pathways in the muscles, liver, pancreas, gut, fat cells, kidneys and brain. These core pathophysiological pathways are called the 'ominous octet'; insulin resistance in the muscles and liver, ßeta cell failure, α-cell hyperplasia with glucagonoma, gastrointestinal incretin resistance/failure, accelerated lipolysis in fat cells, increased uptake of glucose via SGLT2 receptors in the kidneys and insulin resistance in the brain [2–4]. Additionally, cardiovascular risk factors such as smoking, high blood pressure, and depression are also known to be associated with the increased risks in the development of T2DM [5].

Treatment of T2DM essentially aims to address the environmental risk factors with lifestyle modifications (LSM). Primary and secondary preventative approaches with dietary, exercise and combined interventions have been shown to reduce T2DM among those at high risk and even remit T2DM in those with overt diabetes [6–9]. Pharmacological treatment of T2DM, on the other hand, aims at reversing the core

 IntechOpen

pathological mechanisms through a multidrug therapeutic approach [2] recommended by the current international diabetes guidelines on pharmacotherapy of T2DM.

The development of newer oral hypoglycaemics, the sodium-glucose transporters 2 receptor inhibitors (SGLT2R-i), oral glucagon-like peptide 1 receptor agonists (GLP1-RA), the injectables, the dipeptidyl peptidase-4 inhibitors (DPP4-i) and the analogue insulins have expanded the pharmacological armamentarium of the treatment of T2DM. In addition to their targeted actions on the core pathophysiology of T2DM, the SGLT2R-i, GLP1-RA and DPP4-i classes of drugs provide pleiotropic benefits in reducing the comorbidities associated with T2DM, such as obesity, hypertension and dyslipidaemia [10–13]. Moreover, studies have also shown that these drugs, especially the SGLT2R-i and the GLP1-RA protect and improve renal and cardiac functions [14–17].

The insulin analogues also have better efficacies and safety and offer patients greater flexibility in the management of diabetes [18–20]. Additionally, the improvement in the different insulin delivery systems has made insulin easy for patients to use to achieve optimal glycaemic control in both types of diabetes [21–23].

This chapter reviews the treatment modalities of T2DM (LSM + pharmacotherapy) with specific emphasis on pharmacotherapy (oral, injectables and insulin) and their roles and hierarchy in the contemporary pharmacological management of T2DM and their modes of delivery to reverse the pathophysiological mechanisms, achieve effective glycaemic control and reduce complications and comorbidities.

2. Pillars of treatment

The great diabetologist of the century, Elliot Joslin said "The three pillars of T2DM are Dieting, Exercise and Pharmacotherapy." Dieting and exercise prescriptions are collectively called 'lifestyle modifications' (LSM) and are fundamental to the management of T2DM. Recent preventative trials among the prediabetic populations have shown that glycaemic control is achievable with LSM [6–9] and improves glycaemic control among overt T2DM patients [24–26]. Combined exercise and dieting have more pronounced effects on the glycaemic control, comorbidities and patient's quality of life (QoL) than individually. The effects are more prominent with supervised exercise than with the unsupervised exercise regimen [27–29].

2.1 Dietary prescription

Dietary prescription is an integral part of the LSM strategy for all T2DM patients; however, there is no standardised dietary regimen. Therefore, dietary prescription is personalised according to the local availability with the caveat of eating healthy (more vegetables, less carbohydrates and alcohol). The Mediterranean diet is a dietary practise prevalent among the countries bordering the Mediterranean Sea. Whilst it has no specific definition, it is rich in vegetables, fruits, nuts, whole grains and olive oil. This diet has been extensively studied, and a meta-analysis of these studies shows that it is associated with reduced blood pressure, cholesterol and heart attacks [30]. Another meta-analysis shows that it significantly prevents diabetes among those at high risk of developing T2DM and confers optimal control of those with established T2DM [31]. Diet alone, however, has minimal effect [6] but dietary prescription with exercise does have a greater impact on the glycaemic control, improvement of other comorbidities and the quality of life (QoL) of patients [7]. The Mediterranean diet, therefore, provides a great dietary option for people with diabetes (**Figure 1**).

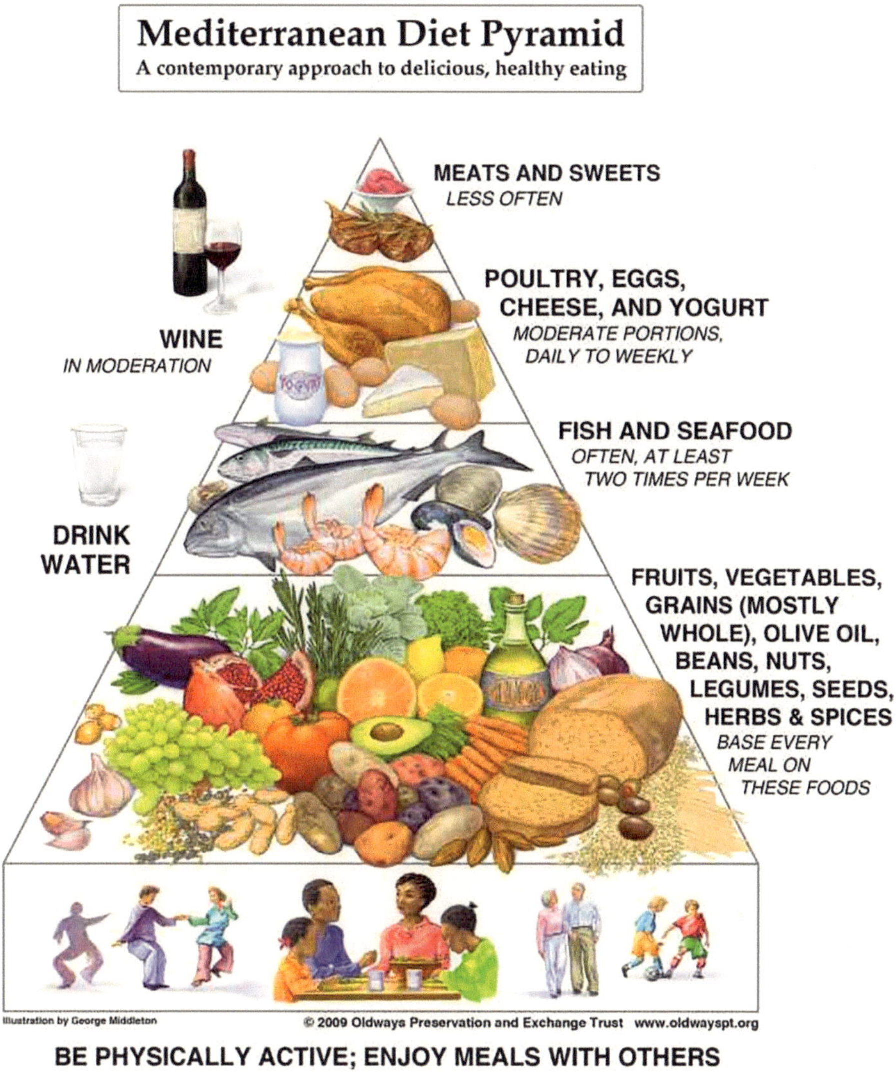

Figure 1.
Mediterranean diet pyramid. Image adapted from Oldways.

2.2 Exercise prescription

Although supervised and unsupervised exercise regimens have been shown to reduce T2DM among those with impaired fasting glucose (IFG), the Italian Diabetes Exercise Study (IDES) showed that the supervised group had significant improvement in blood sugar, blood pressure, cholesterol control, weight reduction and improved physical fitness [27]. These are further supported by a meta-analysis showing that supervised aerobic or resistance exercises improve glycaemic control in T2DM regardless of dietary prescription [28]. Supervised exercise, therefore, leads to better outcomes, lending the term 'exercise prescription' for the management of T2DM.

2.3 Pharmacotherapy

Studies have shown that optimal pharmacological management of T2DM based on the HBA1c leads to the reduction in chronic complications [32–34]. Treatment guidelines recommend that management of T2DM also consider the management of cardiovascular risk factors and other comorbidities [35–37] as shown in **Figure 2**. However, the guidelines do not provide specific recommendations on the selection and titration of the pharmacological therapeutics [35, 36] but rather a multifactorial management approach and thereby provide a hierarchy of pharmacological escalation [37, 38] as shown in **Figure 3**, with the choice of diabetic drug selection and titration dependent on the patient's clinical profile, preferences, comorbidities and the likelihood of its long-term benefits [37].

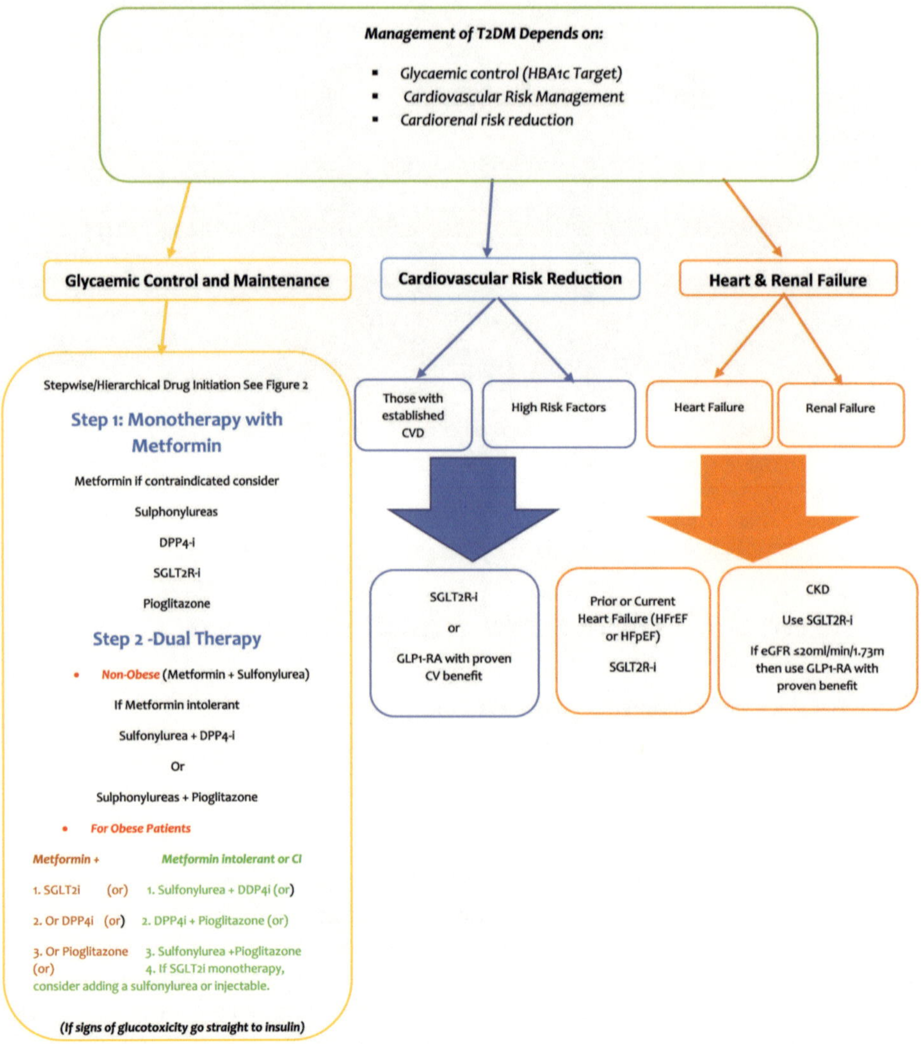

Figure 2.
Pharmacological management of T2DM according to patient profile.

DOI: http://dx.doi.org/10.5772/intechopen.1002478

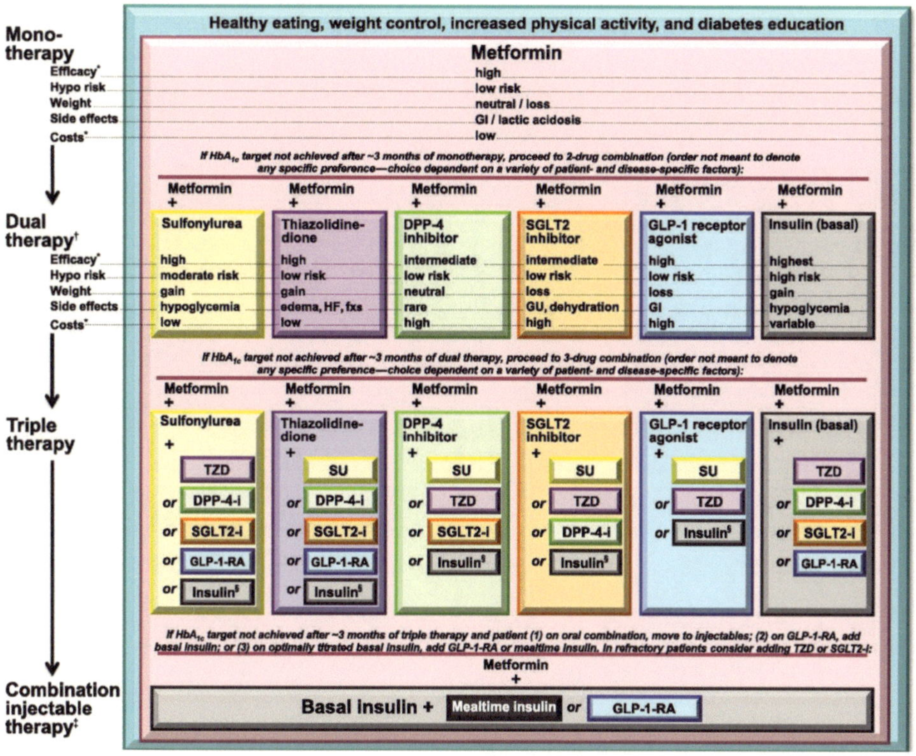

Figure 3.
Hierarchical of treatment escalation. Adapted from Inzucchi et al. [39].

The drugs in this section are reviewed as traditional or new hypoglycemic agents in order of their guideline hierarchy (**Table 1**).

2.3.1 Hypoglycaemic agents

The hypoglycaemic agents have been the mainstay of the pharmacological management of the T2DM for over half a century and remain relevant today. In fact, they are either first and or second-line treatments according to current treatment guidelines.

2.3.1.1 Traditional oral hypoglycaemic agents (OHGA)

The traditional classes of OHGA have been in use since the 1960s for their glycaemic control. In 1998, the United Kingdom Prospective Diabetes Study (UKPDS) showed that sulfonylurea, metformin, and human insulin could reduce the chronic complications of T2DM [32] and demonstrated long-term metabolic benefits of metformin. Studies of the thiazolidinediones class of drugs have also shown significant glycaemic control and conferred other benefits, including the reduction of cardiovascular events [40–42]. The current traditional classes of the OHGA in practice are, in their order of hierarchy on the guidelines, biguanide, sulfonylureas and thiazolidinediones.

Class	Agents (route of administration)	Cellular mechanisms	Primary physiological actions	Advantages	Disadvantages	Cost
Biguanides	Metformin Metformin XR (oral)	Activates AMP—kinase (others!)	• Reduces hepatic glucose production	• Extensive experiences • Rare hypoglycaemia • Reduces CV events [39] • High HBA1c efficacy	• Gastric distress (nausea, vomiting, abdominal cramps) • Vitamin B12 deficiency • CI in eGFR <30 ml/min/1.73 m^2, acidosis, hypoxia, dehydration etc. • Lactic acidosis (rare)	Low
GLP1-RAs	*Albiglutide* *Dulaglutide* *Exenatide* *Exenatide XR* *Liraglutide* *Lixisenetide* *(Subcutaneous injection)*	Activates GLP1-R	• ↑ insulin secretion (glucose-dependent) • Reduces gluca-gon secretion (glucose-dependent) • Slows gastric emptying. • Increases satiety	• Rare hypoglycaemia • Reduces weight • Reduces PPG excursion • Reduces some CV risk factors • Reduces CV events in patients with CVD [10, 11]	• Gastric distress (nausea, vomiting, abdominal pain) • ↑Heart rate • Acute pancreatitis? • C-cell hyperplasia/med-ullary thyroid tumours in animals • Injectable • Training required	High
SGLT2-i	Canagliflozin Dapagliflozin Empagliflozin Ertugliflozin Sotagliflozin (oral)	Inhibits SGLT2R in proximal renal tubule	• Blocks glucose reabsorption in the kidneys increasing glucosuria	• Rare hypoglycaemia • Reduce weight • Reduce BP • Reduce HFH, mortality [14–16]	• Genitourinary infection • Polyuria • Volume depletion/hypotension/dizziness • ↑LDL-C • Transient hypercreatinemia • Euglycemic DKA	High

DOI: http://dx.doi.org/10.5772/intechopen.1002478

Class	Agents (route of administration)	Cellular mechanisms	Primary physiological actions	Advantages	Disadvantages	Cost
DPP4-i	*Vildagliptin* *Alogliptin* *Linagliptin* *Sitagliptin* *Saxagliptin* *(Oral)*	Inhibits DPP4 activity. Increasing postprandial incretins (GLP1, GIP) concentration	• ↑insulin secretion (Glucose-dependent) • ↑glucagon secretion (Glucose-dependent)	• Rare hypoglycaemia • Well tolerated	• Angioedema/Urticaria • Acute pancreatitis? • HFH (Saxaglitin, Alogliptin?)	High
Sulfonylurea	Second generation Glibenclamide Glipizide Gliclazide Glimepiride (Oral)	Closes KATP channels on beta cell membrane	• ↑insulin secretion	• Extensive experiences • Reduces microvascular risks [32] • High HBA1c efficacy	• Hypoglycaemia • ↑weight	Low
TZDs	Pioglitazone Rosiglitazone (oral)	Activates the nuclear transcription factor (PPAR-y)	• ↑Insulin sensitivity	• Rare hypoglycaemia • High HBA1c efficacy • Durability • Reduces Triglycerides • Reduces CV events [40] • Reduces risks of stroke and MI in patients without diabetes and insulin resistance and with recent stroke or TIA [41, 42]	• ↑weight • Edema/HFH • Bone fracture • ↑LDL-C (Rosiglitazone)	Low
Biagonist	Tirzepatide® [43, 44]	GLP1-RA and GIPRA	• Increase exogenous GLP1 and GIP levels and effects	• Single weekly dose • Provides same but better benefits as GLP1RA	• Mild gastrointestinal symptoms	Not known

Class	Agents (route of administration)	Cellular mechanisms	Primary physiological actions	Advantages	Disadvantages	Cost
Trigonist	Retatrutide® [45–48]	GLP1-RA, GIPRA and a glucagon agonist	Increase exogenous GLP1, GIP and glucagon levels and effects.	• Provides the same but benefits as GLP1RA. • Single weekly dose	• Mild gastrointestinal symptoms	Not known

Reproduced from Thrasher.
AMP = adenosine mono phosphate, CV = cardiovascular, DKA = diabetes ketoacidosis, HFH = heart failure hospitalisation, CI = contraindications, LDL-C = low density lipoprotein- cholesterol, KATP = potassium adenosine phosphate channel, PPP-y = peroxisome proliferator-activated receptor gamma.
® Combination compound received approval. Not on the current diabetic guidelines.
GLP1-RA = glucagon-like peptide 1-receptor agonist, GIPRA = glucagon insulinotropic dependent peptide receptor agonist.

Table 1.
Non-insulin drugs used in the treatment of type 2 diabetes mellitus.

2.3.1.1.1 Metformin

Metformin is a traditional oral hypoglycaemic agent and the only biguanide currently in use in the management of T2DM. It is the first drug recommended by all guidelines for the treatment of T2DM and the prevention of overt diabetes among the high-risk prediabetes population [49]. It is cheap and readily available in all healthcare systems.

It inhibits hepatic gluconeogenesis, increases insulin sensitivity, decreases glycogenolysis, reduces fatty acid oxidation, facilitates glucose disposal, and protects the cardiovascular system from effects of hyperglycaemia [50–52]. Metformin in the intensive arm with sulphonylureas/insulin vs. standard arm in the UKPDS showed a significant reduction in the microvascular complication (retinopathy, nephropathy, and neuropathy) by 25% with a median HBA1c of 7% compared with the conventional therapy with a median HBA1c of 7.9% [32]. The 10-year follow-up epidemiological analysis of the patient's taken metformin showed persistent correlation between glycaemic control and their clinical outcomes [39]. For every percentage decrease in HBA1c, there was a 25% reduction in diabetes-related deaths and 7% reduction in both fatal and non-fatal myocardial infarction and an 18% reduction in all-cause lending the term 'metformin's metabolic memory' [39]. Additionally, metformin shows pleiotropic effects in the improvement of endothelial function, redistribution in lipid and fat metabolisms, stress oxidation and homeostasis [53].

The common side effect of metformin relates to gastric distress (nausea and vomiting). This can be overcome by slow titration of the doses over weeks or by using the slow-release form called glucophage. Metformin can be used in patients with an eGFR of <60mls/min/1.73m^2 but it is advised that benefits versus risks must be weighted in those with eGFR of 30 – 45mls/min/1.73m^2 [54].

2.3.1.1.2 Sulphonylurea

Sulphonylurea is a class of traditional oral hypoglycaemic drugs used in the treatment of T2DM since the 1960s. It binds on the K+ channel of the pancreatic beta-cell and prevents K+ exit. This depolarises the cell, causing an influx of Ca2+, which causes the fusion of insulin granules with the cell membrane, leading to the exudation of insulin into the blood [55]. The sulphonylureas, unlike many other oral Type 2 Diabetes hypoglycaemic agents, are 'glucose independent' meaning they can cause hypoglycaemia even in the stage of low plasma glucose.

They are categorised into two generational classes based on their efficacies, hypoglycaemic and cardiovascular effects [56]. The first generation is no longer in use because of increased adverse effects.

First generation

- Chlorpropamide
- Tolbutamide

Second generation

- Glibenclamide
- Glipizide

- Gliclazide
- Glimepiride

The sulphonylureas only work in patients who have preserved ßeta cell function, but they do not have any effects on those with declining and or absent functions. They are recommended as a second-class oral hypoglycaemic agent on the ADA/EASD guideline to be used either as an alternative to metformin if contraindicated as monotherapy or either as dual or triple therapy [11, 36, 38].

Their use with metformin and insulin in the UKPDS shows significant reduction of microvascular complications, underscoring the importance of early intensive management [32]. However, whether the effect is specific of sulfonylurea is not known. Their effects wane over 6 months of continuous treatment and return if restarted after a pause. Furthermore, there were some cardiovascular concerns about their effects of negating the protective effects of preconditioning [57–61]. However, systematic reviews do not show any such effects [62]. Their other adverse effects include a modest weight gain [62]. They are, however, cheap, accessible, and readily available in many under resourced healthcare systems and remain fundamental in the management of T2DM.

2.3.1.1.3 Thiazolidinediones (glitazones)

The glitazones are insulin sensitisers and have a high glucose efficacy [63] with an internuclear mechanism of action. They bind on peroxisome proliferator-activated receptors (PPARγ) in the nucleus, leading to the translation of increased GLUT-4 receptors on adipocytes, liver and muscle cells, which increases the glucose uptake [64]. The PRoActive study suggested that pioglitazone reduces cardiovascular diseases [40] and stroke [41, 42] and has a beneficial effect on non-alcoholic fatty liver disease. The risks and benefits must be weighed out before initiation. The risks include weight gain, bone fracture, fluid retention and heart failure.

Rosiglitazone was shown to precipitate an increased incidence of heart failure [65]. This led to the withdrawal of rosiglitazone from the market in 2008. Consequentially, the FDA released new criteria to all pharmaceutical companies to ensure all diabetic drugs are tested for cardiovascular safety as an integral safety assurance for meeting the FDA criteria. The data from the study by Nissen et al. was later reviewed, and restriction has now been relaxed [66] with an FDA recommendation for the use of rosiglitazone together with lifestyle modification in the management of T2DM.

The glitazones are second and or third line of drugs on the treatment guidelines recommendations. However, pioglitazone and rosiglitazone can still be used as a monotherapy if metformin is contraindicated or not tolerated as the first option. The decision must be balanced between glycaemic efficacy and its side effect profile.

2.3.1.2 New Hypoglycaemic agents

The incretin mimetics, SGLT2R-i, biagonist tirzapatide and the investigational triagonist rezatrutide are four new classes of diabetic drugs that possess pleiotropic effects in addition to their hypoglycaemic effects.

The incretin mimetics includes the GLP1-RA and the DPP4-i. The incretin mimetics specifically the GLP1-RA negate some of the pathophysiological processes of T2DM at the gut, pancreas and at the brain levels. They have better glycaemic efficacies and are safe. Additionally, they have cardiorenal protective effects and reduce obesity, hypertension and dyslipidaemia associated with T2DM.

The SGLT2R-i is a glucosuric class with extended pleiotropic effects. It reduces cardiovascular risk factors, heart failure hospitalisation in both the diabetic and the non-diabetic patients. Additionally, it reduces the progression of renal failure in chronic renal failure patients, though with an initial 'permissive hypercreatinemia'. This class, however, has not been studied in patients with eGFR $\leq$20mls/min/1.73m^2.

The groundbreaking combined drugs (Tirzepatitde and investigational Rezatrutide) offer optimism of a new era in the pharmacological treatment of T2DM with extended-spectrum over and above the incretin mimetics.

These new classes of hypoglycaemic agents in their order of hierarchy are GLP1-RA, SGLT2R-i, DPP4-i, Bi-agonist—Tirzepatitide and Triagonist—Rezatrutide.

2.3.1.2.1 Glucagon-like peptide 1 receptor agonists (GLP1-RA)

GLP1 is an incretin peptide secreted from the L-cells of the distal ileum and colon in response to glucose in the stomach. It has pleiotropic effects on many organs including stimulation of pancreatic insulin release, reduction in glucagon, delays gastric emptying, causes early satiety through its effect on the satiety centre in the hypothalamus and reduces liver glycogenolysis [67]. Its effects are terminated by the dipeptidyl peptidase 4 enzyme (DPP4) within 2 minutes of secretion.

The GLP1-RA are synthetic analogues of the native GLP1 that are stable and have improved biological and pharmacokinetic effects [68]. They are mostly injectables with one oral preparation (semaglutide), and they have a glucose-dependent action, which reduces the risks of hypoglycaemia unless used concomitantly with sulphonylureas or insulin. They are two classes of GLP_1-RA based on their duration of actions:

a. Short acting GLP1-RA (half-life 2–5 h)

- Lixisenatide
- Exenatide
- Dulaglutide

b. Long acting GLP1-RA (half-life >12 h)

- Albiglutide
- Liraglutide
- Exenatide extended release
- Semaglutide
- Dulaglutide

The long-acting GLP1-RA have a predominant effect on the fasting plasma glucose (FPG) whilst the short-acting acts predominantly on the postprandial glucose excursion [68].

The head-to-head trials of the short- and long-acting GLP1-RA show that the long-acting class achieves better glycaemic control and cardiovascular risk factor reduction in addition to reducing the major adverse cardiovascular events (MACE) compared with the shorter class [10, 11]. A meta-analysis of all studies further suggests that the long-acting GLP1-RA has effective HBA1c reduction, with more patients achieving their HBA1c targets, increased weight loss, and fewer hypoglycaemic episodes compared with the short-acting GLP1-RA [69].

The commonest side effect of the GLP1-RA is gastric distress (nausea, vomiting and diarrhoea), which tends to diminish as treatment progresses into the second week [70]. Education on mindful eating (eating small at a time, only when hungry and stopping when full) and gradual titration of drug dosages help overcome these effects. Preclinical studies have suggested increased thyroid malignancies [71–73], but no human trials have demonstrated any trends. Post-marketing pancreatitis has also been reported as a complication, but no causal relationship has been established [70]. However, it is prudent not to prescribe in those with a history of pancreatitis or acute pancreatitis. Caution should be exercised in prescribing GLP1-RA for those with moderate renal failure. It is not recommended for those with end-stage renal failure [74, 75].

2.3.1.2.1.1 Personalised management of T2DM using GLP1-RA

The GLP1-RA is now used in combination therapy with other treatments for both glycaemic control and management of other comorbidities. For example, liraglutide 3 mg once weekly and semaglutide 2.4 mg once weekly are currently recommended for chronic weight management [12, 13]. Liraglutide and semaglutide can be used to reduce major adverse cardiovascular events (MACE) as shown in the LEADER and SUSTAIN-6 studies respectively [10, 11]. The PIONEER study, however, showed that oral semaglutide was non-inferior to injectable liraglutide in glycaemic control but was superior in reducing weight [76]. This finding shows that oral semaglutide can be used earlier in T2DM to provide comparative glycaemic control, used as a weight reducing drug among those with T2DM with obesity and reduce patient's needle phobia to overcome patient's clinical inertia. The initial dose of semaglutide is 3 mg oral daily for 30 days. If more glycaemic control is required, then the dose is escalated to 7 mg daily for another 30 days. Further escalation to 14 mg once daily if more glycaemic and weight control is required [77]. The initiation dose is 3 mg and maintenance doses are 7 and 14 mg oral once daily.

The use of GLP1-RA with insulin as a fixed-dose combination is a novel strategy that offers several potential benefits for patients with T2DM whereby weight gain and hypoglycaemic effects of insulin are negated and insulin doses are often reduced. In November 2016, the US Food and Drug Authority (FDA) approved two fixed-dose combinations of insulin and GLP1-i for this purpose.

- IDeGLira/Xutolpy (Degludec + Liraglutide)
- iGlarLixi (Glargine + Lixisenatide)

2.3.1.2.2 Sodium-glucose transporters 2 receptor inhibitors (SGLT2R-i)

The SGLT2R-i is a new class of oral hypoglycaemia drug approved for use in patients with T2DM as dual and or triple therapy. Canagliflozin was the first in the class to be approved in 2013 [78, 79] followed by others. The SGLT2R-i drugs currently on the market are:

- Dapagliflozin
- Empagliflozin
- Canagliflozin
- Ertugliflozin
- Sotagliflozin

The sodium glucose transporters 2 receptors (SGLT2R) in the kidneys reabsorbed all filtered glucose. 90% of the receptors are in the proximal convoluted tubules and 10% in the distal convoluted tubules. Evidence suggests that they are increased in patients with T2DM, which leads to increased plasma glucose reabsorption [79]. The SGLT2R-i binds to these SGLT2R in the proximal convoluted renal tubules and prevents the reabsorption of 90% of the filtered glucose from the blood. They have a high glycaemic efficacy in non-renal failure patients.

They gained prominence when the EMPA-Reg trial in 2015, using empagliflozin with standard care in patients with T2DM at high risk of cardiovascular events, showed a relative risk reduction (RRR) of 38% in cardiovascular mortality, 35% RRR in heart failure hospitalisation (HFH) and 32% RRR in all-cause mortality [14]. This was supported by the DECALRE-TIMI 58 trial, which showed that dapagliflozin although not inferior to placebo in the reduction of the MACE, did reduce cardiovascular death by 4.9%, HFH by 5.8% and improved cardiovascular risk factors among the T2DM with high risk of cardiovascular events [15]. Further, the use of this class in heart failure has shown that even those T2DM patients with heart failure derive significant clinical benefits compared with standard care. The DAPA-HF trial among T2DM patients with chronic heart failure with reduced ejection fraction (HFrEF) showed a 16% RRR in heart failure mortality and HFH by 3.7% [16]. Similar findings were noted among those without diabetes. Additionally, the EMPEROR Reduced trial attested to the findings of the DAPA-HF trial with additional findings of reduction in the deterioration of renal function [17]. These studies, therefore, demonstrate that the SGLT2R-i offers high-risk T2DM patients with or without heart failure, significant benefit of reduction of HFH and mortality with additional renoprotective effect in those with chronic renal failure. Patients with eGFR $\leq$20 ml/min/1.73 m^2 however, were not included in these trials.

The common side effects of the SGLT2R-i are uncomplicated urethral mycotic infection. Education with basic advice to patients before initiation such as the slogan "wee, wash and dry" will help reduce the risk. Another notable side effect is euglycemic ketoacidosis, noted as a class effect. The incidence is very low [80] and the CV outcome trials report DKA rates between 0.1% and 0.6% compared with < 0.1-0.3% among the placebo [79–83]. Although the FDA has raised concerns about foot amputation and reduced mineral bone density with canagliflozin, these have not been demonstrated in the heart failure trials.

2.3.1.2.3 Dipeptidyl peptidase 4 inhibitors (DPP4-i)

The DPP4-i is a new class of drug used in T2DM. They are available as single drugs and or fixed-dose combinations to be used as monotherapy or combination therapy. The following are currently on the market:

- Vildagliptin
- Alogliptin
- Linagliptin
- Sitagliptin
- Saxagliptin Fixed-dose combinations are:
- Kazano = alogliptin/metformin (12.5 mg/50 or 1000 mg) bd daily.
- Janumet = sitagliptin/metformin has various strengths (50 mg/500 mg, 50 mg/ 1000 mg, 100 mg/1000 mg) bd daily.
- Galvus Met = vildagliptin/metformin (50 mg/500 mg or 50 mg/1000 mg).

Their mechanism of action is based on the reduction of the DPP4 enzymatic degradation of the GLP_1 and GIP [84], which thereby prolongs the duration of actions of these incretins. Although they have effects on both the fasting plasma glucose (FPG) and the postprandial glucose (PPG), their effect on the PPG is prominent. They are glucose-dependent and therefore do not cause hypoglycaemia unless combined with other hypoglycaemic agents. They reduce blood pressure by a mean of 2.5 mmHg and have modest effect on the HBA1c reduction by 0.5–1% [85]. A meta-analysis of 80 trials has shown a mean change of HBA1c from −0.6% to −1.1% [12]. They are weight neutral [86] but reduce albuminuria progression with linagliptin [87]. Whilst generally tolerated, saxagliptin has been shown to increase HFH [88] and thus has precautionary warning. Arthralgia and hypersensitivity reactions are rare and are reported as class effect [89].

2.3.1.2.4 Biagonist—Tirzepatide

Tirzepatide is a novel bi-agonist composed of GLP1-RA and glucagon-dependent insulinotropic peptide (GIP) engineered from the native GIP. It has effects on both the GLP1R and glucagon-dependent insulinotropic receptor (GIPPR). It was approved by the Food Drug Administration (FDA) for T2DM in March 2022 [90] and the European Medicine Agency in September 2022 [91]. A phase III randomised controlled trial comparing Tirzepatide doses of 5 mg, 10 mg and 15 mg weekly injection with semaglutide 1 mg once weekly injection showed that Tirzepatide at all doses was superior in glycaemic control and weight reduction compared with semaglutide [92]. Another phase III randomised controlled trial among the non-diabetic obese patients with body mass index (BMI) of ≥ 30 or ≥ 27 + one obesity complication showed that all doses of Tirzepatide (5 mg, 10 mg, 10 mg) once weekly injection showed a significant and sustained reduction in body weight of 33.9% compared with placebo in the intention to treat analysis [43]. As suggested by Chavda et al., Tirzepatide could set the stage for a new era of dual-targeted therapy for diabetes and obesity [44].

2.3.1.2.5 Trigonist—Retatrutide

Retatrutide is another novel investigational therapy recently presented in the 83rd American Diabetes Association Scientific Session in San Diego on the 26th of June 2023. It is a triple therapy that is composed of a GLP1-RA, GIPR agonist and a glucagon agonist. It is one of the game-breaking agents in clinical trials for the treatment of T2DM with obesity [45–47]. It has also been shown to improve fat oxidation, mitochondrial function and reduces fibrosis in those with non-alcoholic steatohepatitis (NASH), a condition common among 5–7% of patients with T2DM. Nine out of ten patients with diabetes with concomitant NASH had normalised liver fats on MRI after 48 weeks of high doses of retatrutide [48]. This suggests that retatrutide has the potential to treat T2DM with obesity and NASH [93, 94].

3. Insulin therapy of Type 2 diabetes mellitus

Insulin is secreted in a bimodal fashion by the pancreatic beta cells to control the basal and the postprandial glucose excursion. Exogenous insulin is administered in different regimens such as the basal bolus and the basal plus regimens to simulate the physiological secretion.

Therapy for T2DM patients is indicated for those whose glycaemic control is poor despite being on other treatments. Other criteria include clinical symptoms and signs of glucotoxicities (polyuria, polydipsia, polyphagia and weight loss), HBA1c ≥9%, RBSL 16 mmol/L, uncontrolled glycemia despite optimal glycaemic therapy and acute myocardial infarction [95].

Insulin therapy in T2DM has traditionally been thought of as the last-line therapy. In fact, the current treatment guidelines categorise insulin therapy for T2DM as either second or third-line therapy [96, 97]. Recent studies have however shown that early insulinisation of T2DM patients results in beta cell preservation and clinical remission [32, 96, 98]. Therefore, insulin therapy can be initiated early in T2DM. There are, however, no specific recommendations for the initiation, titration and maintenance of insulin therapy in those with T2DM.

3.1 Insulin types, dosages and regimens

Insulins are categorised according to their duration of action (**Table 2**).

Human insulins have generally been shown to improve glycaemic control in diabetes [32–34]. The new analogue insulin, however, has better safety and efficacy compared with human insulins. Chlup et al. have shown that short-acting analogue insulin aspart was efficacious with better patient's acceptance than regular human insulin [18]. Further, studies show that a basal plus insulin regimen with aspart insulin was better [19] and more effective [20] in glycaemic control compared with basal insulin.

Intensive insulin treatment of T2DM has significantly reduced chronic complications [33, 34]. The Diabetes Control and Complication Trial (DCCT) among the T1Dm patient showed that patients with multiple drug injections (MDI)

Insulin class*	Onset of action	Peak	Duration of action	When to use
Ultra short acting*	15 min	1 h	2–4 h	Administered at mealtimes, just before or after the meals
Lispro (Humalog)†	15 min	30–90 min	3 – 5 h	
Aspart (Novarapid)†	15 min	1–3 h	4 – 5 h	
Glulisine (Aphidra)	15–30 min	30–60 min	4 h	
Short-acting*	30 min	2–3 h	3–6 h	Administered 30 min before meals or after if unpredictable
Humulin S (Actrapid)	30 min	1.5–2.5 h		
Insuman Rapid	30 min			
Intermediate acting* Humulin Human insulatard Isophane	2–4 h	4–12 h	12–18 h	Administered twice daily. Not dependent on meals
Long acting*	2 h	Do not peak	*Up to 24 h*	Administered once a day and not dependent on meals
Glargine	6 h	No peak	24 h	
Determir	1–2 h	No peak	14–24 h	
Degludec	1–2 h	No peak	>40 h	
Fixed dose*	5–6mins	Variable peaks	10–16 h	Administered twice daily with food as basal insulin plus regimen
Humalog mix • 25 (Lispro + Protamine) • Humalog Mix 50 (Lispro + Protamine)	30–60 min	(Lispro +Protamine)	10–16 h	
Novamix (Aspart + Protamine) • Novamix 30 • Novamix 50	5–15 min	Dual (Protamine + Aspart)	10–16 min	
NPH (Isophane + Regular insulin) • 70/30 • 50/50	30–60 min	Dual (NPH/ Regular)	10–16 h	
Mixtard (soluble insulin + Isophane) • 30/70 • 40/60 • 50/50	30 min	Dual (soluble insulin + isophane)	10–16 h	
Degludec/Aspart (70/30)	15 min	Dual (Degludec + Aspart)	>40 h	

**Times are approximate and assume subcutaneous. The effects can vary depending on several factors such as injection technique and factors affecting absorption.*
†Lispro and aspart are also available in premixed forms with intermediate-acting insulins.

Table 2.
Pharmacokinetics of different classes of insulins and time to use.

although had greater glycaemic control with a significant reduction of the rates of chronic complications, the episodes of severe hypoglycaemia were significant [97]. Many patients with MDI continue to have erratic fluctuations of plasma glucose.

Criteria	Definition	Dosage
Argumentation	Argumentation of relative insulin deficiency with basal or bolus insulin	0.1–0.5 units/kg
Replacement	Replacement of absolute insulin deficiency with either in T1DM or T2DM with, basal, premix or bolus insulin	0.6–1 units/kg
Carbohydrate Count	Amount of insulin units estimated to cover ingested carbohydrate	500 g of carbohydrate divided by total daily insulin requirement
Insulin sensitivity/correction factor	1 unit of insulin estimated to normalise glucose to defined level	100 divided by total daily insulin dose

Table 3.
Insulin dose calculation.

The OpT2Mis study suggested that continuous insulin infusion via insulin pump for patients with erratic blood sugar fluctuations was safe, effective [21], and a durable system of insulin delivery for patients with T2DM [22]. A meta-analysis demonstrated the superior glycaemic control and a 26% insulin reduction by continuous insulin infusion compared with MDI [23]. In the United Kingdom, the continuous insulin infusion pump costs between £2000 and £3000 depending on the supplier.

Simultaneous delivery of multiple insulins is another method of improving insulin delivery and reducing MDI. Studies suggest that improvement of the delivery systems of multiple insulins simultaneously could potentially improve patient insulin inertia, needle phobia and improve compliance. An intensive insulin regimen with a simple manual-operated injector pen for MDI was found to be less painful and very convenient for patients with T2DM [23]. Further, a small Danish study also showed that multiple insulin injection regimens using a self-contained injection device Novopen showed good glycaemic control and patient satisfaction. Out of ten patients who completed the study, eight expressed satisfaction with continuing to use the self-injection device [99].

3.1.1 Insulin initiation

Insulin initiation is based on the clinical profiles of the patients and their preferences. Overcoming patient's barriers to insulin is important in the process of insulinisation. Pre-insulin education is important in overcoming patients' insulin inertia [100]. Improvements in insulin delivery systems have also made a significant impact on the management of diabetes [23, 99–102].

Insulin is initiated in T2DM patients for the purpose of augmentation or replacement for those who meet the criteria. Augmentation dose at 0.3–0.5 units/kg to support those patients with some degree of endogenous insulin secretion. Basal long-acting insulin used in augmentation resulted in better glycaemic control with minimal weight gain and fewer hypoglycaemic episodes compared with the pre-mix and bolus insulins [34]. Replacement insulin is initiated at the dose of 0.1–0.6 units/kg for those who have reached the burnt-out stage. Insulin dose calculation is shown in **Table 3**.

3.1.2 Insulin titration and maintenance

Titration of insulin is critical to achieve glycaemic target and to reach a maintenance dose which is important to reduce the chronic complications. Education of the patient's and their careers to escalate and deescalate insulin dosages according to prevailing glucose levels are important to archive glycaemic control and in addition, give patients confidence in their own management.

4. Conclusion

Pharmacotherapy is an integral part of the management of T2DM since the 1960s. Recent developments of many new drugs have increased the pharmacological armamentarium in addressing the ominous octet. These drugs have variable mechanisms of action, better efficacies and safety profiles. They have pleiotropic effects which have translated into better glycaemic control with the reduction of the chronic complications of T2DM. Additionally, they reduce other cardiovascular risk factors such as obesity, hypertension and dyslipidaemia and have protective cardiorenal effects.

Insulin therapy for T2DM is initiated in those meeting the criteria using an augmentation and replacement principle. The new analogue insulins provide effective glycaemic control compared with the human insulin. They have less weight gain and hypoglycaemic effects than the human insulins. Improvement in their delivery systems improves patient compliance and outcomes.

Two new investigational drugs are on the origin: Tirzepatitide, a biagonist and Rezatrutide, a triagonist. Both are impressive, with similar effects of the GLP1RA and GIP effects but a once-weekly dose. They could provide a new era for pharmacotherapy of T2DM.

Funding

There were no funding sources for this paper.

Conflict of interest

The author declares no conflict of interest in writing this paper.

Author details

Leslie Bahn Kawa
Internal Medicine Division, Port Moresby General Hospital, Papua New Guinea

*Address all correspondence to: lesliebahnkawa740@gmail.com

References

[1] World Health Organization. Diabetes Program. Available from: http://www.who.int/diabetes/goal/en

[2] Defronzo RA. Banting Lecture. From the triumvirate to the ominous octet: A new paradigm for the treatment of type 2 diabetes mellitus. Diabetes. 2009;**58**(4):773-795. DOI: 10.2337/db09-9028

[3] Chlup R, Kaňa R, Hanáčková L, Zálešáková H, Doubravová B. Pathophysiologic Approach to Type 2 Diabetes Management: One Centre Experience 1980-2020. London, UK, London, UK: IntechOpen.; 2021. DOI: 10.5772/intechopen.96237

[4] Alonge KM, D'Alessio DA, Schwartz MW. Brain control of blood glucose levels: Implications for the pathogenesis of type 2 diabetes. Diabetologia. 2021;**64**:5-14. DOI: 10.1007/s00125-020-05293-3

[5] Yuan S, Larsson SC. An atlas on risk factors for type 2 diabetes: A wide-angled Mendelian randomisation study. Diabetologia. 2020;**63**(11):2359-2371. DOI: 10.1007/s00125-020-05253-x

[6] Pan XR, Li GW, Hu YH, Wang JX, Yang WY, An ZX, et al. Effects of diet and exercise in preventing NIDDM in people with impaired glucose tolerance. The Da Qing IGT and Diabetes Study. Diabetes Care. 1997;**20**(4):537-544. DOI: 10.2337/diacare.20.4.537

[7] Tuomilehto J, Lindstřom J, Erisson JG, Valle TT, Hämäläinen H, Ilanne-Parikka P, et al. Finnish Diabetes Prevention Study Group. Prevention of type 2 diabetes mellitus by changes in lifestyle among subjects with impaired glucose tolerance. The New England Journal of Medicine. 2001;**344**(18):1343-1350. DOI: 10.1056/NEJM200105033441801

[8] Knowler WC, Connor EB, Fowler SE, Hamman RF, Lachin JF, Walker EA, et al. The Diabetes Prevention Program Research Group. Reduction in the incidence of type 2 diabetes with lifestyle intervention or metformin. The New England Journal of Medicine. 2002;**346**:393-403. DOI: 10.1056/NEJMoa012512

[9] Ramachandran A, Snehalatha C, Mary S, et al. Indian Diabetes Prevention Program (IDPP). The Indian Diabetes Prevention Program shows that lifestyle modification and metformin prevent type 2 diabetes in Asian Indian subjects with impaired glucose tolerance (IDPP-1). Diabetologia. 2006;**49**:289-297. DOI: 10.1007/s00125-005-0097-z

[10] Marso SP, Daniels GH, Brown-Frandsen K, et al. Liraglutide and cardiovascular outcomes in type 2 diabetes. The New England Journal of Medicine. 2016;**375**(4):311-322. DOI: 10.1056/NEJMoa1603827

[11] Marso SP, Bain SC, Consoli A, et al. Semaglutide and cardiovascular outcomes in patients with type 2 diabetes. The New England Journal of Medicine. 2016;**375**(19):1834-1844. DOI: 10.1056/NEJMoa1607141

[12] Aroda VR, Henry RR, Han J, Huang W, DeYoung MB, Darsow T, et al. Efficacy of GLP1 receptor agonists and DPP-4 inhibitors: Meta-analysis and systematic review. Clinical Therapeutics. 2012;**34**(6):1247-1258.e22. DOI: 10.1016/j.clinthera.2012.04.013

[13] Semaglutide for managing overweight and obesity. NICE appraisal 2023. Available from: https://www.nice.org.uk/guidance/TA875

[14] Zinman B, Wanner C, Lachin JM, et al. Empagliflozin, cardiovascular outcomes, and mortality in type 2 diabetes. The New England Journal of Medicine. 2015;**373**(22):2117-2128. DOI: 10.1056/NEJMoa1504720

[15] Wiviott SD, Raz I, Bonaca MP, Mosenzon O, et al. Dapagliflozin and cardiovascular outcomes in type 2 diabetes. The New England Journal of Medicine. 2019;**380**(4):347-357. DOI: 10.1056/NEJMoa1812389

[16] McMurray JJV, DeMets DL, Inzucchi SE, et al. A trial to evaluate the effect of the sodium-glucose co-transporter 2 inhibitor dapagliflozin on morbidity and mortality in patients with heart failure and reduced left ventricular ejection fraction (DAPA-HF). European Journal of Heart Failure. 2019;**21**(5):665-675. DOI: 10.1002/ejhf.1432

[17] Packer M, Anker SD, Butler J, Filippatos G, Ferreira JP, Pocock SJ, et al. Effect of empagliflozin on the clinical stability of patients with heart failure and a reduced ejection fraction: The EMPEROR-reduced trial. Circulation. 2021;**143**(4):326-336. DOI: 10.1161/CIRCULATIONAHA.120.051783

[18] Chlup R, Zapletalová J, Seckar P, Malá E, Doubravová B, Táncosová S, et al. Benefits of complementary therapy with insulin aspart versus human regular insulin in persons with type 2 diabetes mellitus. Diabetes Technology & Therapeutics. 2007;**9**(3):223-231. DOI: 10.1089/dia.2006.0018

[19] Holman RR, Thorne KI, Farmer AJ, Davies MJ, Keenan JF, Paul S, et al. Addition of biphasic, prandial, or basal insulin to oral therapy in type 2 diabetes. The New England Journal of Medicine. 2007;**357**(17):1716-1730. DOI: 10.1056/NEJMoa075392

[20] Bretzel RG, Eckhard M, Landgraf W, Owens DR, Linn T. Initiating insulin therapy in type 2 diabetic patients failing on oral hypoglycemic agents: Basal or prandial insulin? The APOLLO trial and beyond. Diabetes Care. 2009;**32**(Suppl 2):S260-S265. DOI: 10.2337/dc09-S319

[21] Aronson R, Reznik Y, Conget I, Castañeda JA, Runzis S, Lee SW, et al. Sustained efficacy of insulin pump therapy compared with multiple daily injections in type 2 diabetes: 12-month data from the OpT2mise randomized trial. Diabetes, Obesity & Metabolism. 2016;**18**(5):500-507. DOI: 10.1111/dom.12642

[22] Pickup JC, Reznik Y, Sutton AJ. Glycemic control during continuous subcutaneous insulin infusion versus multiple daily insulin injections in type 2 diabetes: Individual patient data meta-analysis and meta-regression of randomized controlled trials. Diabetes Care. 2017;**40**(5):715-722. DOI: 10.2337/dc16-2201

[23] Updike SJ, Shults MC, Cornwell ST, Tuffli GA, Zografi GD. Facilitating intensive conventional insulin management using a manually operated syringe injector. Diabetes Research (Edinburgh, Scotland). 1984;**1**(3):135-141

[24] Eriksson KF, Lindgärde F. No excess 12-year mortality in men with impaired glucose tolerance who participated in the Malmö Preventive Trial with diet and exercise. Diabetologia. 1998;**41**(9):1010-1016. DOI: 10.1007/s001250051024

[25] Boulé NG, Haddad E, Kenny GP, Wells GA, Sigal RJ. Effects of exercise on glycemic control and body mass in type 2 diabetes mellitus: A meta-analysis of controlled clinical trials. JAMA. 2001;**286**(10):1218-1227. DOI: 10.1001/jama.286.10.1218

[26] Thomas DE, Elliott EJ, Naughton GA. Exercise for type 2 diabetes mellitus. The Cochrane Database of Systematic Reviews. 2006;**2006**(3):CD002968. DOI: 10.1002/14651858.CD002968.pub2

[27] Balducci S, Zanuso S, Nicolucci A, et al. Effect of an intensive exercise intervention strategy on modifiable cardiovascular risk factors in subjects with type 2 diabetes mellitus: A randomized controlled trial: The Italian Diabetes and Exercise Study (IDES). Archives of Internal Medicine. 2010;**170**(20):1794-1803. DOI: 10.1001/archinternmed.2010.380

[28] Umpierre D, Ribeiro PA, Kramer CK, Leitão CB, Zucatti AT, Azevedo MJ, et al. Physical activity advice only or structured exercise training and association with HbA1c levels in type 2 diabetes: A systematic review and meta-analysis. JAMA. 2011;**305**(17):1790-1799. DOI: 10.1001/jama.2011.576

[29] Myers VH, McVay MA, Brashear MM, Johannsen NM, Swift DL, Kramer K, et al. Exercise training and quality of life in individuals with type 2 diabetes: A randomized controlled trial. Diabetes Care. 2013;**36**(7):1884-1890. DOI: 10.2337/dc12-1153

[30] Esposito K, Maiorino MI, Bellastella G, Chiodini P, Panagiotakos D, Giugliano D. A journey into a Mediterranean diet and type 2 diabetes: A systematic review with meta-analyses. BMJ Open. 2015;**5**(8):e008222. DOI: 10.1136/bmjopen-2015-008222

[31] Milenkovic T, Bozhinovska N, Macut D, Bjekic-Macut J, Rahelic D, Velija Asimi Z, et al. Mediterranean diet and type 2 diabetes mellitus: A perpetual inspiration for the scientific world. A review. Nutrients. 2021;**13**(4):1307. DOI: 10.3390/nu13041307

[32] Intensive blood-glucose control with sulphonylureas or insulin compared with conventional treatment and risk of complications in patients with type 2 diabetes (UKPDS 33). UK Prospective Diabetes Study (UKPDS) Group. Lancet (London, England). 1998;**352**(9131):837-853

[33] Shichiri M, Kishikawa H, Ohkubo Y, Wake N. Long-term results of the Kumamoto Study on optimal diabetes control in type 2 diabetic patients. Diabetes Care. 2000;**23**(Suppl 2):B21-B29

[34] ADVANCE Collaborative Group, Patel A, MacMahon S, Chalmers J, Neal B, Billot L, et al. Intensive blood glucose control and vascular outcomes in patients with type 2 diabetes. The New England Journal of Medicine. 2008;**358**(24):2560-2572. DOI: 10.1056/NEJMoa0802987

[35] Inzucchi SE, Bergenstal RM, Buse JB, Diamant M, Ferrannini E, Nauck M, et al. Management of hyperglycaemia in type 2 diabetes, 2015: A patient-centred approach. Update to a position statement of the American Diabetes Association and the European Association for the Study of Diabetes. Diabetologia. 2015;**58**(3):429-442. DOI: 10.1007/s00125-014-3460-0

[36] American Diabetes Association. 8. Pharmacologic Approaches to Glycemic Treatment. Diabetes Care. 2017;**40**(Suppl 1):S64-S74. DOI: 10.2337/dc17-S011

[37] Davies MJ, Aroda VR, Collins BS, Gabbay RA, Green J, Maruthur NM, et al. Management of hyperglycaemia in type 2 diabetes, 2022. A consensus report by the American Diabetes Association (ADA) and the European Association for the Study of Diabetes (EASD). Diabetologia. 2022;**65**(12):1925-1966. DOI: 10.1007/s00125-022-05787-2

[38] Garber AJ, Abrahamson MJ, Barzilay JI, et al. Consensus statement

by the American Association of Clinical Endocrinologists and American College of Endocrinology on the comprehensive type 2 diabetes management algorithm—2017 executive summary. Endocrine Practice: Official Journal of the American College of Endocrinology and the American Association of Clinical Endocrinologists. 2017;**23**(2):207-238. DOI: 10.4158/EP161682.CS

[39] Holman RR, Paul SK, Bethel MA, Neil HA, Matthews DR. Long-term follow-up after tight control of blood pressure in type 2 diabetes. The New England Journal of Medicine. 2008;**359**(15):1565-1576. DOI: 10.1056/NEJMoa0806359

[40] Dormandy JA, Charbonnel B, Eckland DJ, et al. Secondary prevention of macrovascular events in patients with type 2 diabetes in the PROactive Study (PROspective pioglitAzone Clinical Trial In macroVascular Events): A randomised controlled trial. Lancet (London, England). 2005;**366**(9493):1279-1289. DOI: 10.1016/S0140-6736(05)67528-9

[41] Kernan WN, Viscoli CM, et al. Pioglitazone after ischemic stroke or transient ischemic attack. The New England Journal of Medicine. 2016;**374**(14):1321-1331. DOI: 10.1056/NEJMoa1506930

[42] Spence JD, Viscoli CM, Inzucchi SE, Dearborn-Tomazos J, Ford GA, Gorman M, et al. Pioglitazone therapy in patients with stroke and prediabetes: A post hoc analysis of the IRIS randomized clinical trial. JAMA Neurology. 2019;**76**(5):526-535. DOI: 10.1001/jamaneurol.2019.0079

[43] Jastreboff AM, Aronne LJ, Ahmad NN, Wharton S, Connery L, Alves B, et al. Tirzepatide once weekly for the treatment of obesity. The New England Journal of Medicine. 2022;**387**(3):205-216. DOI: 10.1056/NEJMoa2206038

[44] Chavda VP, Ajabiya J, Teli D, Bojarska J, Apostolopoulos V. Tirzepatide, a new era of dual-targeted treatment for diabetes and obesity: A mini-review. Molecules (Basel, Switzerland). 2022;**27**(13):4315. DOI: 10.3390/molecules27134315

[45] Jastreboff AM, Kaplan LM, Frías JP, Wu Q, Du Y, Gurbuz S, et al. Triple-hormone-receptor agonist retatrutide for obesity—A phase 2 trial. The New England Journal of Medicine. 2023;**389**(6):514-526. DOI: 10.1056/NEJMoa2301972

[46] Zhang J, Zhang Z, Ma C, Zeng L, Zhang Y, Wang P, et al. A novel thrombin-based triagonist with diabetes-protective and weight-lowering potential. Life Sciences. 2020;**256**:117853. DOI: 10.1016/j.lfs.2020.117853

[47] Urva S, Coskun T, Loh MT, Du Y, Thomas MK, Gurbuz S, et al. LY3437943, a novel triple GIP, GLP1, and glucagon receptor agonist in people with type 2 diabetes: A phase 1b, multicentre, double-blind, placebo-controlled, randomised, multiple-ascending dose trial. Lancet (London, England). 2022;**400**(10366):1869-1881. DOI: 10.1016/S0140-6736(22)02033-5

[48] Retatrutide (LY3437943), a Novel GIP/GLP 1/Glucagon Receptor Triagonist—Obesity, NAFLD, and T2D Phase 2 Trial Results. American Diabetes Association 83rd Scientific Meeting. Available from: https://www.diabetes.org/newsroom/press-release/2023/american-diabetes-highlights-novel-agent-retatrutide-results-substantial-weight-reduction-people-with-obesity-type-2-diabetes-during-late-breaking-symposium.

[49] Nathan DM, Davidson M, DeFronzo RA, et al. Impaired fasting

glucose and impaired glucose tolerance: Implications for care. a consensus statement from the American Diabetes Association. Diabetes Care. 2007;**30**:753-759. DOI: 10.2337/dc07-9920

[50] Kirpichnikov D, McFarlane SI, Sowers JR. Metformin: An update. Annals of Internal Medicine. 2002;**137**(1):25-33. DOI: 10.7326/0003-4819-137-1-200207020-00009

[51] Gong L, Goswami S, Giacomini KM, Altman RB, Klein TE. Metformin pathways: Pharmacokinetics and pharmacodynamics. Pharmacogenetics and Genomics. 2012;**22**(11):820-827. DOI: 10.1097/FPC.0b013e3283559b22

[52] An H, He L. Current understanding of metformin effect on the control of hyperglycemia in diabetes. The Journal of Endocrinology. 2016;**228**(3):R97-R106. DOI: 10.1530/JOE-15-0447

[53] Rojas LB, Gomes MB. Metformin: An old but still the best treatment for type 2 diabetes. Diabetology & Metabolic Syndrome. 2013;**5**(1):6. DOI: 10.1186/1758-5996-5-6

[54] US Food and Drug Administration. Drug Safety Communication (April 8, 2016): FDA Revises Warnings Regarding Use of the Diabetes Medicine Metformin in Certain Patients with Reduced Kidney Function. Available from: http://www.fda.gov/downloads/Drugs/DrugSafety/UCM494140.pdf

[55] Panten U, Schwanstecher M, Schwanstecher C. Mode of action of sulfonylureas. In: Kuhlmann J, Puls W, editors. Oral Antidiabetics. Handbook of Experimental Pharmacology. Vol. 119. Berlin, Heidelberg: Springer; 1996. DOI: 10.1007/978-3-662-09127-2_6

[56] Sola D, Rossi L, Schianca GP, Maffioli P, Bigliocca M, Mella R, et al. Sulfonylureas and their use in clinical practice. Archives of Medical Science. AMS. 2015;**11**(4):840-848. DOI: 10.5114/aoms.2015.53304

[57] Speechly-Dick ME, Grover GJ, Yellon DM. Does ischemic preconditioning in the human involve protein kinase C and the ATP-dependent K+ channel? Studies of contractile function after simulated ischemia in an atrial in vitro model. Circulation Research. 1995;**77**(5):1030-1035. DOI: 10.1161/01.res.77.5.1030

[58] Cleveland JC Jr, Meldrum DR, Cain BS, Banerjee A, Harken AH. Oral sulfonylurea hypoglycemic agents prevent ischemic preconditioning in human myocardium. Two paradoxes revisited. Circulation. 1997;**96**(1):29-32. DOI: 10.1161/01.cir.96.1.29

[59] Tomai F, Crea F, Gaspardone A, Versaci F, De Paulis R, Penta de Peppo A, et al. Ischemic preconditioning during coronary angioplasty is prevented by glibenclamide, a selective ATP-sensitive K+ channel blocker. Circulation. 1994;**90**(2):700-705. DOI: 10.1161/01.cir.90.2.700

[60] O'Keefe JH, Blackstone EH, Sergeant P, McCallister BD. The optimal mode of coronary revascularization for diabetics. A risk-adjusted long-term study comparing coronary angioplasty and coronary bypass surgery. European Heart Journal. 1998;**19**(11):1696-1703. DOI: 10.1053/euhj.1998.1153

[61] Danchin N, Charpentier G, Ledru F, Vaur L, Guéret P, Hanania G, et al. Role of previous treatment with sulfonylureas in diabetic patients with acute myocardial infarction: Results from a nationwide French registry. Diabetes/Metabolism Research and Reviews. 2005;**21**(2):143-149. DOI: 10.1002/dmrr.498

[62] Khunti K, Chatterjee S, Gerstein HC, Zoungas S, Davies MJ. Do sulphonylureas still have a place in clinical practice? Lancet Diabetes & Endocrinology. 2018;**6**(10):821-832. DOI: 10.1016/S2213-8587(18)30025-1

[63] Davies MJ, D'Alessio DA, Fradkin J, Kernan WN, Mathieu C, Mingrone G, et al. Management of hyperglycaemia in type 2 diabetes, 2018. A consensus report by the American Diabetes Association (ADA) and the European Association for the Study of Diabetes (EASD). Diabetologia. 2018;**61**(12):2461-2498. DOI: 10.1007/s00125-018-4729-5

[64] Monsalve FA, Pyarasani RD, Delgado-Lopez F, Moore-Carrasco R. Peroxisome proliferator-activated receptor targets for the treatment of metabolic diseases. Mediators of Inflammation. 2013;**2013**:549627. DOI: 10.1155/2013/549627

[65] Nissen SE, Wolski K. Effect of rosiglitazone on the risk of myocardial infarction and death from cardiovascular causes. The New England Journal of Medicine. 2007;**356**(24):2457-2471. DOI: 10.1056/NEJMoa072761

[66] Mitka M. FDA eases restrictions on the glucose-lowering drug rosiglitazone. JAMA. 2013;**310**(24):2604. DOI: 10.1001/jama.2013.284788

[67] Tahrani AA, Barnett AH, Bailey CJ. Pharmacology and therapeutic implications of current drugs for type 2 diabetes mellitus. Nature Reviews. Endocrinology. 2016;**12**(10):566-592. DOI: 10.1038/nrendo.2016.86

[68] Lorenz M, Pfeiffer C, Steinsträsser A, Becker RH, Rütten H, Ruus P, et al. Effects of lixisenatide once daily on gastric emptying in type 2 diabetes--relationship to postprandial glycemia. Regulatory Peptides. 2013;**185**:1-8. DOI: 10.1016/j.regpep.2013.04.001

[69] Huthmacher JA, Meier JJ, Nauck MA. Efficacy and safety of short- and long-acting glucagon-like peptide 1 receptor agonists on a background of basal insulin in type 2 diabetes: A meta-analysis. Diabetes Care. 2020;**43**(9):2303-2312. DOI: 10.2337/dc20-0498

[70] Handelsman Y, Bloomgarden ZT, Grunberger G, et al. American association of clinical endocrinologists and American college of endocrinology—Clinical practice guidelines for developing a diabetes mellitus comprehensive care plan—2015. Endocrine Practice: Official Journal of the American College of Endocrinology and the American Association of Clinical Endocrinologists. 2015;**21**(Suppl 1):1-87. DOI: 10.4158/EP15672.GL

[71] AstraZeneca Pharmaceuticals LP. Prescribing Information (09/2015): BYDUREON (Exenatide Extended Release), for Injectable Suspension. Available from: http://www.accessdata.fda.gov/drugsatfda_docs/label/2015/022200s015s016s017s018lbl.pdf

[72] Eli Lilly and Company. Prescribing Information (03/2017): TRULICITYTM (Dulaglutide) Injection, for Subcutaneous Use. Available from: http://pi.lilly.com/us/trulicity-uspi.pdf

[73] GlaxoSmithKline. Prescribing Information (09/2016): TANZEUM (Albiglutide) Injection, for Subcutaneous Use. Available from: https://www.gsksource.com/gskprm/htdocs/documents/TANZEUM-PI-MG-IFUCOMBINED.PDF

[74] AstraZeneca Pharmaceuticals LP. Prescribing Information (02/2015): BYETTA (Exenatide) Injection. Available from: http://www.accessdata.fda.gov/drugsatfda_docs/label/2015/021773s040lbl.pdf

[75] Novo Nordisk A/S. Prescribing Information (04/2016): VICTOZA

(Liraglutide [rDNA origin]) Injection, for Subcutaneous Use. Available from: http://www.novo-pi.com/victoza.pdf

[76] Aroda VR, Rosenstock J, Terauchi Y, Altuntas Y, Lalic NM, Morales Villegas EC, et al. PIONEER 1: Randomized clinical trial of the efficacy and safety of oral semaglutide monotherapy in comparison with placebo in patients with type 2 diabetes. Diabetes Care. 2019;**42**(9):1724-1732. DOI: 10.2337/dc19-0749

[77] Rybelsus. Uses, Dosages, Side Effects, Warnings. Available from: https://www.drugs.com/rybelsus.html

[78] Invokana EPAR. European Medicines Agency (EMA). Available from: http://www.ema.europa.eu/en/medicine/human/EPAR/invokana

[79] Abdul-Ghani MA, DeFronzo RA. Inhibition of renal glucose reabsorption: A novel strategy for achieving glucose control in type 2 diabetes mellitus. Endocrine Practice: Official Journal of the American College of Endocrinology and the American Association of Clinical Endocrinologists. 2008;**14**(6):782-790. DOI: 10.4158/EP.14.6.782

[80] McGuire DK, Shih WJ, Cosentino F, et al. Association of SGLT2 inhibitors with cardiovascular and kidney outcomes in patients with type 2 diabetes: A meta-analysis. JAMA Cardiology. 2021;**6**(2):148-158. DOI: 10.1001/jamacardio.2020.4511

[81] Neal B, Perkovic V, Mahaffey KW, de Zeeuw D, Fulcher G, Erondu N, et al. Canagliflozin and cardiovascular and renal events in type 2 diabetes. The New England Journal of Medicine. 2017;**377**(7):644-657. DOI: 10.1056/NEJMoa1611925

[82] Cannon CP, Pratley R, Dagogo-Jack S, et al. Cardiovascular outcomes with ertugliflozin in type 2 diabetes. The New England Journal of Medicine. 2020;**383**(15):1425-1435. DOI: 10.1056/NEJMoa2004967 147

[83] Bhatt DL, Szarek M, Pitt B, et al. Sotagliflozin in patients with diabetes and chronic kidney disease. The New England Journal of Medicine. 2021;**384**(2):129-139. DOI: 10.1056/NEJMoa2030186

[84] Drucker DJ, Nauck MA. The incretin system: Glucagon-like peptide-1 receptor agonists and dipeptidyl peptidase-4 inhibitors in type 2 diabetes. Lancet (London, England). 2006;**368**(9548):1696-1705. DOI: 10.1016/S0140-6736(06)69705-5

[85] Blonde L, Russell-Jones D. The safety and efficacy of liraglutide with or without oral antidiabetic drug therapy in type 2 diabetes: An overview of the LEAD 1-5 studies. Diabetes, Obesity & Metabolism. 2009;**11**(Suppl 3):26-34. DOI: 10.1111/j.1463-1326.2009.01075.x

[86] Scheen AJ. Safety of dipeptidyl peptidase-4 inhibitors for treating type 2 diabetes. Expert Opinion on Drug Safety. 2015;**14**(4):505-524. DOI: 10.1517/14740338.2015.1006625

[87] Perkovic V, Toto R, Cooper ME, et al. Effects of linagliptin on cardiovascular and kidney outcomes in people with normal and reduced kidney function: Secondary analysis of the CARMELINA randomized trial. Diabetes Care. 2020;**43**(8):1803-1812. DOI: 10.2337/dc20-0279

[88] Scirica BM, Bhatt DL, Braunwald E, et al. Saxagliptin and cardiovascular outcomes in patients with type 2 diabetes mellitus. The New England Journal of Medicine. 2013;**369**(14):1317-1326. DOI: 10.1056/NEJMoa1307684

[89] American Diabetes Association Professional Practice Committee. 9.

Pharmacologic approaches to glycemic treatment: Standards of medical care in diabetes-2022. Diabetes Care. 2022;**45**(Suppl 1):S125-S143. DOI: 10.2337/dc22-S009

[90] FDA Approves Novel, Dual-Targeted Treatment for Type 2 Diabetes. US Food and Drug Administration (FDA) (Press Release). Available from: http://www.gov./news-events/press-announcements/fda-approves-novel-dual-targettedtreatment-tyep-2-diabetes

[91] Mounjaro European Medicine Agency. Available from: https://www.ema.europa.eu/en/medicines/human/EPAR/mounjaro.

[92] Frías JP, Davies MJ, Rosenstock J, et al. Tirzepatide versus semaglutide once weekly in patients with type 2 diabetes. The New England Journal of Medicine. 2021;**385**(6):503-515. DOI: 10.1056/NEJMoa2107519

[93] ElSayed NA, Aleppo G, Aroda VR, Bannuru RR, et al. 9. Pharmacologic approaches to glycemic treatment: Standards of care in diabetes-2023. Diabetes Care. 2023;**46**(Suppl 1):S140-S157. DOI: 10.2337/dc23-S009

[94] Davies MJ, D'Alessio DA, Fradkin J, Kernan WN, Mathieu C, Mingrone G, et al. Management of hyperglycemia in type 2 diabetes, 2018. A consensus report by the American Diabetes Association (ADA) and the European Association for the Study of Diabetes (EASD). Diabetes Care. 2018;**41**(12):2669-2701. DOI: 10.2337/dci18-0033

[95] Ritsinger V, Malmberg K, Mårtensson A, Rydén L, Wedel H, Norhammar A. Intensified insulin-based glycaemic control after myocardial infarction: Mortality during 20 year follow-up of the randomised Diabetes Mellitus Insulin Glucose Infusion in Acute Myocardial Infarction (DIGAMI 1) trial. The Lancet. Diabetes & Endocrinology. 2014;**2**(8):627-633. DOI: 10.1016/S2213-8587(14)70088-9

[96] Pennartz C, Schenker N, Menge BA, Schmidt WE, Nauck MA, Meier JJ. Chronic reduction of fasting glycemia with insulin glargine improves first- and second-phase insulin secretion in patients with type 2 diabetes. Diabetes Care. 2011;**34**(9):2048-2053. DOI: 10.2337/dc11-0471

[97] Diabetes Control and Complications Trial Research Group, Nathan DM, Genuth S, Lachin J, Cleary P, Crofford O, et al. The effect of intensive treatment of diabetes on the development and progression of long-term complications in insulin-dependent diabetes mellitus. The New England Journal of Medicine. 1993;**329**(14):977-986. DOI: 10.1056/NEJM199309303291401

[98] Weng J, Li Y, Xu W, et al. Effect of intensive insulin therapy on beta-cell function and glycaemic control in patients with newly diagnosed type 2 diabetes: A multicentre randomised parallel-group trial. Lancet (London, England). 2008;**371**(9626):1753-1760. DOI: 10.1016/S0140-6736(08)60762-X

[99] Jefferson IG, Marteau TM, Smith MA, Baum JD. A multiple injection regimen using an insulin injection pen and pre-filled cartridged soluble human insulin in adolescents with diabetes. Diabetic Medicine: A Journal of the British Diabetic Association. 1985;**2**(6):493-495. DOI: 10.1111/j.1464-5491.1985.tb00690.x

[100] Giugliano D, Maiorino MI, Bellastella G, Esposito K. Clinical inertia, reverse clinical inertia, and medication non-adherence in type 2 diabetes. Journal of Endocrinological Investigation. 2019;**42**(5):495-503. DOI: 10.1007/s40618-018-0951-8

[101] Chlup R, Janü K, Venháčová J, Bartek J. Six models of a new insulin pen (MADI): Description and first clinical trial. Practical Diabetes International. 1995;**12**:32-35

[102] Gudiksen N, Hofstätter T, Rønn BB, Sparre T. FlexTouch: An insulin pen-injector with a low activation force across different insulin formulations, needle technologies, and temperature conditions. Diabetes Technology & Therapeutics. 2017;**19**(10):603-607. DOI: 10.1089/dia.2017.0121

Chapter 11

Paradigm of Complementary and Alternative Medicine in Type 2 Diabetes

Mohammed Zaid Aljulifi

Abstract

Complementary and alternative medicine (CAM) is increasingly used by patients nowadays. The pooled prevalence of CAM use is about 51%. Many types of CAM have been practiced by patients with diabetes. Some of them showed promising results on blood glucose and other cardiometabolic parameters such as blood pressure, body mass, and lipid profile. This chapter explores two main types of CAM: Herbs and mind–body therapy. Different types of mind–body therapy and plants, plant extracts, and herbal substances have been utilized for an extended period and are sometimes favored by many individuals with T2D. Those practices and compounds found in these natural remedies are believed to have the potential to benefit the body in several ways, including the reduction of symptoms, alleviation of pain, and promotion of overall health. This chapter includes a summary of the findings of the available systematic reviews and meta-analyses regarding the most used medicinal herbs and body–mind therapies. In conclusion, as some of these interventions are promising, it is unclear to what extent glucose metabolism and certain substances can help mitigate complications in late-stage diabetes. Healthcare providers should be aware about them.

Keywords: type 2 diabetes mellitus, conventional, alternative medicine, complementary medicine, CAM, herbal medicine, mind–body therapy

1. Introduction

Type 2 diabetes mellitus (T2D) is a chronic condition, where the body's metabolic pathways for carbohydrates, proteins, and fat are disrupted due to various factors. These factors include defects in insulin secretion, reduced production of incretins in the gut, high levels of glucagon, increased production of glucose by the liver, issues with the endocrine function of adipose tissue, insulin resistance, increased activity of specific glucose transporter in the kidneys called sodium-glucose transporter-2 (SGLT2), and dysfunction in the hypothalamic centers that regulate hunger and fullness. All these lead to hyperglycemia, which carries risks to many organs of the human body [1]. The number of patients with T2D is expected to increase as long as there is no definitive treatment. It is expected to be around 578 million patients with T2D by 2030 and 700 million by 2045 worldwide [2].

Complementary and alternative medicine (CAM) has been defined as any healthcare practice that is not part of the nation's standard medical care [3–5]. However, it is important to say there is no unified definition, and the terms "complementary" and "alternative" has been used interchangeably [5]. Each institute has its term and definition for such practices, for example, traditional or integrative medicine. The first terms used to describe unconventional medicine were "alternative" in 1975, "unconventional" in 1980, "complementary" in 1984, "complementary and alternative" in 1994, and "integrated/integrative" in 1995 [6]. CAM is widely spread and popular all over the world [3]. The pooled prevalence of CAM use is about 51%, with a wide range in prevalence between studies (8–93%) [7]. At present, traditional and complementary medicine (T&CM) has a user base of over 100 million in Europe. About one-fifth of these people use T&CM regularly, and the same amount of people prefer healthcare options that include T&CM. The number of united states adults using herbs and supplements went up from 38.2 million in 2002 to 40.6 million in 2012 [8]. Chinese medication was valued at approximately $83.1 in 2012. This was a 20% increase compared to the previous year [3]. According to research in Saudi Arabia, people typically spend about $560 per year from their own money on T&CM services [9].

Generally, patients with chronic diseases tend to use CAM because they are looking for any measure that could help to treat, control, or reduce the severity of their medical problems [10, 11]. According to the 2012 National Health Interview Survey and the Adult Alternative Medicine supplement, they collected the data of about 15 thousand patients who have one or more of the following diseases: hypertension, diabetes, hypercholesterolemia, or obesity. They found that 29.5% of the patients had used a CAM before [12]. The percentage of people who reported using T&CM (products and/or practitioners/therapies) in the past year ranged from 24 to 71.3% [13]. CAM is frequently utilized by a considerable percentage of individuals in Saudi Arabia, varying from a few to as many as 96%, who experience chronic mental and physical illnesses [14]. However, in Eastern Mediterranean countries members of the World Health Organization, the prevalence of CAM use among patients with T2D within the 14 countries ranged between 9 and 88.4% [15]. American diabetes association advised asking every patient with diabetes about any CAM use every visit [16].

There are some predictors to use CAM among patients such as affordability of the CAM, cultural beliefs, the cost of the healthcare services, loss of trust in healthcare workers and hospitals, and the belief in the importance and value of one's inner life and experiences [3, 14, 17].

This chapter includes a summary of the findings of the available systematic reviews and meta-analyses regarding the most used medicinal herbs and body–mind therapies. It also includes suggestions for healthcare providers, stakeholders, and researchers in the field of CAM therapy in the management of type 2 diabetes.

2. Herbal medicine

Herbal medicine refers to the use of plants or plant extracts for their medicinal properties to promote healing and well-being. It is a traditional form of medicine that has been practiced for thousands of years in various cultures around the world. Herbal medicines often involve the use of leaves, flowers, stems, roots, or seeds of specific plants, which are prepared as teas, tinctures, capsules, or topical applications.

These natural remedies are believed to contain bioactive compounds that can have therapeutic effects on the body such as reducing symptoms, alleviating pain, or supporting overall health. However, number of them have been studied, and their use is not strictly controlled, so it is hard to know what side effects they might have. This makes it difficult to figure out which therapies are the safest and most effective and to know how to prescribe such therapies [18]. One study was conducted on outpatients with chronic disease in Turkey and found that the level of adherence is affected by the use of herbal medicine [19]. About 7 out of 100 people had purchased natural herbal products online [20]. Although there is insufficient evidence to definitively confirm the effectiveness of specific herbs and supplements for diabetes, they generally appear to be safe [21]. Many herb consumers mistakenly believe that natural remedies are always safe and have no risks. However, some medicinal plants are toxic. Like all medicines, herbal remedies can have adverse side effects. Some of these side effects are caused by quality issues, such as the inclusion of undisclosed medications or potent pharmaceutical substances. Adverse events can also occur due to the incorrect use of herbal medicines, interactions with other medications, and the use of contaminated products. In the following sections, we will go through a review of the herbs used in T2D management.

2.1 Curcumin

Curcumin, also known as diferuloylmethane, is a natural substance found in the roots of the turmeric plant and other related plants. Curcuma longa is a plant that has been used as a medicine in Asia for a long time [22]. A randomized controlled trial was conducted to determine whether curcumin could help in diabetes prevention and found that after 9 months of curcumin intervention in prediabetic patients. The participants were asked to take six capsules of either curcumin or a placebo, each capsule containing a curcuminoid content of 250 mg. A significantly lower number of prediabetic individuals eventually developed T2D [23]. Another study on nano curcumin (as nano-micelle 80 mg/day) has found that it could help in reducing glycated hemoglobin (HbA1C), fasting plasma concentration (FPC), and 2-hour postprandial sugar (2hPP) in patients with T2D [24]. Combining Curcuma longa with hypoglycemic drugs, especially ones that are processed by the CYP2C19 and CYP2C9 enzymes and have a narrow therapeutic range, can alter their functionality within the body. Also, the combination can potentially interact in significant ways. However, additional research is needed to determine the advantages of using these things together [25].

In conclusion, Curcumin is one of the most extensively studied food-driven substances and is generally safe. The allowed daily intake is 0–3 mg/kg body mass. Curcumin might help in the prevention of diabetes complications; however, more studies are needed [26–28]. Moreover, it could help in reducing the non-high-density lipoprotein cholesterol (HDL-C) and lipoprotein(a) [Lp(a)] [29]. There are few side effects reported with higher doses such as diarrhea, skin rash, yellow stool, and an increase in serum alkaline phosphatase and lactate dehydrogenase [22].

2.2 Aloe vera

Aloe vera is a type of plant that belongs to the Asphodelaceae family. It is a type of plant that can survive in dry environments. For a long time, people in South Africa have been using traditional medicine, including Aloe vera to treat skin problems and other illnesses. This practice has been around for thousands of years [30]. Patients have used it for a long time to help lower plasma glucose concentration in people with diabetes or prediabetes. Some substances found in Aloe vera called chromium and alprogen can help fix damaged insulin cells in the pancreas, improve the working of insulin, and reduce high blood sugar levels [31].

A systematic review and meta-analysis was published in 2022 and included 642 patients, and found reduced FPC in patients with prediabetes and T2D. However, the sample size of the clinical trials was small in size, and most of the studies' periods were short [31]. The previous clinical studies did not notice any negative herb-drug interaction [25].

There is still a need for more well-established and longer-duration studies. The patients need to consult with a healthcare provider before using Aloe vera as a supplement or adjunctive treatment for T2D.

2.3 Moringa oleifera

In the past, Moringa oleifera had been grown and consumed within its original regions. In the 1990s, some researchers began studying how it could be used to purify water. They later found out its nutritional and medical benefits, and now it is grown in almost all tropical and subtropical areas [32]. A systematic review covering the studies between 2008 and 2018 and found that moringa leaf powder intake showed statistical evidence of reduced plasma glucose concentration [33].

Moringa oleifera is not very safe because it has been found that there are certain compounds that can cause serious problems in the liver, kidneys, blood, and other parts of the body. Roasted Moringa oleifera seeds have substances that might lead to genotoxicity. The leaf contains a lot of saponins, which can be potentially harmful to vegetarians. These saponins can lower the amount of divalent and trivalent metals, such as zinc (Zn) and magnesium (Mg) that the body could absorb. Alkaloids in the tree's root and bark, such as Spirochin and Benzothiocyanate, are toxic substances that are mostly present in the root and bark. As a result, the leaf was deemed the safest part to eat [34].

Moringa oleifera could help patients with diabetes when used with certain medications that are metabolized by CYP1A2 and CYP3A4 enzymes, such as pioglitazone. This combination can have a positive effect and allow for a lower dosage of antihyperglycemic medications [25]. There is still a need for well-constructed RCT to know the best way to prepare, use, and know the effect on plasma glucose concentration.

2.4 Fenugreek

Fenugreek (Trigonella foenum-graecum) is a plant found in various countries, with yellow flowers and pods containing seeds. The term "Trigonella" refers to its triangular flower shape, while "foenum-graecum" means Greek hay. It has been used in cooking and traditional medicine for a long time [35].

A recent systematic review of 14 clinical trial studies found a significant effect of fenugreek on HbA1c. However, the reduction in FPC and postprandial glucose (PPG) was not statistically significant [36]. A previous systematic review study found a significant effect of fenugreek on FPC, 2hPP, and HbA1c. Moreover, it concluded that the amount of fenugreek used was different for each person. Some participants used as little as 1 gram per day, while others used as much as 100 grams per day. The impact of using different amounts of fenugreek varied greatly. Studies using low doses of fenugreek (less than 5 g per day) showed no effects, while studies using a higher dose showed stronger effects [37]. The way the fenugreek supplement is made also affects how it affects glucose levels [37, 38]. As shown, using fenugreek for a long duration (180 days) does not add more benefit to blood glucose [38]. All the published systematic review papers addressed the heterogeneity and the problems in the quality of the clinical studies. There are a few side effects reported by the participants, such as abdominal pain and dyspepsia. However, all these symptoms subside after a 2-day withdrawal of fenugreek without any specific treatment [37]. More studies are required considering the fenugreek dose, as well as other factors that could affect the glucose level.

2.5 Urtica dioica (nettle)

Urtica dioica or stinging nettle is a plant that grows in many places around the world, including Asia, Europe, North Africa, and North America [39]. It is believed that it affects the glucose level through the induction of insulin secretion and proliferation of pancreatic B cells [40]. Ziaei et al. found that ingestion of Urtica dioica by patients with T2D reduced FPC but did not affect HbA1c or insulin levels [41]. One of the limitations of the systematic review by Ziaei et al. is the mode of preparation of Urtica dioica was varying between the studies. Moreover, all the studies were conducted in one country [41]. In another study, Tabrizi et al. found that Urtica dioica improved FPC, HbA1c, triglycerides, and SBP in patients with T2D [42]. There is limited scientific evidence regarding the specific effects of Urtica dioica (commonly known as stinging nettle) on type 2 diabetes. While some studies suggest that stinging nettle may exhibit antidiabetic properties, more research is needed to establish its effectiveness and determine the appropriate dosage.

2.6 Salvia officinalis

Salvia officinalis (Sage) is a plant that grows all over the world and has been used for a long time in cooking and medicine. It is also used in traditional medicine to help with different health problems such as seizures, ulcers, diarrhea, and inflammation [43]. Abdollahi et al. found that S. officinalis reduced 2hPP, FPC, and HbA1c in patients with T2D in a systematic review that included three studies only [44]. Overuse or excessive consumption of the ethanolic extract and volatile oil of S. officinalis can result in adverse effects on health. S.Officinalis can cause vomiting, excessive saliva, tachycardia, dizziness, hot flashes, allergic reactions, swelling of the tongue, bluish skin, and even seizures. Officinalis oil affects the nervous system directly, especially at doses higher than 0.5 grams per kilogram. Camphor, thujone, and terpene ketones are the most dangerous substances in Salvia oil. These substances might cause harm to the developing baby during pregnancy and after birth [43]. More studies are needed for longer durations to assess the effects on glycemic control considering the possible side effects of S. officinalis.

2.7 Sesamum indicum L. (sesame)

Sesame is a type of plant that produces seeds that people use to make oil. It is one of the oldest crops that humans have grown and eaten. In China, people have been using sesame seeds for over 5000 years. The biggest producers of sesame seeds are

India, Sudan, Myanmar, China, and Tanzania. Tanzania has become the top producer in recent years, surpassing India. In 2017, the whole world produced about 5.9 million tons of sesame seeds, with Tanzania producing the most followed by China [45]. Ramírez-Coronel et al. and Sohouli et al. found that sesame help in reducing FPC and HbA1c significantly in patients with T2D [46, 47]. For people with certain health conditions, such as T2D and Metabolic syndrome, taking a certain amount of sesame oil or adding it to their food every day can help improve their health. They can have 30–35 ml of sesame oil each day or include it in their meals so that it makes up 30% of all the energy they get from food for 8–12 weeks. They can also take a supplement called sesamin, which is a special kind of sesame oil, by taking 200 mg of it every day for eight weeks [48].

2.8 Nigella sativa (black seed)

Nigella sativa, also known as black seed, that has been used for a long time in medicine. It comes from places such as Southern Europe, North Africa, and Southwest Asia. People have used the seeds and their oil to treat different sicknesses all around the world. It is even mentioned in religious texts as a special healing plant. People who follow the Islamic faith believe it is a very important medicine and should be used regularly [49]. It has been found that Nigella sativa improves FPC, HbA1c, total cholesterol, and LDL in patients with T2D [50–52]. When thymoquinone, Nigella sative derivative, was taken alongside metformin daily, it resulted in a more significant decrease in HbA1c and plasma glucose concentrations compared to taking metformin alone [53]. The effects of Nigella sativa on diabetes might be related to antioxidants and anti-inflammatory effects. It may also help in improving the levels of good cholesterol while reducing the levels of LDL and body mass [54].

2.9 Psyllium fiber (Isabgol)

Psyllium seeds, also known as Isabgol, come from the Plantago ovata plant and are highly valued for their nutrient-rich husk [55]. The first scientific article discussing psyllium was published in 1927, and since then, there have been over 1200 articles related to psyllium. Psyllium fiber was significantly reducing FPC, HbA1c, LDL, and triglyceride [56]. Dietary fibers in general significantly reduced TG, LDL, FPC, and HbA1c [57, 58]. A systematic review found that adding viscous fiber reduced HbA1c levels by 0.58% following a median dose of about 13.1 g/day over 8 weeks [58]. Individuals who have diabetes or are susceptible to diabetes should aim to consume a minimum of 14 grams of fiber per 1000 calories consumed. Half of the grains they eat should be whole grains. Eating enough fiber regularly can lower the risk of death for people with diabetes. Studies have shown that eating more fiber is also linked to a lower risk of getting type 2 diabetes [59].

2.10 Nopal

Nopal, which is also referred to as prickly pear cactus, has been proposed as having potential advantages for people diagnosed with (T2D). There are different types of Nopal, such as Opuntia streptacantha and Opuntia ficus-indica. Gouws et al. found no benefit for peaky fruit on glucose or insulin levels. However, the cladode exhibits potential glucose-lowering effects that are deserving further research and exploration [60]. The results of animal experiments demonstrated the potential of fruit extracts in the effective regulation of blood sugar levels [61].

Prickly pear seeds helped diabetic rats by increasing muscle and liver glycogen levels while also reducing plasma glucose concentration and increasing insulin sensitivity. It was observed in one study that the prickly pear cactus pad had led to a decrease in blood sugar levels in people with T2D on glipizide and metformin [62]. However, more studies are needed to confirm if using this herb together with standard diabetic medications is effective.

2.11 Astragalus membranaceus

Astragalus membranaceus, which is a member of the Fabaceae/Leguminosae family. The dried root of this plant is widely used and is recognized in both Chinese and Japanese pharmacopeia [55]. Tian et al. found that FPC, postprandial glucose, and HbA1c were significantly reduced after using Astragalus membranaceus in people with T2D [63]. One systematic review found a positive effect of Astragalus membranaceus on people with diabetic kidney disease [64]. Astragalus membranaceus has the ability to lower blood sugar levels by helping in increasing glucose transporter (GLUT4) in cells, preserving the function of beta cells, and increasing the release of insulin [65].

2.12 Momordica charantia (bitter gourd/bitter melon)

Momordica charantia, also known as bitter gourd or bitter melon, is a plant from the Cucurbitaceae family that is often utilized for its medicinal properties [66]. It helps in regulating the secretion of insulin and the synthesis of glycogen [25]. Momordica charantia was found to decrease FPC, PPG, and HbA1c significantly in people with T2D [67, 68]. No side effects were reported.

2.13 Olive oil

Olive oil is obtained from olives (Olea europaea, family Oleaceae). Mediterranean nations heavily rely on olive oil, which serves as a significant fat source. The quality of olive oil depends on various factors and processes involved in extracting it. During the time it is stored, it can additionally experience alterations before it is put to use [69]. Olive oil intake was associated with a significant reduction in FPC and HbA1c [70]. Increasing olive oil consumption by 25 grams per day was linked to a notable 22% decrease in the risk of developing T2D [71]. However, extra-virgin olive oil (EVOO) did not show any significant glycemic effect on people with T2D. However, animal studies showed a good hypoglycemic effect after EVOO use [72]. More RCT studies on EVOO with different doses are required to assess the hypoglycemic effect on people with T2D.

2.14 Allium sativum (garlic)

Garlic, Allium sativum, is a type of aromatic plant that is used in cooking. It was first found in places, such as Kazakhstan and China a long time ago, and people have been growing it ever since. Many different kinds of garlic can grow in different places around the world. Garlic was found to reduce the FPC and HbA1c significantly in people with diabetes [73, 74]. The inclusion of garlic in the diet had a notable impact on reducing HbA1c levels, and this effect was more pronounced among individuals who consumed garlic for a period of 24 weeks compared to those who consumed it for only 12 weeks [75]. Garlic was found to decrease blood pressure readings as well. Studies conducted on animals have provided evidence suggesting that aged garlic extract can inhibit the rise in plasma glycated albumin levels in mouse models with T2D. This beneficial effect is believed to be attributed, at least partially, to the activation of AMP-activated protein kinase, which subsequently leads to the suppression of both free fatty acid production and monocyte chemoattractant protein 1 (MCP1) gene expression in adipose tissue [76]. Garlic can help with common symptoms of diabetes such as polydipsia, polyuria, weight loss, and especially polyphagia. The consumption of garlic can regulate hunger and satiety, maintaining healthy energy levels of metabolism [77].

2.15 Zingiber officinale (ginger)

Ginger (Zingiber officinale) is a type of plant, that is, in the same family as other ginger plants. For hundreds of years, people have been using ginger to add flavor to their food and as a traditional medicine. We first learned about the medical use of ginger root in the sixth century BC. In the beginning, this plant was mostly used in countries, such as India and China. Over time, it started being sent to the Mediterranean region. The Greeks also used ginger to help with digestive problems [78]. Ginger reduced HbA1c and FPC significantly [79]. This was supported by previous studies that found that ginger could affect FPC, HbA1c, and lipid parameters positively [80–82]. No major differences in HbA1C levels were found in the trials when ginger was given as a supplement to research participants over the age of 50 [79]. Ginger aids in the management of diabetes by restoring the functionality of pancreatic β-cells and improving the utilization of glucose within the body. Other mechanisms involve enhancing the liver's glycogen synthesis, promoting increased insulin release from the pancreas, and inhibiting the liver's glucose production [25].

2.16 Panax spp. (ginseng)

Ginseng is a highly valued plant that can help treat many different illnesses. The ancient Chinese used ginseng in their medicine about 5000 years ago. Ginseng can be made from different types of Panax plants. These plants are used to make botanical preparations. There are 13 different types of ginseng, but the ones that are mostly used are Panax ginseng (also known as Korean ginseng) which is grown in China and Korea, and Panax quinquefolius (also known as American ginseng) which is grown in the United States and Canada. Multiple research studies have demonstrated the potential benefits of Panax ginseng and Panax quinquefolius with various health-related issues such as neurological, metabolic, infectious, and cancerous diseases [83].

One systematic review looked at the impact of taking a dose ranging from 200 mg to 8 g of Panax ginseng compared to a placebo, it found that the amount of blood glucose decreased by 1.77 mmol/L*hr. [84]. Another study showed that the ingestion of ginseng supplements for a duration of 8 weeks or more resulted in a significant improvement in fasting blood sugar (FSB) levels. However, the heart rate increased by about 2.65 beats per minute in patients taking ginseng compared to the control group [85].

No significant effect of ginseng on HbA1c level [84–87]. Ginseng has been found in extensive research *in vitro* and on animal and human subjects to have the potential in regulating insulin levels, glucose absorption, and glucose processing in the body. It does this by preventing the death of beta cells and increasing the production of glucagon-like peptide-1 (GLP-1), which helps reduce the effects of diabetes [86].

2.17 Other herbs with promising effects on T2D

Cinnamon reduced FPC but did not affect HbA1c or insulin levels significantly [88, 89]. On the other side, Camellia sinensis, which belongs to the Camellia genus, is a type of plant that is used to make green and other types of tea, where assessed by Wang et al. found a statistically significant reduction of FPC and HbA1c in people with T2D by Camellia sinensis use [90, 91]. These findings are contradicting previous studies that failed to show any benefit on blood glucose in people with T2D [92, 93]. The studies are still inconclusive and advise for more well-organized RCT to assess the green tee effectiveness. Another plant called Coccinia grandis belongs to the Cucurbitaceae family, which includes 960 different species. This herb was assessed by a double-blind RCT. The patients were advised to take 20 g of leaves of Coccinia grandis with the breakfast. It found that the postprandial glucose was significantly reduced compared to the control group [94]. The need for more RCT is required to prove the effect of this plant.

2.18 Common herbs with no significant effect on blood glucose levels

2.18.1 Ginkgo Biloba

Ginkgo biloba L. is a valuable source for developing new herbal medicines, also known as the maidenhair tree. It is a living fossil that has impressed scientists worldwide due to its abundance of bioactive compounds and medicinal value. This type of species is commonly used to treat some central nervous system diseases, such as Alzheimer's disease and memory problems. The Ginkgo tree is grown a lot in many countries such as Asia, Europe, North America, New Zealand, and Argentina. This tree has been used in Chinese medicine for a very long time, around 2000 years. Many people use Ginkgo leaf extracts in herbal medicine, food supplements, and natural remedies [95]. Ginkgo biloba was found to increase HbA1c levels in people with T2D [96]. However, the extract from the Ginkgo biloba tree reduced the amount of albumin in urine, lowered the fasting blood sugar levels, and decreased levels of creatinine, blood urea, and nitrogen [97]. Moreover, it might help in treating diabetic retinopathy alongside conventional medicine [98]. More studies are required to assess the effect of Ginkgo biloba on plasma glucose concentration.

2.18.2 Walnut

It has been found by two systematic review studies that the consumption of walnuts did not significantly impact fasting blood sugar levels or HbA1c. That means the positive effect of walnut on the cardiovascular system is not related to the improvement of blood sugar levels. The current evidence has a high risk of bias, so we need more randomized well-conducted clinical trials to get reliable results on the walnut effect on blood sugar [99, 100]. Moreover, the walnut increased leptin and adiponectin levels but does not affect the body mass of people with T2D [101, 102].

2.18.3 Capsicum frutescens or annuum

Pepper, also known as Capsicum, is a widely cultivated crop with a long history of use. It originated in America and there are over 200 species of pepper, each with different tastes and levels of heat. Pepper is commonly used as a condiment or food ingredient and has various medicinal uses in Indian, American, and Chinese traditions. It belongs to the Solanaceae family and is highly valued for its spiciness and flavor [103]. A systematic review and meta-analysis study found no effect of Capsicum annuum on plasma glucose concentration. However, the number of the studies is small with high heterogeneity [104]. Moreover, studies have shown that using capsaicin cream with a low concentration of 0.075% can help reduce pain in people with diabetic neuropathy. This cream can be applied to painful areas for around 8 weeks. It is well tolerated by patients and is effective in improving pain levels, mobility, ability to work and sleep, and participation in recreational activities. Similarly, giving a higher amount of topical capsaicin, specifically 8%, also works well in reducing pain for people with diabetic neuropathy [105].

2.18.4 Homeopathy

Homeopathic medicine follows two main ideas. First, the principle of similarity says that something that causes a problem can also cure it. Second, it believes that the more diluted a substance is, the stronger its healing power becomes. However, these ideas have not been proven and go against what doctors and scientists know about medicine [106]. The prevalence of using homeopathy in adults over the last 12 months across 11 countries is between 0.2–8.2% for the period 1990–2012 [107]. A systematic review tried to assess homeopathy in people with T2D and no studies were found comparing homeopathic remedies to either a placebo or an active drug for treating diabetes or obesity [108].

One study tried to track the case reports and series that are related to the adverse effects of homeopathy. It found that there are about 1159 patients who experienced direct or indirect adverse effects of homeopathy. The direct adverse effects of homeopathy use lead to serious outcomes such as cancer, death, dialysis, toxic polyneuropathy, and quadriparesis. Indirect adverse effects included deterioration of pulmonary allergy, hypertensive heart failure, encephalopathy, and others. Most cases of adverse effects in homeopathy are caused by allergic reactions or ingestion of toxic substances. Heavy metals, such as arsenic, cadmium, mercury, and iron, commonly used in homeopathy, can be toxic if not properly diluted. Other poisons used in homeopathy, such as aconitum, kerosene, or thallium, can also pose serious health risks if not adequately diluted [109].

The National Health and Medical Research Council (NHMRC) in Australia has determined that there is no reliable evidence to support the effectiveness of homeopathy in treating any health conditions. Therefore, it is not recommended to use homeopathy for chronic, serious, or potentially serious conditions. People who rely solely on homeopathy may jeopardize their health by rejecting or delaying treatments that have been proven safe and effective [110].

3. Conclusion regarding the medicinal herbs

Some herbs, such as Sesame, Aloe vera leaf gel, Psyllium fiber, and Fenugreek seeds demonstrated a significant impact on the levels of HbA1c compared to other studied herbs. Other herbs decreased HbA1c by at least 0.5%, such as Nigella sativa and Astragalus membranaceus. Some herbal remedies had not been assessed by a meta-analysis [111].

Traditional dietary and lifestyle recommendations for people with diabetes rarely include information on natural remedies, herbs, and spices that can help control blood sugar levels. However, this review guides patients interested in using herbal supplements and foods as part of their self-care and diet, as well as clinicians consulting them. Some of the tested remedies are both effective and safe, and many of these herbs and spices are commonly used in food and considered very safe. Some can easily be incorporated into the diet, while others can be purchased without a prescription. However, it is important to ensure that the most effective preparations are used in adequate dosages. Additionally, it is important to inform patients and clinicians about remedies that are ineffective or lack sufficient evidence of effectiveness [111].

Regarding the clinical trials on the herbs, the discussion is focused on how both environmental and individual factors can influence the outcomes achieved. It is difficult to determine whether the results are due to natural treatments or accompanying medicines. Unhealthy habits, such as a poor diet, can have negative consequences when using natural products. Each patient's unique qualities, including lifestyle, genetics, existing health issues, and previous treatments, can lead to different outcomes. Therefore, it is important to consider these personal characteristics when conducting such studies. Most of the trials encountered a couple of issues. An obstacle is presented by the differences among the clinical trial participants. Furthermore, the trials' poor design has resulted in different results for different individuals. Moreover, both the inadequate number of participants and brief durations characterize these trials. Additionally, the limited amount of data available can impact the application of the results to a larger population or special population, such as pregnant ladies or patients with diminished renal or liver functions [112, 113]. The summary for all systematic reviews and meta-analysis regarding medicinal herbs are shown in **Table 1**.

4. Mind-body therapies

4.1 Yoga

Yoga is a type of exercise that focuses on both body and mind. It requires both physical movement and mindful focus on one's thoughts, feelings, breathing, and energy [115]. One systematic review and meta-analysis published in 2022, tried to assess whether yoga training could affect diabetes-related indicators compared to usual care. It included 13 studies with a sample size of 1335 people with T2D. The study found a significant effect of yoga on HbA1c, FPC, PPBG, and TG. In the coming years, it is recommended to undertake extensive studies involving a higher number of participants to examine the prolonged effects of yoga on individuals diagnosed with T2D [116]. These findings are similar to previous systemic reviews, which were published in 2010 and 2016 and found that positive effect of yoga on HbA1c and FPC. However, the risk of bias and heterogeneity among the included studies is high [117, 118].

Study's First author	Herb	No. of included studies/patients	Study period	The main findings	The effect on glucose level
Budiastutik et al. [31]	Aloe vera	13 / 642	2011–2021	• Aloe vera reduced FBS significantly. • There is high heterogeneity between the included clinical trial	FBG: (−1.238 mg/dl, 95% CI: −1.853, −0.623)
Owens et al. [33]	Moringa oleifera	30 / 158	May 1, 2008 - May 1, 2018	• Moringa significantly decreased blood glucose levels • In some cases, increased insulin levels in diabetic patients.	It is a systematic review paper, not a meta-analysis
Shabil et al. [36]	Fenugreek	14 / 894	Up to November 18, 2022	• There is a reduction in FBS, and PPG, but was not statistically significant. • There is a statistically significant reduction in HbA1c • There is high heterogeneity between the included studies	FBS: (MD: 3.70, 95% CI of −27.02, 19.62) PPG: (MD: −10.61, 95% CI of −68.48, 47.26) HbA1c (MD: −0.88, 95% CI −1.49, −0.27)
Neelakantan et al. [37]	Fenugreek	10 / 278	up to 29 Nov 2013	• significant reduction in FBS, 2-hr glucose, and HbA1c. • There was a large variation between the included studies in the dose of fenugreek seeds used ranging from 1 g per day to 100 g/day. • The quality of the included clinical trials was generally poor	FBS: (−0.96 mmol/l (95% CI: −1.52, −0.40) 2-hPP: (−2.19 mmol/l (95% CI: −3.19, −1.19) HbA1c: (−0.85% (95% CI: −1.49%, −0.22%)
Khodamoradi et al. [38]	Fenugreek	12 / 823	2000 to 31 July 2019	• Fenugreek reduces FBS, LDL-C, and HbA1c levels significantly. • Fenugreek did not affect BMI	FBS: (−12.94 mg/dL, 95%CI: −21.39, −4.49) HbA1c: (−0.58%, 95% CI: −0.99, −0.17%)
Ziaei et al. [41]	Urtica dioica	8 / 266	2012 and 2017	• Effective in reducing FBS • No effect on HbA1C or insulin level	FBS [WMD]: (−18.01 mg/dl, 95% CI: −30.04 to −5.97) HbA1c: [WMD]: (−0.77%, 95% CI: −1.77 to 0.22)

Study's First author	Herb	No. of included studies/patients	Study period	The main findings	The effect on glucose level
Tabrizi et al. [42]	Urtica dioica	13 studies	Up to December 2019	• improvement in levels of FBS, HbA1c, CRP, triglycerides, and SBP • No significant change in serum levels of insulin, TC, LDL-C, HDL-C, BMI, and diastolic blood pressure (DBP)	FBG [WMD]: (− 17.17 mg/dl, 95% CI: −26.60, −7.73) HbA1c [WMD]: (−0.93, 95% CI: - 1.66, −0.17)
Abdollahi et al. [44]	Salvia officinalis	3 / 85	Up to March 2021	• Salvia officinalis reduced 2hPP, HbA1c, TC, LDL. • No significant effect on TG, and HDL. • No specific side effects were reported	FBS [MD]: (−31.15 mg/dL; 95% CI: −37.56 to −24.73) HbA1c [MD]: (−0.94%; 95% CI: −1.25 to −0.63)
Ramírez-Coronel et al. [46]	Sesamum indicum L.	8 / 395	Up to December 2022	• Sesame consumption significantly reduced serum FBS and HbA1c percentage in patients with T2D	FBS [WMD]: (−28.61 mg/dL, 95% CI: −36.07 to −21.16) HbA1C [WMD]: (−0.99%, 95% CI: −1.22 to −0.76)
Sohouli et al. [47]	Sesamum indicum L.	8 / 510	Up to February 2021	• Sesame consumption significantly reduced serum FBS and HbA1c percentage in patients with T2D	FBG [WMD]: (−21.31 mg/dl, 95% CI: −41.23, −1.39) HbA1c [WMD]: (−0.75, 95% CI: −1.16, −0.34)
Khotbehsara et al. [50]	Nigella sativa	7 / 255	Up to February 2017	• Significantly improved FBS, HbA1c, TC and LDL • The overall effects of TG and HDL-c were insignificant	FBS: (−17.84 mg/dl, 95% CI: −21.19 to −14.49) HbA1c: (−0.71%, 95% CI: −1.04, −0.39)
Hamdan et al. [51]	Nigella sativa	7 / 447	2009 and 2015	• Concluded that there is Improvement of FBS, 2hPP, HbA1c, insulin level and insulin resistance	It is a systematic review paper, not a meta-analysis
Hallajzadeh et al. [52]	Nigella sativa	50 / 3679	Up to October 30, 2019	Significantly reduced FBS, HbA1c, TG, TC, VLDL, LDL. No effect on insulin level or insulin resistance	FBS [WMD]: (−15.18 mg/dl; 95% CI: −19.82, −10.55) HbA1C [WMD]: (−0.45%; 95% CI: −0.66, −0.23)

Study's First author	Herb	No. of included studies/patients	Study period	The main findings	The effect on glucose level
Mahomoodally et al. [53]	Nigella sativa	17 / 3679	Up to January 2022	• Concluded that there is improvement of FBG, PPBG, HbA1c, HOMA-IR, and HOMA-β	It is a systematic review paper, not a meta-analysis
Xiao et al. [56]	Psyllium fiber	8 / 395	from 1998 to August 2019	• Significant reduction in TG, LDL, FBS, and HbA1c using about 10 g/day • No significant change in weight • No side effects were reported	HbA1c [MD]: (−0.91%, 95% CI −1.31, −0.51) FBS [MD]: (−31.71 ml/dl, 95% CI −50.04, −13.38)
Ting Mao et al. [57]	Dietary fiber	22 / 911	Up to March 23, 2021	• Significant reduction in FBS, HbA1c, fasting insulin, and HOMA-IR using about 10 g/day • No significant effect on BMI	FBS [WMD]: (−0.80 mmol/L, 95% CI −1.14, −0.46) HbA1c: (−0.66%, 95% CI −0.94, −0.38)
Jovanovski et al. [58]	Viscous fiber including psyllium	28 /1394	Up to 15 June 2018	• Significant reduction in FBS, HbA1c, and HOMA-IR • HbA1c levels were reduced by 0.58% following a median dose of about 13.1 g/day over 8 weeks	HbA1c [MD]: (−0.58% [95% CI −0.88, −0.28) FBS [MD]: (−0.82 mmol/L, 95% CI −1.32, −0.31)
Gouws et al. [60]	Opuntia spp. cacti	20 / 450	Up to September 2018	• Prickly Pear fruit was predominately reported to have no significant effects on glucose or insulin. • The cladode does however show promise in potential glucose-lowering effects which warrant further investigation	It is a systematic review paper, not a meta-analysis
Tian et al. [63]	Astragalus membranaceus	13 / 1054	Up to December 2015	• reduced FBS, PPG, and HbA1C • no adverse reactions were reported	FBS [WMD]: (−0.28, 95% CI −0.46 to −0.10) PPG [WMD]: (−0.47, 95% CI −0.77 to −0.17) HbA1c [WMD]: (−1.77, 95% CI −3.06 to −0.47)

Study's First author	Herb	No. of included studies/patients	Study period	The main findings	The effect on glucose level
Peter et al. [67]	Momordica charantia	10 / 1045	1st January 1960–30th April 2018	• reduced significantly FBS, PPG, and HbA1C • There is an overall moderate to high risk of bias • No serious adverse effects were reported	FBS [MD]: (– 0.72 mmol/L, 95% CI: −1.33, −0.12) PPG [MD]: (– 1.43 mmol/L, 95% CI: −2.18, −0.67) HbA1c [MD]:(– 0.26%, 95% CI: −0.49, −0.03)
Phimarn et al. [68]	Momordica charantia	8 / 507	Up to June 2016	• Significant reduction in FBS, HbA1C, LDL-C, TC, TG, and body weight	FBS [WMD]: (−25.03 mg/dL; 95% CI −41.17, −8.89) HbA1c [WMD]: (−0.20%; 95% CI −0.36, −0.04)
Schwingshackl et al. [70]	Olive oil	33 / 187,068	Up to August 2016	Olive oil reduced HbA1c and FBS significantly It is associated with a 16% risk reduction of T2D	HbA1c [MD]: (−0.27%; 95% CI: −0.37, −0.17) FBS [MD]: (−0.44 mmol l – 1; 95% CI −0.66, −0.22)
Dehghani et al. [72]	Olive oil	13 / 633	Up to 1 September 2020	• Extra-virgin olive oil did not show any effect on blood glucose	FBS [SMD]: (−0.07; 95% CI: −0.20, −0.07)
Shabani et al. [73]	Allium sativum (Garlic)	33 / 1273	1988 and 2016	• Garlic reduced HbA1c, FBS, TC, LDL, and TG. • Moderate risk of publication bias may exist in HbA1c.	FBS: (10.90 mg/dl, 95% CI, −16.40, −5.40) HbA1c: (0.60 mg/dl, 95% CI, −0.98, −0.22)
Wang et al. [74]	Allium sativum (Garlic)	9 / 768	up to April 2017	• Significant improvement of FBS, HbA1c and fructosamine • Improved TC and LDL	After 24 weeks: FBS [SMD]: (−21.02, 95%CI −32.47, −9.57) HbA1c [SMD] = (−13.25, 95%CI −15.83, −10.68)
Ebrahimzadeh et al. [79]	Zingiber officinale (Ginger)	10 / 597	2013 - September 2021	Significant reduction in FBS and HbA1c Significant effect on SBP and DBP No significant effect on lipid profile	FBS (WMD) = (– 18.81; 95% CI: – 28.70, – 8.92) HbA1C (WMD) = (−0.57; 95% CI: −0.93, −0.20)

Study's First author	Herb	No. of included studies/patients	Study period	The main findings	The effect on glucose level
Jafarnejad et al. [80]	Zingiber officinale (Ginger)	9 studies	up to 30 October 2016	• Reduced FBG, TG, and TC and significantly increased HDL-C • No serious side effects	FBS (WMD) = (−14.93; 95% CI: −19.83 to −10.04)
Zhu et al. [82]	Zingiber officinale (Ginger)	10 / 608	Up to May 19, 2017	• Significant reduction of HbA1c. FBS and fasting insulin • Positive significant effect on TG, TC, LDL, and HDL • No serious side effect	HbA1c [MD]: (−1.00, (95% CI: −1.56, −0.44) FBS [MD]: (−21.24; 95% CI: −33.21, −9.26)
Fy Huang et al. [81]	Zingiber officinale (Ginger)	8 / 454	Up to July 2018	• No significant effect of FBS • Significant reduction of HbA1c	FBS [WMD]: −0.27, 95% CI: (−5.09–4.54) HbA1c [WMD]: (−0.46, 95% CI: 0.09–0.84)
Park et al. [84]	Panax quinquefolius (Ginseng)	23 /224	Up to September 2020	• No significant improvement in FBS, HbA1c, and 2hpp • Statistically significant effect on TC, TG, and LDL • Improvement of blood pressure	FBS [AUC]: −1.77 mmol/L*hr. (95% CI: −2.97 to −0.57)
Naseri et al. [85]	Panax quinquefolius (Ginseng)	20 /1295	Up to 10 April 2022	• Significant reduction of FBS, HOMA-IR, and TC. • No significant effect on OGTT, HbA1,c, TG and BMI	FBS [WMD]:(−7.03 mg/dL; 95% CI: −10.89, −3.17)
Gui et al. [114]	Panax quinquefolius (Ginseng)	8 / 90	Up to March 2, 2015	• No significant effect on HbA1c, FBS or postprandial glucose	HbA1c: std. diff in means: (−0.148, 95% CI: −0.637 to 0.228) FBS, std. diff in means: (−0.306, 95% CI: −0.539 to −0.074)

Study's First author	Herb	No. of included studies/patients	Study period	The main findings	The effect on glucose level
Shishtar et al. [87]	Panax quinquefolius (Ginseng)	16 / 770	Up to July 3, 2013	• Significant effect on FBS • No significant effect on HbA1c, or postprandial glucose	FBS: MD = (−0.31 mmol/L [95% CI: −0.59 to −0.03])
Namazi et al. [88]	Cinnamomum verum	18 studies	Up to 31 February 2018	• Significant reduction of FBS • No statistically significant reduction in HbA1c, insulin levels, waist circumference, and BMI.	FBS: (−19.26 mg/dL, 95% CI: −28.08, −10.45) HbA1C (−0.24%; 95% CI: −0.48, −0.01; I2: 76.8%)
Wang. [91]	Camellia sinensis	16 / 832	up to January 30, 2021	• Statistically significant reduction of FBS, HbA1c, and TG • No positive effect on LDL • The tea preparations were different between the studies. • No serious adverse events were reported	FBS [MD]: (−0.50 mmol/L 95%CI, −0.99, −0.01) HbA1c [MD]: (−0.37%, 95%CI -0.47, −0.26)
Yu. [93]	Camellia sinensis	6 / 382	up to April 2017	• No significant effect on fasting insulin, FBS, or HbA1C • The included studies are small	HbA1c [SMD]: (−0.32; 95% CI −0.86 to 0.23) FBS [SMD]: (−0.10; 95% CI, −0.50 to 0.30)
Tabrizi et al. [96]	Ginkgo biloba	7 / 768	Up to September 2, 2019	• Ginkgo biloba can significantly improve HDL-cholesterol levels; however, it increases HbA1c levels.	HbA1c [WMD]: (−0.26, 95% CI -0.02, −0.50) FBS [WMD]: (−4.15, 95% CI −8.99, 0.70)
Mateș et al. [99]	Walnut	17 / 871	Up to November 2021	• statistically significant decreasing effects for triglyceride, total cholesterol, and LDL cholesterol concentrations • No consequences on anthropometric or glycemic parameters.	FBS [SMD]: (−0.01; 95% CI: 0–0.02) HbA1c [SMD]: (0.08; 95% CI: −0.04–0.2)

Study's First author	Herb	No. of included studies/patients	Study period	The main findings	The effect on glucose level
Neale et al. [100]	Walnut	16 / 1283	Up to 2 March 2019	• No positive effect on blood sugar levels	FBS [WMD]: (−0·331 mg/ dl; 95% CI −0·817, 1·479) HbA1c [WMD]: (−0.03, 95% cl −0.00,0.06)
Jang et al. [104]	Capsicum annuum	3 studies	up to April 2020	• BMI reduced but not statistically significant • No effect on blood glucose TC, or BP • Had a significant effect on LDL	Blood glucose [SMD]: (− 0.58; 95% CI − 1.62, 0.45)

FBS: fasting blood sugar, PPG: postprandial glucose, HbA1c: glycated hemoglobin, MD: mean difference, WMD: Weighted mean difference, HDL: high-density lipoprotein, LDL: low-density lipoprotein, VLDL: very low-density lipoprotein, TC: total cholesterol, TG: triglyceride, BMI: body mass index, 2hPP: 2-hour postprandial, BP: blood pressure. HOMA-IR: Homeostatic Model Assessment for Insulin Resistance, SMD: standardized mean differences. AUC: area under the curve.

Table 1.
Summary of systematic review and meta-analysis papers of the studied herbs.

4.2 Meditation

Meditation involves engagement in activities that promote relaxation and contentment for the mind and body. It helps people feel better overall. Meditation usually involves focusing on breathing, feeling relaxed, staying focused, and being mindful of the thoughts and body at the same time. A survey reveals that the number of American adults who engaged in meditation with mantras, mindfulness, or for spiritual motives had tripled between 2012 and 2017. It went from 4.1 to 14.2% [119]. One systematic review and meta-analysis study was conducted to assess the effects of meditation interventions on the self-management of people with T2D. It found that mindfulness-based meditation reduced hemoglobin A1c levels but not fasting blood sugar levels [120]. There were problems with the randomization in some studies and with missing information about the results. Variations in the duration of follow-up, group size, and measured outcomes were prominent among the included studies [120].

4.3 Hydrotherapy

Hydrotherapy means using water as medicine to improve health. It involves using hot or cold water and sometimes adding minerals or herbs to directly affect the flow of blood and hormones in the body, which helps alleviate symptoms of certain illnesses [121]. Hydrotherapy was found to have a positive effect on high blood sugar as shown in a systematic review study [122]. The patients need to be cautious about the water temperature since patients with neuropathy may not have the ability to perceive if they are burning themselves. When recommending hot-tub therapy to people with diabetes, it is important to treat the water properly and give them the right instructions [123].

4.4 Muscle relaxation

Progressive muscle relaxation (PMR) was tried by quasi-experiment with pre-and posttest randomized control study. The study involved 48 inpatients with high plasma sugar concentration. The people in the study practiced relaxation exercises two times a day for three days in a row. Each session lasted about 25 to 30 minutes. Participants in the control group engaged in breathing exercises. There were big differences in the average plasma sugar levels of T2D people who received treatment compared to the other group [124]. PMR and mindfulness meditation were found to alleviate diabetic neuropathy in people with T2D [125].

4.5 Acupuncture

A systematic review showed a positive effect of acupuncture on plasma glucose concentration and HbA1C. However, most of these studies were conducted in China, and some of them have a bias in the methodology [126]. Other systematic review research showed that acupuncture, when used alongside medication for diabetes, can slightly but statistically significantly help in lowering fasting plasma glucose concentration and improving insulin resistance. The effects of acupuncture on HbA1c, 2hBG, and fasting insulin levels were uncertain [127]. One study reviewed the side effects on 229,230 patients who received on average 10.2 ± 3.0 acupuncture treatments. It found that 19,726 patients (8.6%) had at least one adverse effect and 4963

(2.2%) reported one which required treatment. The most commonly reported side effects were hematoma or bleeding [128].

Acupuncture is generally considered safe for individuals who have mild diabetes and should be performed by trained specialists to minimize the side effects. However, there is still a need for more well-conducted clinical trials to show how acupuncture affects T2D either in the short or long term.

4.6 Therapeutic massage

Therapeutic massage aims to enhance overall well-being by gently manipulating and stroking the body's soft tissues, to facilitate relaxation and improve sleep quality. It can also help with specific issues, such as reducing muscle pains or discomfort. Most cultures have created ways to use therapeutic massage. Massage methods are significant in traditional Chinese and Indian healthcare [129]. There are different types and techniques of massage therapy such as Swedish, tactile, and compressed air. Bayat et al. found that therapeutic massage could decrease FBS and HbA1c. Also, it could help in improving neuropathic pain in patients with diabetic neuropathy [130].

4.7 Tai chi

Tai chi sessions involve various physical movements, such as slow, flowing motions resembling a dance. It can also include sitting or standing meditation postures and gentle or vigorous body shaking. The focus is on deliberately controlling both breath and thoughts while coordinating with the body's movements [131].

A meta-analysis showed that doing tai chi for 4000–5999 minutes can help improve blood sugar and HbA1c levels for people with type 2 diabetes. Doing tai chi exercise for 80–120 minutes each week for over a year, or 160–240 minutes each week for over six months, can help control their blood sugar and HbA1c levels. The recommended quantity of tai chi exercise aligns with the amount of moderate-intensity exercise suggested in the clinical practice guidelines, which is around 150 minutes weekly [132]. Moreover, practicing tai chi could help people with T2D to reduce triglyceride, improve HDL-C cholesterol, lower their BMI, and improve their quality of life [133–135].

4.8 Moxibustion

Moxibustion is a traditional treatment method that has been used in Eastern Asian countries for thousands of years to alleviate various ailments, with a particular focus on pain conditions. This therapy involves stimulating specific acupuncture points on the body using dried Mugwort leaves, which are burned and applied directly or indirectly to the skin. In a study conducted by Kim et al. the effectiveness of moxibustion in the treatment of T2D was investigated. However, the researchers faced challenges in drawing definitive conclusions about the efficacy of moxibustion for controlling T2D due to the limited number of trials available and the overall poor quality of the included studies [136].

4.9 Conclusion regarding the mind-body therapies

Mind–body interventions encompass various practices and methods that promote the integration of the mind, body, thoughts, and actions to enhance physical

Study's First author	CAM modality	No. of included studies/ patients	Study period	The finding
Chen et al. [116]	Yoga	13 / 1335	Up to July 2021	• Good and significant effect on FBS, HbA1c, and TG • No effect on TC or BMI
Aljasir et al. [117]	Yoga	5 / 362	Up to May 2007	• Good effect on FBS, and lipid profile • Reduction of Hb1c and BMI but was not significant in the trials. • No calculated pooled effect because of the high level of heterogeneity between the characteristics of the studies
Kumar et al. [118]	Yoga	17 / 1521	Up to December 17, 2014	• Good effect of yoga as an additional intervention to the treatment • Good effect on FBS and HbA1c • risk of bias was overall high
Heo et al. [120]	Meditation	9 / 698	Up to March 2022	• Improved hemoglobin A1c but not fasting blood glucose
Yogapriya Chidambaram et al. [122]	Hydrotherapy	6 studies	Up to December 20, 2022	• Hydrotherapy is effective in reducing blood sugar level • Two studies used hot treatments, two used cold treatments, and two used both ht and cold treatments.
Chen et al. [126]	Acupuncture	21 / 1943	2001 - June 4, 2018	• Acupuncture plus baseline treatments yield a reduction in FBG, 2hPP, and HbA1c. • There are many pitfalls in the method of the involved clinical trials.
Qing et al. [127]	Acupuncture	21 / 1188	Up to July 5, 2020	• Improved fasting blood glucose and insulin resistance. • No clear improvement in HbA1c or 2hPP levels
Bayat et al. [130]	Massage	12 /581	January 1, 2000 - May 13, 2018	• Statistically significant improvement in FBS, and HbA1c • Improvement in neuropathic pain • Low sample size of the RCTs
Chao et al. [132]	Tai chi	14 / 798	Up to June 2016	• Tai chi reduces FBS and HbA1c • The quality of included papers was low

Study's First author	CAM modality	No. of included studies/ patients	Study period	The finding
Xinzheng et al. [133]	Tai chi	18 / 1220	2008 and 2020	• Tai Chi exercise therapy shows significant superiority in improving the FBG, HbA1c, TG, and HDL-C
Cai et al. [135]	Tai chi	24 / 1314	Up to December 2021	• Tai Chi improved HbA1c, FBG, fasting insulin, DBP, BMI, and the quality of life (QoL) in patients with T2DM. • There was no difference between Tai Chi and other exercise types in the HbA1c, FBG, TC, TG, HDL, LDL, BMI, and (WC).

FBS: fasting blood sugar, PPG: postprandial glucose, HbA1c: glycated hemoglobin,, HDL: high-density lipoprotein, LDL: low-density lipoprotein, VLDL: very low-density lipoprotein, TC: total cholesterol, TG: triglyceride, BMI: body mass index, 2hPP: 2-hour postprandial, BP: blood pressure DBP: diastolic blood pressure. WC: waist circumference.

Table 2.
Summary of systematic review and meta-analysis papers of the studied mind–body therapies.

well-being and overall health. Practices, such as yoga, meditation, and tai chi, have been found to improve glycemic control, reduce stress, and enhance overall well-being in individuals with T2D. Based on all the above-mentioned studies, it seems like we need more research studies in the field of T2D treatment to determine if using (CAM), including mind–body therapies, on a regular basis is effective and safe. These studies should have to include a large number of participants and reliable data to make strong conclusions. Experienced experts are in a great position to create, carry out, and explain integrative research for common use. The summary for all systematic reviews and meta-analysis regarding mind–body therapies are shown in **Table 2**.

5. Suggested actions for stakeholders and healthcare providers

World health organization published a guideline entitled "WHO guidelines on safety monitoring of herbal medicines in pharmacovigilance systems" and encouraged the national health supervision centers to keep people safe when using herbal medicines by application of the followings:

1. Recognizing the adverse events has occurred.

2. Management of the risks.

3. Putting rules and regulations in place to prevent the adverse events.

4. Explaining clearly the advantages and risks of herbal remedies in an easy-to-understand manner.

WHO published another strategy named (WHO traditional medicine strategy 2014–2023) to face the challenges facing traditional and complementary medicine T&CM. This strategy includes [3]:

1. build the knowledge base that will allow T&CM to be managed actively through appropriate national policies that understand and recognize the role and potential of T&CM.

2. strengthen the quality assurance, safety, proper use, and effectiveness of T&CM by regulating products, practices, and practitioners through T&CM education and training, skills development, services, and therapies.

3. promote universal health coverage by integrating T&CM services into health service delivery and self-health care by capitalizing on their potential contribution to improve health services and health outcomes, and by ensuring users are able to make informed choices about self-health care.

Moreover, Healthcare providers need to be aware of the reliability and accuracy of online information regarding CAM treatments for T2D. In over half (56%) of the websites surveyed, the sources utilized for information gathering were deemed unreliable [137]. Healthcare providers need to communicate with their patients about the various treatment options. They also should understand how their patients search for information and direct them to reliable resources for health information. Furthermore, researchers, healthcare providers, and educators must establish guidelines addressing emerging and significant concerns associated with online health information. They should also be aware people about the false information on the internet and social media and help patients find trustworthy online sources.

Author details

Mohammed Zaid Aljulifi
Family and Community Medicine Department, College of Medicine, Majmaah University, Majmaah, Saudi Arabia

*Address all correspondence to: m.aljulifi@mu.edu.sa

References

[1] Chlup R, Kaňa R, Hanáčková L, Zálešáková H, Doubravová B. In: Stoian AP, editor. Pathophysiologic Approach to Type 2 Diabetes Management: One Centre Experience 1980-2020. Rijeka: IntechOpen; 2021. p. Ch. 1. DOI: 10.5772/intechopen.96237

[2] Saeedi P, Petersohn I, Salpea P, Malanda B, Karuranga S, Unwin N, et al. Global and regional diabetes prevalence estimates for 2019 and projections for 2030 and 2045: Results from the international diabetes federation diabetes atlas. Diabetes Research and Clinical Practice. 2019;**157**:107843

[3] World Health Organization. WHO Traditional Medicine Strategy: 2014-2023. Geneva: World Health Organization; 2013

[4] Defining and describing complementary and alternative medicine. Panel on definition and description, CAM research methodology conference, April 1995. Alternative Therapies in Health and Medicine. 1997;**3**(2):49-57

[5] National Center for Complementary and Integrative Health (NCCIH). Complementary, Alternative, or Integrative Health: What's In a Name? [Internet]. 2021. Available from: https://www.nccih.nih.gov/health/complementary-alternative-or-integrative-health-whats-in-a-name

[6] Ng JY, Boon HS, Thompson AK, Whitehead CR. Making sense of "alternative", "complementary", "unconventional" and "integrative" medicine: Exploring the terms and meanings through a textual analysis. BMC Complementary and Alternative Medicine. 2016;**16**(1):134. DOI: 10.1186/s12906-016-1111-3

[7] Alzahrani AS, Price MJ, Greenfield SM, Paudyal V. Global prevalence and types of complementary and alternative medicines use amongst adults with diabetes: Systematic review and meta-analysis. European Journal of Clinical Pharmacology. 2021;**77**(9):1259-1274. DOI: 10.1007/s00228-021-03097-x

[8] Wu CH, Wang CC, Tsai MT, Huang WT, Kennedy J. Trend and pattern of herb and supplement use in the United States: Results from the 2002, 2007, and 2012 National Health Interview Surveys. Evidence-Based Complement Alternative Medicine. 2014;**2014**:872320. DOI: 10.1155/2014/872320

[9] AlBedah AMN, Khalil MKM, Elolemy AT, Al Mudaiheem AA, Al Eidi S, Al-Yahia OA, et al. The use of and out-of-pocket spending on complementary and alternative medicine in Qassim province, Saudi Arabia. Annals of Saudi Medicine. 2013;**33**(3):282-289

[10] Kesavadev J, Saboo B, Sadikot S, Das AK, Joshi S, Chawla R, et al. Unproven therapies for diabetes and their implications. Advances in Therapy. 2017;**34**(1):60-77. DOI: 10.1007/s12325-016-0439-x

[11] Hasan SS, Ahmed SI, Bukhari NI, Loon WCW. Use of complementary and alternative medicine among patients with chronic diseases at outpatient clinics. Complementary Therapies in Clinical Practice. 2009;**15**(3):152-157

[12] Mbizo J, Okafor A, Sutton MA, Leyva B, Stone LM, Olaku O. Complementary and alternative medicine use among persons with multiple chronic conditions: Results from the 2012 National Health Interview Survey. BMC Complementary and Alternative

Medicine. 2018;**18**(1):281. DOI: 10.1186/s12906-018-2342-2

[13] Lee EL, Richards N, Harrison J, Barnes J. Prevalence of use of traditional, complementary and alternative medicine by the general population: A systematic review of national studies published from 2010 to 2019. Drug Safety. 2022;**45**(7):713-735

[14] Qureshi NA, Khalil AA, Alsanad SM. Spiritual and religious healing practices: Some reflections from Saudi National Center for Complementary and Alternative Medicine, Riyadh. Journal of Religion and Health. 2020;**59**:845-869

[15] Adib-Hajbaghery M, Fattahi Ardakani M, Sotoudeh A, Asadian A. Prevalence of complementary and alternative medicine (CAM) among diabetic patients in eastern Mediterranean country members of the World Health Organization (WHO): A review. Journal of Herbal Medicine. 2021;**29**:100476

[16] ElSayed NA, Aleppo G, Aroda VR, Bannuru RR, Brown FM, Bruemmer D, et al. Comprehensive medical evaluation and assessment of comorbidities: Standards of Care in Diabetes—2023. Diabetes Care. 2022;**46**(Supplement_1):s49-s67.2. DOI: 10.2337/dc23-S004

[17] Astin JA. Why patients use alternative medicine results of a National Study. Journal of the American Medical Association. 1998;**279**(19):1548-1553. DOI: 10.1001/jama.279.19.1548

[18] Bhat MDA, Malik R. Challenges in monitoring the safety of herbal medicines-an appraisal. Journal of Pharmacovigilance and Drug Research. 2022;**3**(4):3-8

[19] Islamoglu MS, Borku Uysal B, Yavuzer S, Cengiz M. Does the use of herbal medicine affect adherence to medication - a cross sectional study of outpatients with chronic disease? European Journal of Integrative Medicine. 2021;**44**:101326

[20] Ang JY, Ho RY, Tong SF, Aziz F, Ooi GS. The prevalence of online natural health products purchase: A systematic review. The Malaysian Journal of Medicine and Health Sciences. 2023;**19**(2):250-258

[21] Yeh GY, Eisenberg DM, Kaptchuk TJ, Phillips RS. Systematic review of herbs and dietary supplements for glycemic control in diabetes. Diabetes Care. 2003;**26**(4):1277-1294. DOI: 10.2337/diacare.26.4.1277

[22] Hewlings SJ, DS K. Curcumin: A review of its effects on human health. Food. 2017;**6**(10):92. DOI: 10.3390/foods6100092

[23] Chuengsamarn S, Rattanamongkolgul S, Luechapudiporn R, Phisalaphong C, Jirawatnotai S. Curcumin extract for prevention of type 2 diabetes. Diabetes Care. 2012;**35**(11):2121-2127. DOI: 10.2337/dc12-0116

[24] Rahimi HR, Mohammadpour AH, Dastani M, Jaafari MR, Abnous K, Mobarhan MG, et al. The effect of nano-curcumin on HbA1c, fasting blood glucose, and lipid profile in diabetic subjects: A randomized clinical trial. Avicenna Journal of Phytomedicine. 2016;**6**(5):567-577

[25] Thikekar AK, Thomas AB, Chitlange SS. Herb-drug interactions in diabetes mellitus: A review based on pre-clinical and clinical data. Phytotherapy Research. 2021;**35**(9):4763-4781. DOI: 10.1002/ptr.7108

[26] Asadi S, Gholami MS, Siassi F, Qorbani M, Khamoshian K, Sotoudeh G.

Nano curcumin supplementation reduced the severity of diabetic sensorimotor polyneuropathy in patients with type 2 diabetes mellitus: A randomized double-blind placebo-controlled clinical trial. Complementary Therapies in Medicine. 2019;**43**:253-260

[27] Muthenna P, Suryanarayana P, Gunda SK, Petrash JM, Reddy GB. Inhibition of aldose reductase by dietary antioxidant curcumin: Mechanism of inhibition, specificity and significance. FEBS Letters. 2009;**583**(22):3637-3642

[28] Sharma S, Kulkarni SK, Chopra K. Curcumin, the active principle of turmeric (Curcuma longa), ameliorates diabetic nephropathy in rats. Clinical and Experimental Pharmacology & Physiology. 2006;**33**(10):940-945

[29] Panahi Y, Khalili N, Sahebi E, Namazi S, Reiner Ž, Majeed M, et al. Curcuminoids modify lipid profile in type 2 diabetes mellitus: A randomized controlled trial. Complementary Therapies in Medicine. 2017;**33**:1-5

[30] Kumar R, Singh AK, Gupta A, Bishayee A, Pandey AK. Therapeutic potential of Aloe vera—A miracle gift of nature. Phytomedicine. 2019;**60**:152996

[31] Budiastutik I, Subagio WH, Kartasurya IM, Widjanarko B, Kartini A, Soegiyanto B, et al. The effect of Aloe vera on fasting blood glucose levels in pre-diabetes and type 2 diabetes mellitus: A systematic review and meta-analysis. Journal of Pharmacy & Pharmacognosy Research. 2022;**10**(4):737-747

[32] Leone A, Spada A, Battezzati A, Schiraldi A, Aristil J, Bertoli S. Cultivation, genetic, Ethnopharmacology, Phytochemistry and pharmacology of Moringa oleifera leaves: An overview. International Journal of Molecular Sciences. 2015;**16**:12791-12835

[33] Owens FS III, Dada O, Cyrus JW, Adedoyin OO, Adunlin G. The effects of Moringa oleifera on blood glucose levels: A scoping review of the literature. Complementary Therapies in Medicine. 2020;**50**:102362

[34] Milla PG, Peñalver R, Nieto G. Health benefits of uses and applications of Moringa oleifera in bakery products. Plants. 2021;**10**:318

[35] Singletary KW. Fenugreek: Overview of potential health benefits. Nutrition Today. 2017;**52**(2):93-111

[36] Shabil M, Bushi G, Bodige PK, Maradi PS, Patra BP, Padhi BK, et al. Effect of fenugreek on hyperglycemia: A systematic review and meta-analysis. Medicina. 2023;**59**:248

[37] Neelakantan N, Narayanan M, de Souza RJ, van Dam RM. Effect of fenugreek (Trigonella foenum-graecumL.) intake on glycemia: A meta-analysis of clinical trials. Nutrition Journal. 2014;**13**(1):7. DOI: 10.1186/1475-2891-13-7

[38] Khodamoradi K, Khosropanah MH, Ayati Z, Chang D, Nasli-Esfahani E, Ayati MH, et al. The effects of fenugreek on Cardiometabolic risk factors in adults: A systematic review and meta-analysis. Complementary Therapies in Medicine. 2020;**52**:102416

[39] Devkota HP, Paudel KR, Khanal SBA, Panth N, Adhikari-Devkota A, Jha NK, et al. Stinging nettle (Urtica dioica L.): Nutritional composition, bioactive compounds, and food functional properties. Molecules. 2022;**27**(16):5219. DOI: 10.3390/molecules27165219

[40] Samakar B, Mehri S, Hosseinzadeh H. A review of the effects

of Urtica dioica (nettle) in metabolic syndrome. Iranian Journal of Basic Medical Sciences. 2022;**25**(5):543

[41] Ziaei R, Foshati S, Hadi A, Kermani MAH, Ghavami A, Clark CCT, et al. The effect of nettle (Urtica dioica) supplementation on the glycemic control of patients with type 2 diabetes mellitus: A systematic review and meta-analysis. Phytotherapy Research. 2020;**34**(2):282-294. DOI: 10.1002/ptr.6535

[42] Tabrizi R, Sekhavati E, Nowrouzi-Sohrabi P, Rezaei S, Tabari P, Ghoran SH, et al. Effects of Urtica dioica on metabolic profiles in type 2 diabetes: A systematic review and meta-analysis of clinical trials. Mini Reviews in Medicinal Chemistry. 2022;**22**(3):550-563

[43] Ghorbani A, Esmaeilizadeh M. Pharmacological properties of Salvia officinalis and its components. Journal of Traditional and Complementary Medicine. 2017;**7**(4):433-440

[44] Abdollahi A, Adelibahram F, Ghassab-Abdollahi N, Araj-khodaei M, Parsian Z, Mirghafourvand M. The effect of Salvia officinalis on blood glycemic indexes and blood lipid profile in diabetic patients: A systematic review and meta-analysis. Journal of Complementary and Integrative Medicine. 2022. DOI: 10.1515/jcim-2021-0425 l

[45] Wei P, Zhao F, Wang Z, Wang Q, Chai X, Hou G, et al. Sesame (Sesamum indicum L.): A comprehensive review of nutritional value, phytochemical composition, health benefits, development of food, and industrial applications. Nutrients. 2022;**14**:4079

[46] Ramírez-Coronel AA, Ali Alhilali KA, Basheer Ahmed Y, Almalki SG, Karimian J. Effect of sesame (Sesamum indicum L.) consumption on glycemic control in patients with type 2 diabetes: A systematic review and meta-analysis of randomized controlled trials. Phytotherapy Research. 2023:1-11 DOI: 10.1002/ptr.7918

[47] Sohouli MH, Haghshenas N, Hernández-Ruiz Á, Shidfar F. Consumption of sesame seeds and sesame products has favorable effects on blood glucose levels but not on insulin resistance: A systematic review and meta-analysis of controlled clinical trials. Phytotherapy Research. 2022;**36**(3):1126-1134. DOI: 10.1002/ptr.7379

[48] Mahmoodi MR, Abbasi MM. Therapeutic effectiveness of sesame preparations and its bioactive ingredients in Management of Cardiometabolic Syndrome in diabetes mellitus: A systematic review. Current Diabetes Reviews. 2023;**19**(3):79-93

[49] Ahmad A, Husain A, Mujeeb M, Khan SA, Najmi AK, Siddique NA, et al. A review on therapeutic potential of Nigella sativa: A miracle herb. Asian Pacific Journal of Tropical Biomedicine. 2013;**3**(5):337-352

[50] Daryabeygi-Khotbehsara R, Golzarand M, Ghaffari MP, Djafarian K. Nigella sativa improves glucose homeostasis and serum lipids in type 2 diabetes: A systematic review and meta-analysis. Complementary Therapies in Medicine. 2017;**35**:6-13

[51] Hamdan A, Haji Idrus R, Mokhtar MH. Effects of nigella sativa on Type-2 diabetes mellitus: A systematic review. International Journal of Environmental Research and Public Health. 2019;**16**(24):4911

[52] Hallajzadeh J, Milajerdi A, Mobini M, Amirani E, Azizi S, Nikkhah E, et al. Effects of Nigella sativa on glycemic control, lipid profiles, and biomarkers of inflammatory and oxidative stress:

A systematic review and meta-analysis of randomized controlled clinical trials. Phytotherapy Research. 2020;**34**(10):2586-2608. DOI: 10.1002/ptr.6708

[53] Mahomoodally MF, Aumeeruddy MZ, Legoabe LJ, Montesano D, Zengin G. Nigella sativa L. and its active compound Thymoquinone in the clinical Management of Diabetes: A systematic review. International Journal of Molecular Sciences. 2022;**23**(20):12111.

[54] Yimer EM, Tuem KB, Karim A, Ur-Rehman N, Anwar F. *Nigella sativa* L. (black cumin): A promising natural remedy for wide range of illnesses. Evidence-Based Complement Alternative Medicine. 2019;**2019**:1528635. DOI: 10.1155/2019/1528635

[55] Belorio M, Gómez M. Psyllium: A useful functional ingredient in food systems. Critical Reviews in Food Science and Nutrition. 2022;**62**(2):527-538. DOI: 10.1080/10408398.2020.1822276

[56] Xiao Z, Chen H, Zhang Y, Deng H, Wang K, Bhagavathula AS, et al. The effect of psyllium consumption on weight, body mass index, lipid profile, and glucose metabolism in diabetic patients: A systematic review and dose-response meta-analysis of randomized controlled trials. Phytotherapy Research. 2020;**34**(6):1237-1247. DOI: 10.1002/ptr.6609

[57] Mao T, Huang F, Zhu X, Wei D, Chen L. Effects of dietary fiber on glycemic control and insulin sensitivity in patients with type 2 diabetes: A systematic review and meta-analysis. Journal of Functional Foods. 2021;**82**:104500

[58] Jovanovski E, Khayyat R, Zurbau A, Komishon A, Mazhar N, Sievenpiper JL, et al. Should viscous fiber supplements Be considered in diabetes control? Results from a systematic review and meta-analysis of randomized controlled trials. Diabetes Care. 2019;**42**(5):755-766. DOI: 10.2337/dc18-1126

[59] ElSayed NA, Aleppo G, Aroda VR, Bannuru RR, Brown FM, Bruemmer D, et al. 5. Facilitating positive health behaviors and well-being to improve health outcomes: Standards of Care in Diabetes—2023. Diabetes Care. 2022;**46**(Supplement_1):S68-S96. DOI: 10.2337/dc23-S005

[60] Gouws CA, Georgousopoulou EN, Mellor DD, McKune A, Naumovski N. Effects of the consumption of prickly pear cacti (Opuntia spp.) and its products on blood glucose levels and insulin: A systematic review. Medicina. 2019;**55**(5):138

[61] Giraldo-Silva L, Ferreira B, Rosa E, Dias ACP. Opuntia ficus-indica fruit: A systematic review of its phytochemicals and pharmacological activities. Plants. 2023;**12**:543

[62] Gupta RC, Chang D, Nammi S, Bensoussan A, Bilinski K, Roufogalis BD. Interactions between antidiabetic drugs and herbs: An overview of mechanisms of action and clinical implications. Diabetology and Metabolic Syndrome. 2017;**9**(1):1-12

[63] Tian H, Lu J, He H, Zhang L, Dong Y, Yao H, et al. The effect of Astragalus as an adjuvant treatment in type 2 diabetes mellitus: A (preliminary) meta-analysis. Journal of Ethnopharmacology. 2016;**191**:206-215

[64] Zhang L, Shergis JL, Yang L, Zhang AL, Guo X, Zhang L, et al. Astragalus membranaceus (Huang Qi) as adjunctive therapy for diabetic kidney disease: An updated systematic

review and meta-analysis. Journal of Ethnopharmacology. 2019;**239**:111921

[65] Venkatakrishnan K, Chiu HF, Wang CK. Popular functional foods and herbs for the management of type-2-diabetes mellitus: A comprehensive review with special reference to clinical trials and its proposed mechanism. Journal of Functional Foods. 2019;**57**:425-438

[66] Grover JK, Yadav SP. Pharmacological actions and potential uses of Momordica charantia: A review. Journal of Ethnopharmacology. 2004;**93**(1):123-132

[67] Peter EL, Kasali FM, Deyno S, Mtewa A, Nagendrappa PB, Tolo CU, et al. Momordica charantia L. lowers elevated glycaemia in type 2 diabetes mellitus patients: Systematic review and meta-analysis. Journal of Ethnopharmacology. 2019;**231**:311-324

[68] Phimarn W, Sungthong B, Saramunee K, Caichompoo W. Efficacy of Momordica charantia L. on blood glucose, blood lipid, and body weight: A meta-analysis of randomized controlled trials. Pharmacognosy Magazine. 2018;**14**(56):351-358

[69] Taticchi A, Selvaggini R, Esposto S, Sordini B, Veneziani G, Servili M. Physicochemical characterization of virgin olive oil obtained using an ultrasound-assisted extraction at an industrial scale: Influence of olive maturity index and malaxation time. Food Chemistry. 2019;**289**:7-15

[70] Schwingshackl L, Lampousi AM, Portillo MP, Romaguera D, Hoffmann G, Boeing H. Olive oil in the prevention and management of type 2 diabetes mellitus: A systematic review and meta-analysis of cohort studies and intervention trials. Nutrition & Diabetes. 2017;7(4):e262-e262. DOI: 10.1038/nutd.2017.12

[71] Martínez-González MA, Sayón-Orea C, Bullón-Vela V, Bes-Rastrollo M, Rodríguez-Artalejo F, Yusta-Boyo MJ, et al. Effect of olive oil consumption on cardiovascular disease, cancer, type 2 diabetes, and all-cause mortality: A systematic review and meta-analysis. Clinical Nutrition. 2022;**41**:2659-2682

[72] Dehghani F, Morvaridzadeh M, Pizarro AB, Rouzitalab T, Khorshidi M, Izadi A, et al. Effect of extra virgin olive oil consumption on glycemic control: A systematic review and meta-analysis. Nutrition, Metabolism, and Cardiovascular Diseases. 2021;**31**(7):1953-1961

[73] Shabani E, Sayemiri K, Mohammadpour M. The effect of garlic on lipid profile and glucose parameters in diabetic patients: A systematic review and meta-analysis. Primary Care Diabetes. 2019;**13**(1):28-42

[74] Wang J, Zhang X, Lan H, Wang W. Effect of garlic supplement in the management of type 2 diabetes mellitus (T2DM): A meta-analysis of randomized controlled trials. Food & Nutrition Research. 2017;**61**(1):1377571. DOI: 10.1080/16546628.2017.1377571

[75] Wan Q, Li N, Du L, Zhao R, Yi M, Xu Q, et al. Allium vegetable consumption and health: An umbrella review of meta-analyses of multiple health outcomes. Food Science & Nutrition. 2019;7(8):2451-2470. DOI: 10.1002/fsn3.1117

[76] Miki S, Ichi IK, Takashima M, Nishida M, Sasaki Y, Ushijima M, et al. Aged garlic extract suppresses the increase of plasma glycated albumin level

and enhances the AMP-activated protein kinase in adipose tissue in TSOD mice. Molecular Nutrition & Food Research. 2017;**61**(5):1600797. DOI: 10.1002/mnfr.201600797

[77] Jiang Y, Yue R, Liu G, Liu J, Peng B, Yang M, et al. Garlic (Allium sativum L.) in diabetes and its complications: Recent advances in mechanisms of action. Critical Reviews in Food Science and Nutrition. 2022:1-51. DOI: 10.1080/10408398.2022.2153793

[78] Antoniewicz J, Jakubczyk K, Gutowska I, Janda K. Ginger (Zingiber officinale) – A spice with therapeutic properties TT - Imbir lekarski (*Zingiber officinale*) – Surowiec o właściwościach terapeutycznych. Med Ogólna i Nauk o Zdrowiu. 2021;**27**(1):40-44

[79] Ebrahimzadeh A, Ebrahimzadeh A, Mirghazanfari SM, Hazrati E, Hadi S, Milajerdi A. The effect of ginger supplementation on metabolic profiles in patients with type 2 diabetes mellitus: A systematic review and meta-analysis of randomized controlled trials. Complementary Therapies in Medicine. 2022;**65**:102802

[80] Jafarnejad S, Keshavarz SA, Mahbubi S, Saremi S, Arab A, Abbasi S, et al. Effect of ginger (Zingiber officinale) on blood glucose and lipid concentrations in diabetic and hyperlipidemic subjects: A meta-analysis of randomized controlled trials. Journal of Functional Foods. 2017;**29**:127-134

[81] Huang F-Y, Deng T, Meng L-X, Ma X-L. Dietary ginger as a traditional therapy for blood sugar control in patients with type 2 diabetes mellitus: A systematic review and meta-analysis. Medicine (Baltimore). 2019;**98**(13):e15054

[82] Zhu J, Chen H, Song Z, Wang X, Sun Z. Effects of ginger *(Zingiber officinale roscoe)* on type 2 diabetes mellitus and components of the metabolic syndrome: A systematic review and meta-analysis of randomized controlled trials. Evidence-Based Complement Alternative Medicine. 2018;**2018**:5692962, 10.1155/2018/5692962

[83] Mancuso C, Santangelo R. Panax ginseng and Panax quinquefolius: From pharmacology to toxicology. Food and Chemical Toxicology. 2017;**107**:362-372

[84] Park SH, Chung S, Chung MY, Choi HK, Hwang JT, Park JH. Effects of Panax ginseng on hyperglycemia, hypertension, and hyperlipidemia: A systematic review and meta-analysis. Journal of Ginseng Research. 2022;**46**(2):188-205

[85] Naseri K, Saadati S, Sadeghi A, Asbaghi O, Ghaemi F, Zafarani F, et al. The efficacy of ginseng (Panax) on human prediabetes and type 2 diabetes mellitus: A systematic review and meta-analysis. Nutrients. 2022;**14**:2401

[86] Yuan HD, Kim JT, Kim SH, Chung SH. Ginseng and diabetes: The evidences from in vitro, animal and human studies. Journal of Ginseng Research. 2012;**36**(1):27

[87] Shishtar E, Sievenpiper JL, Djedovic V, Cozma AI, Ha V, Jayalath VH, et al. The effect of ginseng (the genus panax) on glycemic control: A systematic review and meta-analysis of randomized controlled clinical trials. PLoS One. 2014;**9**(9):e107391

[88] Namazi N, Khodamoradi K, Khamechi SP, Heshmati J, Ayati MH, Larijani B. The impact of cinnamon on anthropometric indices and glycemic status in patients with type 2 diabetes: A systematic review and meta-analysis of clinical trials. Complementary Therapies in Medicine. 2019;**43**:92-101

[89] Deyno S, Eneyew K, Seyfe S, Tuyiringire N, Peter EL, Muluye RA, et al. Efficacy and safety of cinnamon in type 2 diabetes mellitus and pre-diabetes patients: A meta-analysis and meta-regression. Diabetes Research and Clinical Practice. 2019;**156**:107815

[90] Namita P, Mukesh R, Vijay KJ. Camellia sinensis (green tea): A review. Global Journal of Pharmacology. 2012;**6**(2):52-59

[91] Wang P, Ma XM, Geng K, Jiang ZZ, Yan PY, Xu Y. Effects of Camellia tea and herbal tea on cardiometabolic risk in patients with type 2 diabetes mellitus: A systematic review and meta-analysis of randomized controlled trials. Phytotherapy Research. 2022;**36**(11):4051-4062. DOI: 10.1002/ptr.7572

[92] Li Y, Wang C, Huai Q, Guo F, Liu L, Feng R, et al. Effects of tea or tea extract on metabolic profiles in patients with type 2 diabetes mellitus: A meta-analysis of ten randomized controlled trials. Diabetes/Metabolism Research and Reviews. 2016;**32**(1):2-10. DOI: 10.1002/dmrr.2641

[93] Yu J, Song P, Perry R, Penfold C, Cooper AR. The effectiveness of green tea or green tea extract on insulin resistance and glycemic control in type 2 diabetes mellitus: A meta-analysis. Diabetes and Metabolism Journal. 2017;**41**(4):251-262

[94] Munasinghe MAAK, Abeysena C, Yaddehige IS, Vidanapathirana T, Piyumal KPB. Blood sugar lowering effect of *Coccinia grandis* (L.) J. Voigt: Path for a new drug for diabetes mellitus. Experimental Diabetes Research. 2011;**2011**:978762. DOI: 10.1155/2011/978762

[95] Belwal T, Giri L, Bahukhandi A, Tariq M, Kewlani P, Bhatt ID, et al. Ginkgo biloba. Nonvitamin and Nonmineral Nutritional Supplements. 2019:241-250. Available from: https://www.sciencedirect.com/science/article/abs/pii/B9780128124918000357

[96] Tabrizi R, Nowrouzi-Sohrabi P, Hessami K, Rezaei S, Jalali M, Savardashtaki A, et al. Effects of Ginkgo biloba intake on cardiometabolic parameters in patients with type 2 diabetes mellitus: A systematic review and meta-analysis of clinical trials. Phytotherapy Research. 2020;**35**(1):246-255

[97] Zhang L, Mao W, Guo X, Wu Y, Li C, Lu Z, et al. *Ginkgo biloba* extract for patients with early diabetic nephropathy: A systematic review. Evidence-Based Complement Alternative Medicine. 2013;**2013**:689142. DOI: 10.1155/2013/689142

[98] Wen XW, Dan Z, Shuang H. Effects of Ginkgo biloba extract on diabetic retinopathy: A meta-analysis and systematic review. TMR Modern Herbal Medicine. 2020;**3**(4):192-201

[99] Mateș L, Popa DS, Rusu ME, Fizeșan I, Leucuța D. Walnut intake interventions targeting biomarkers of metabolic syndrome and inflammation in middle-aged and older adults: A systematic review and meta-analysis of randomized controlled trials. Antioxidants. 2022;**11**:1412

[100] Neale EP, Guan V, Tapsell LC, Probst YC. Effect of walnut consumption on markers of blood glucose control: A systematic review and meta-analysis. The British Journal of Nutrition. 2020;**124**(7):641-653

[101] Yang L, Guo Z, Qi S, Fang T, Zhu H, Santos HO, et al. Walnut intake may increase circulating adiponectin and leptin levels but does not improve

glycemic biomarkers: A systematic review and meta-analysis of randomized clinical trials. Complementary Therapies in Medicine. 2020;**52**:102505

[102] Fernández-Rodríguez R, Martínez-Vizcaíno V, Garrido-Miguel M, Martínez-Ortega IA, Álvarez-Bueno C, Eumann MA. Nut consumption, body weight, and adiposity in patients with type 2 diabetes: A systematic review and meta-analysis of randomized controlled trials. Nutrition Reviews. 2022;**80**(4):645-655

[103] Batiha GE, Alqahtani A, Ojo OA, Shaheen HM, Wasef L, Elzeiny M, et al. Biological properties, bioactive constituents, and pharmacokinetics of some capsicum spp. and Capsaicinoids. International Journal of Molecular Sciences. 2020;**21**:5179

[104] Jang HH, Lee J, Lee SH, Lee YM. Effects of Capsicum annuum supplementation on the components of metabolic syndrome: A systematic review and meta-analysis. Scientific Reports. 2020;**10**(1):20912. DOI: 10.1038/s41598-020-77983-2

[105] Dludla PV, Nkambule BB, Cirilli I, Marcheggiani F, Mabhida SE, Ziqubu K, et al. Capsaicin, its clinical significance in patients with painful diabetic neuropathy. Biomedicine & Pharmacotherapy. 2022;**153**:113439

[106] Grams N. Homeopathy—Where is the science? A current inventory on a pre-scientific artifact. EMBO Reports. 2019;**20**(3):e47761

[107] Katy R, Petter V, Philippa F, Thomas Kate CC. Prevalence of homeopathy use by the general population worldwide: A systematic review. Homeopathy. 2017;**106**(02):69-78

[108] Monami M, Silverii A, Mannucci E. Alternative treatment or alternative to treatment? A systematic review of randomized trials on homeopathic preparations for diabetes and obesity. Acta Diabetologica. 2019;**56**(2):241-243. DOI: 10.1007/s00592-018-1235-7

[109] Posadzki P, Alotaibi A, Ernst E. Adverse effects of homeopathy: A systematic review of published case reports and case series. International Journal of Clinical Practice. 2012;**66**(12):1178-1188. DOI: 10.1111/ijcp.12026

[110] National Health and Medical Research Council (NHMRC). Homeopathy [Internet]. Available from: https://www.nhmrc.gov.au/about-us/resources/homeopathy#block-views-block-file-attachments-content-block-1

[111] Willcox ML, Elugbaju C, Al-Anbaki M, Lown M, Graz B. Effectiveness of medicinal plants for Glycaemic control in type 2 diabetes: An overview of meta-analyses of clinical trials. Frontiers in Pharmacology. 2021;**12**:777561

[112] Vivó-Barrachina L, Rojas-Chacón MJ, Navarro-Salazar R, Belda-Sanchis V, Pérez-Murillo J, Peiró-Puig A, et al. The role of natural products on diabetes mellitus treatment: A systematic review of randomized controlled trials. Pharmaceutics. 2022;**14**:101

[113] Medagama AB, Bandara R. The use of complementary and alternative medicines (CAMs) in the treatment of diabetes mellitus: Is continued use safe and effective? Nutrition Journal. 2014;**13**(1):102. DOI: 10.1186/1475-2891-13-102

[114] Gui QF, Xu ZR, Xu KY, Yang YM. The efficacy of ginseng-related therapies in type 2 diabetes mellitus: An updated systematic review and meta-analysis.

Medicine (Baltimore). 2016;**95**(6):e2584. DOI: 10.1097/MD.0000000000002584

[115] Woodyard C. Exploring the therapeutic effects of yoga and its ability to increase quality of life. International Journal of Yoga. 2011;**4**(2):49-54

[116] Chen S, Deng S, Liu Y, Yin T. Effects of yoga on blood glucose and lipid profile of type 2 diabetes patients without complications: A systematic review and meta-analysis. Frontiers in Sports and Active Living. 2022;**4**:900815

[117] Aljasir B, Bryson M, Al-shehri B. Yoga practice for the Management of Type II diabetes mellitus in adults: A systematic review. Evidence-Based Complement Alternative Medicine. 2010;7:269290. DOI: 10.1093/ecam/nen027

[118] Kumar V, Jagannathan A, Philip M, Thulasi A, Angadi P, Raghuram N. Role of yoga for patients with type II diabetes mellitus: A systematic review and meta-analysis. Complementary Therapies in Medicine. 2016;**25**:104-112

[119] National Centre for Complementary and Integrative Health. Meditation and mindfulness: what you need to know [Internet]. 2022. Available from: https://www.nccih.nih.gov/health/meditation-and-mindfulness-what-you-need-to-know

[120] Heo S, Kang J, Umeakunne E, Lee S, Bertulfo TF, Barbé T, et al. Effects of meditation intervention on self-management in adult patients with type 2 diabetes: A systematic literature review and meta-analysis. The Journal of Cardiovascular Nursing. 2023;**10**:1097

[121] Bahadorfar M. A study of hydrotherapy and its health benefits. International Journal of Research and Review. 2014;**1**(8):294-305

[122] Chidambaram Y, Vijayakumar V, Ravi P, Boopalan D, Anandhan A, Kuppusamy M. Does hydrotherapy influence plasma glucose levels in type 2 diabetes? – A scoping review. Journal of Complementary and Integrative Medicine. 2023. DOI: 10.1515/jcim-2023-0037

[123] Pandey A, Tripathi P, Pandey R, Srivatava R, Goswami S. Alternative therapies useful in the management of diabetes: A systematic review. Journal of Pharmacy & Bioallied Sciences. 2011;**3**(4):504-512

[124] Avianti N, Desmaniarti Z, Rumahorbo H. Progressive muscle relaxation effectiveness of the blood sugar patients with type 2 diabetes. The Open Nursing Journal. 2016;**6**(3):248-254

[125] Izgu N, Gok Metin Z, Karadas C, Ozdemir L, Metinarikan N, Corapcıoglu D. Progressive muscle relaxation and mindfulness meditation on neuropathic pain, fatigue, and quality of life in patients with type 2 diabetes: A randomized clinical trial. Journal of Nursing Scholarship. 2020;**52**(5):476-487. DOI: 10.1111/jnu.12580

[126] Chen C, Liu J, Sun M, Liu W, Han J, Wang H. Acupuncture for type 2 diabetes mellitus: A systematic review and meta-analysis of randomized controlled trials. Complementary Therapies in Clinical Practice. 2019;**36**:100-112

[127] Qing LS, Rong CJ, Lu LM, Ping WY, Zhou X, Sun X. Effect and safety of acupuncture for type 2 diabetes mellitus: A systematic review and meta-analysis of 21 randomised controlled trials. Chinese Journal of Integrative Medicine. 2022;**28**(5):463-471

[128] Witt CM, Pach D, Brinkhaus B, Wruck K, Tag B, Mank S, et al. Safety of acupuncture: Results of a prospective

observational study with 229,230 patients and introduction of a medical information and consent form. Complementary Medicine Research. 2009;**16**(2):91-97

[129] Vickers A, Zollman C. Massage therapies. BMJ. 1999;**319**(7219):1254 LP-1251257

[130] Bayat D, Mohammadbeigi A, Parham M, Mehrandasht A, Hashemi M, Mahlooji K, et al. The effect of massage on diabetes and its complications: A systematic review. Crescent Journal of Medical and Biological Sciences. 2020;**7**(1):22-28

[131] Jahnke R, Larkey L, Rogers C, Etnier J, Lin F. A comprehensive review of health benefits of qigong and tai chi. American Journal of Health Promotion. 2010;**24**(6):e1-e25

[132] Chao M, Wang C, Dong X, Ding M. The effects of tai chi on type 2 diabetes mellitus: A meta-analysis. Journal Diabetes Research. 2018;**2018**:7350567

[133] Xinzheng W, Fanyuan J, Xiaodong W. The effects of tai chi on glucose and lipid metabolism in patients with diabetes mellitus: A meta-analysis. Complementary Therapies in Medicine. 2022;**71**:102871

[134] Qin J, Chen Y, Guo S, You Y, Xu Y, Wu J, et al. Effect of tai chi on quality of life, body mass index, and waist-hip ratio in patients with type 2 diabetes mellitus: A systematic review and meta-analysis. Frontiers in Endocrinology. 2021;**11**:543627

[135] Cai Y, Liu X, Zhao A, Mao J, Guo X, Li G, et al. Effects of tai chi on health outcomes in patients with type 2 diabetes mellitus: A systematic review and meta-analysis. Journal of Traditional Chinese Medical Sciences. 2022;**9**(2):108-120

[136] Kim TH, Choi TY, Shin BC, Lee MS. Moxibustion for managing type 2 diabetes mellitus: A systematic review. Chinese Journal of Integrative Medicine. 2011;**17**(8):575-579. DOI: 10.1007/s11655-011-0811-2

[137] Ng JY, Nayeni M, Gilotra K. Quality of complementary and alternative medicine information for type 2 diabetes: A cross-sectional survey and quality assessment of websites. BMC Complementary Medicine and Therapies. 2021;**21**(1):233. DOI: 10.1186/s12906-021-03390-3

Chapter 12

Pharmacotherapy of Type 2 Diabetes Mellitus

Pankaj Kumar Jha, Heta Shukla, Altaf Makwana and Ashutosh Kakkad

Abstract

This book chapter provides a comprehensive and comparative overview of available pharmacotherapy options for the management of type 2 diabetes mellitus (T2DM). With the increasing prevalence of T2DM worldwide, it is important to understand the effectiveness of all available options for adequate glycemic control and prevention of long-term complications. The chapter begins with a comprehensive overview on different aspects of T2DM, with special attention to details on different pharmacotherapeutic options available for its management. The role of newer antidiabetic medications such as sodium-glucose transporter 2 (SGLT2) inhibitors, glucagon-like peptide-1 (GLP-1) receptor agonist, bile acid sequestrant, and dual GIP/GLP-1 receptor agonist is also emphasized. Additionally, formulations and usage of insulin and non-insulin injectables have been compared. Moreover, the current trends in management of T2DM and drugs in pipeline have also been discussed briefly. In conclusion, this book chapter provides a complete overview along with comparison of oral as well as injectable antidiabetic agents used for the management of T2DM. The healthcare professional will be equipped with the knowledge needed to optimize treatment strategies and improve outcomes for individuals living with T2DM.

Keywords: T2DM, HbA1c, SGLT2i, DPP-4i, sulfonylureas, biguanides, ADA, AACE, GLP-1 RA, alpha-glucosidase inhibitors

1. Introduction

Diabetes mellitus (DM) is a chronic metabolic disorder characterized by persistent hyperglycemia either due to insulin deficiency or resistance or both. Persistent hyperglycemia can lead to long-term microvascular complications such as blindness, end-stage renal disease, and lower limb amputation. It can also lead to macrovascular complications such as coronary artery disease, peripheral vascular disease, and stroke.

2. Epidemiology

Earlier diabetes was once considered a disease of affluent people now afflicting the even middle and poor population. The 10th edition of International Diabetes

Federation (IDF) confirms that diabetes is one of the fastest growing global health emergencies of the twenty-first century. Diabetes is a major health issue that has reached alarming levels. Today, more than half a billion (537 million) people are living with diabetes worldwide [1]. As per 2023 ICMR-INDIAB-17 study, 101 million people are suffering from T2DM and at least 136 million people (15.3% of the population) have prediabetes in India [2]. About 39.4 million (53.1%) adults in India are underdiagnosed and 1 out of 7 diabetic patient in the world is Indian.

One of the contributing factors for future increase in diabetic population in lower- and medium-income countries will be aging population.

3. Etiology

The progression of T2DM is usually slow and following factors increase the risk of development of T2DM [3].

1. Family history of DM
2. Habitual physical inactivity
3. Race or ethnicity
4. Previously identified impaired fasting glucose (IFG), impaired glucose tolerance (IGT), or HbA1c between 5.7% (39 mmol/mol) and 6.4% (46 mmol/mol)
5. Hypertension (blood pressure ≥ 140/90 mmHg or on therapy for hypertension)
6. High-density lipoprotein (HDL) cholesterol <35 mg/dL (0.91 mmol/L) and/or triglyceride level > 250 mg/dL (2.82 mmol/L)
7. History of gestational diabetes mellitus
8. History of cardiovascular disease
9. History of polycystic ovarian syndrome
10. Other conditions associated with insulin resistance (acanthosis nigricans).

4. Pathophysiology

The core pathophysiologic defects in T2DM are beta cell failure and insulin resistance in muscle and liver. In addition to the muscle, liver, and beta cell, other defects are accelerated lipolysis in the fat cell, incretin deficiency or resistance in gastrointestinal tract, hyperglucagonemia due to increased release of glucagon from alpha cells, increased glucose reabsorption in kidney and insulin resistance in brain. All these eight distinct pathophysiological abnormalities play important roles in the development of persistent hyperglycemia in type 2 diabetic individuals [4].

These factors are already well established early in the natural history of T2DM. The activation of inflammatory pathways and impaired insulin-mediated vasodilation

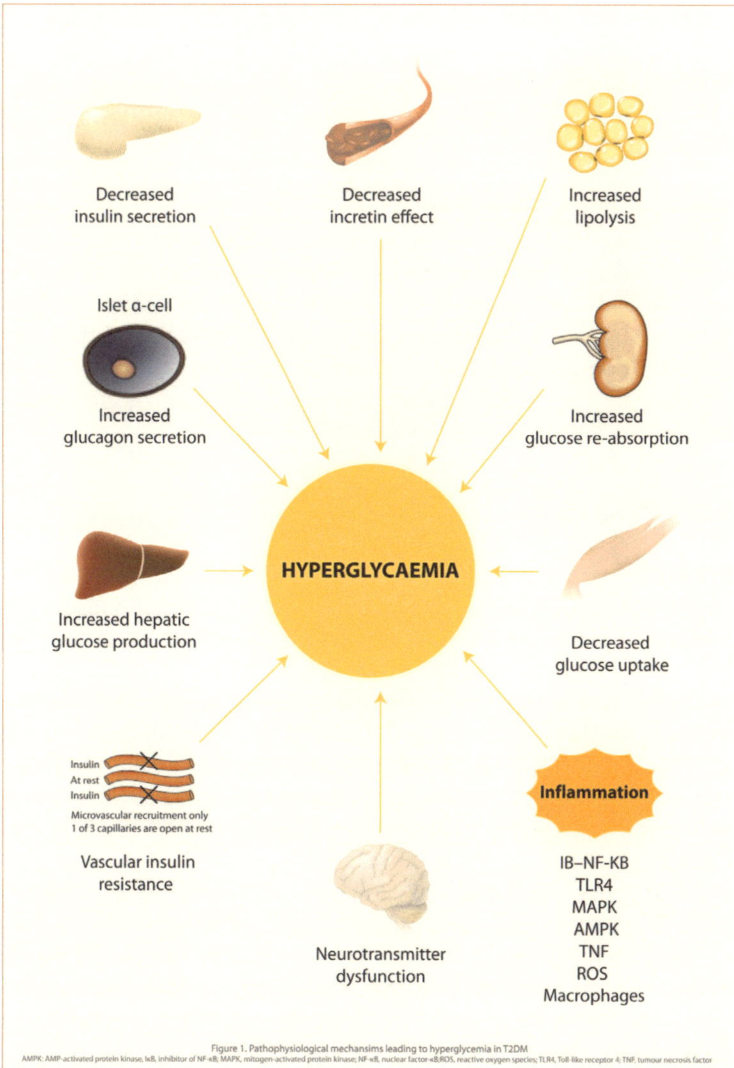

Figure 1.
Pathophysiological mechanisms leading to hyperglycemia in T2DM.

contributing to muscle insulin resistance are two additional pathophysiologic defects [5]. **Figure 1** depicts all pathophysiological abnormalities contributing to persistent hyperglycemia.

5. Treatment

5.1 Goals of therapy

Major goals of T2DM therapy are:

1. Effective glucose control

2. To prevent, reduce, and manage acute and long-term complications

3. To preserve beta cell function

4. To minimize hypoglycemia

5. To maintain overall quality of life

The primary objective in management of diabetes is to achieve near-normal blood glucose level. The Diabetes Control and Complications Trial (DCCT) [6] and the United Kingdom Prospective Diabetes Study (UKPDS) [7] showed that the risk of developing chronic complications is decreased by lowering blood glucose level. With appropriate public education, lifestyle modification, and medications, near-normal blood glucose level can be achieved.

5.2 Pharmacologic therapy

Lifestyle modification along with physical activity and meal planning is the first step in management of individuals with T2DM. However, in individuals who are unable to achieve glycemic control through it, oral and injectable antidiabetic agents are used. Oral agents are summarized in **Table 1** [8, 9].

With the availability of number of glucose-lowering medication, the management of hyperglycemia has become complex. Consistent efforts to improve diet and exercise and individual-centered decision-making and support remain the foundation of all glycemic management. The recommendation of initial use of metformin followed by addition of glucose-lowering medications is based on individual concerns and comorbidities [10].

Non-insulin drug class with site of action and mechanism of action is listed in **Table 2** [8, 10–12] and the expected HbA1c reduction for each non-insulin antiglycemic drug class is listed in **Table 3** [8, 10–12]. The target and mechanism of action of various class of blood glucose-lowering agents is different. Each of these classes may be used individually or in combination with other medications targeting different organs for synergistic effects.

Treatment algorithm for T2DM by American Diabetes Association (ADA) [12] and American Association of Clinical Endocrinology (AACE) [9] prioritizes treatment options based on treatment benefits and patient-specific factors, especially in patients with cardiovascular disease, heart failure, or chronic kidney disease. **Figure 2** shows pharmacologic approaches for glycemic management.

Here are the key points of ADA and AACE Guidelines (**Table 4**).

As T2DM is a progressive disease, many individuals eventually require insulin. ADA favors use of GLP-1RA as an alternative to mealtime insulin in those already maximally titrated with basal regimens. In this scenario, AACE guidelines also suggest DPP-4i or SGLT2i as an option.

5.2.1 Sulfonylureas

There are many antidiabetic drugs available for treatment of T2DM. Despite availability of several treatment options, for nearly 50 years, sulfonylureas have been used extensively and even today widely used for T2DM management [13].

Drug class	Drugs	Site of action	Impact on blood glucose	Dosing strategy (all agents taken orally)	e-GFR 30–50 mL/min	eGFR 30 mL/min	Adjustment of hepatic impairment	Common adverse events
Alpha glucosidase inhibitors	Acarbose, Miglitol	Brush border of small intestine	Postprandial	25 mg t.i.d daily with first bite of each main meal Advance at 4–8 week intervals to maximum of 100 mg t.i.d daily	SCr > 2 mg/dL. Not recommended	SCr > 2 mg/dL. Not recommended	No specific dose adjustment recommended, contraindicated in cirrhosis	GI (flatulence, diarrhea)
	Voglibose	Brush border of small intestine	Postprandial	0.2 mg t.i.d just before each meal Can be increased to 0.3 mg under close observation of the course of disease	Not available	Not available	Not available	GI (flatulence, diarrhea) Abdominal pain
Meglitinides (should not be used in combination with other insulin secretagogues)	Repaglinide	Pancreas	Postprandial	0.5 mg 15–30 min before each meal. Double preprandial dose every 7 days to maximum of 4 mg/dose or 16 mg/day (to be taken only if eating)	20–40 mL/min initial dose: 0.5 mg with careful titration	<20 mL/min. Not studied	Use conservative initial and maintenance doses and use longer intervals between dose adjustments	Hypoglycemia (although less risk than with sulfonylureas)
	Nateglinide	Pancreas	Postprandial	120 mg t.i.d daily before meals (to be taken only if eating)	No specific dose adjustment recommended	Use with caution in severe dysfunction	No dose adjustment needed in mild impairment; use with caution in moderate to severe dysfunction	Hypoglycemia (although less risk than with sulfonylureas)
Second generation sulfonylureas	Glyburide micronized	Pancreas	Fasting and postpradial	1.5–3 mg/day with breakfast. Increase by 1.5 mg weekly to maximum of 12 mg/day	Not recommended	Not recommended	Use conservative dosing and avoid in severe disease	Hypoglycemia and weight gain

Drug class	Drugs	Site of action	Impact on blood glucose	Dosing strategy (all agents taken orally)	e-GFR 30–50 mL/min	eGFR 30 mL/min	Adjustment of hepatic impairment	Common adverse events
	Glyburide	Pancreas	Fasting and postpradial	2.5–5 mg/day with breakfast. Increase by 2.5 mg weekly to maximum of 20 mg/day	Not recommended	Not recommended	Use conservative dosing and avoid in severe disease	Hypoglycemia and weight gain
	Glipizide	Pancreas	Fasting and postpradial	2.5 mg/day 30 min before a meal increase by 2.5–5 mg weekly to maximum of 40 mg/day;divide dose if >15 mg/day	No specific dose adjustment recommended	No specific dose adjustment recommended	Initial dose 2.5 mg/day	Hypoglycemia, weight gain
	Glipizide ER	Pancreas	Fasting and postpradial	2.5–5 mg once daily before a meal increase by 5–10 mg weekly to maximum of 20 mg/day	No specific dose adjustment recommended	No specific dose adjustment recommended	No specific dose adjustment recommended	Hypoglycemia, weight gain
	Glimepiride	Pancreas	Fasting and postpradial	1–2 mg with breakfast increase by 2 mg every 1–2 weeks to maximum of 8 mg/day	No specific dose adjustment recommended	Initial starting dose should be 1 mg < 15 mL/min consider alternative	No specific dose adjustment recommended	Hypoglycemia, weight gain
Biguanides	Metformin Metformin ER	Liver	Fasting and postprandial	500 mg/day to twice daily with meals Advance weekly to maximum of 2000–2500 mg/day	Do not start or, if already taking, continue cautiously if eGFR 30–45 mL/min/1.73 m^2. Consider 50% of maximum doses and monitoring of renal function every 3 months	Contraindicated	Avoid or use cautiously in patients at risk for lactic acidosis (renal impairment or alcohol abuse)	GI (diarrhea, abdominal pain)

DOI: http://dx.doi.org/10.5772/intechopen.1002309

Drug class	Drugs	Site of action	Impact on blood glucose	Dosing strategy (all agents taken orally)	e-GFR 30–50 mL/min	eGFR 30 mL/min	Adjustment of hepatic impairment	Common adverse events
Thiazolidinediones	Pioglitazone	Peripheral tissue	Fasting and postprandial	15–30 mg/day increase after 12 weeks to maximum of 45 mg/day	No adjustment necessary	No adjustment necessary	Clearance lower in Child-Pugh grade B/C; do not start if transaminsases >2.5 X ULN and discontinue if ALT rises to and remains at more than three times ULN	Weight Gain
Dipeptidyl peptidase-4 inhibitors	Sitagliptin	GI tract (increases GLP-1)	Fasting and postprandial	100 mg/day	50 mg once daily	25 mg once daily	Child Pugh No class A and B: No dosage adjustment necessary; Child-Pugh class C: Not studied	Upper respiratory, diarrhea
	Saxagliptin	GI tract (increases GLP-1)	Fasting and postprandial	2.5 or 5 mg/daily	2.5 mg once daily	2.5 mg once daily	No dose adjustment necessary	UTI, Headache
	Linagliptin	GI tract (increases GLP-1)	Fasting and postprandial	5 mg/day	No dose adjustment necessary	No adjustment necessary	No adjustment necessary	Headache, arthralgia, nasopharyngitis
	Alogliptin	GI tract (increases GLP-1)	Fasting and postprandial	25 mg/day	>30 mL/min but < 60 mL/min 12.5 mg/day	>15 mL/min but <30 mL/min 6.25 mg/day; <15 mL/min 6.25 mg/day	No dose adjustment necessary; Child Pugh class C: not studied	Headache, increased ALT greater than three times ULN, nasopharyngitis, upper respiratory tract infections

Drug class	Drugs	Site of action	Impact on blood glucose	Dosing strategy (all agents taken orally)	e-GFR 30–50 mL/min	eGFR 30 mL/min	Adjustment of hepatic impairment	Common adverse events
Selective sodium dependent glucose cotransporter-2 inhibitor	Canagliflozin	Kidney	Fasting and postprandial	100 mg/day in morning, may increase to 300 mg/day	>45 mL/min/1.73 m^2 but <60 mL/min/1.73 m^2:100 mg/day; 30 ml/min/1.73 m^2 with urinary albumin excretion >300 mg/day: 100 mg/day	<30 ml/min/1.73 m^2, contraindicated	Mild to moderate (Child Pugh class A and B) no adjustment necessary severe (Child Pugh class C) not recommended	Hyperkalemia, genitourinary infection, hypovolemia, renal insufficiency, hypotension
	Dapagliflozin	Kidney	Fasting and postprandial	5 mg/day in the morning may increase to 10 mg/day	<45 mL/min/1.73 m^2 not recommended for glycemic control >25 mL/min/1.73 m^2 but <45 mL/min/1.73 m^2 with heart failure or chronic kidney disease: 10 mg/day	<25 ml/min/1.73 m^2 contraindicated	Mild to moderate. No adjustment necessary. Severe not studied	Genitourinary infection, hypovolemia/hypotension, dysuria, polyuria, dyslipidemia, mild hypoglycemia, nasopharyngitis
	Empagliflozin	Kidney	Fasting and postprandial	10 mg/day in the morning; may increase to 25 mg/day	No dosage adjustment	<30 mL/min/1.73 m^2; contraindicated	No dose adjustment necessary	Genitourinary infection, hypovolemia/hypotension, dysuria, polyuria, dyslipidemia, mild hypoglycemia,
	Ertugliflozin	Kidney	Fasting and postprandial	5 mg/day in the morning; may increase to 15 mg/day	<60 mL/min not recommended	<30 mL/min contraindicated		Genitourinary infection, hypovolemia, mild hypoglycemia, polyuria, increased LDL cholesterol, renal insufficiency

Drug class	Drugs	Site of action	Impact on blood glucose	Dosing strategy (all agents taken orally)	e-GFR 30–50 mL/min	eGFR 30 mL/min	Adjustment of hepatic impairment	Common adverse events
GLP1-1 receptor agonist	Semaglutide	GI tract and Pancreas	Fasting and postprandial	3 mg/day in the morning with water 30 min before first food, beverage, or other oral medications for 30 days, increase to 7 mg/day increase to 14 mg/day after 30 days if additional glycemic control needed	No dose adjustment necessary	No dose adjustment necessary	No dose adjustment necessary	GI effects (nausea, diarrhea, flatulence, abdominal pain), risk of pancreatitis, increased heart rate
Dopamine receptor agonist	Bromocriptine mesylate	Hypothalamus	Postprandial	0.8 mg once daily within 2 h of waking, may increase in weekly intervals to 4.8 mg once daily	No dose adjustment necessary	No dose adjustment necessary	No specific dose adjustment recommended, although adjustment may be necessary because of extensive hepatic metabolism	Nausea, headache
Bile acid sequestrant	Colesevelam	Intestinal lumen	Fasting	1.875 g twice daily or 3.75 mg once daily	No dose adjustment necessary	No dose adjustment necessary	No dose adjustment necessary	Constipation

ALT, alanine aminotransferase; eGFR, estimated glomerular filtration rate; ER, extended release; GI, gastrointestinal; GLP-1, glucagon like peptide-1; LDL, low density lipoprotein, SCr, serum creatinine; ULN, upper limit of normal; UTI, urinary tract infection.

Table 1.
Oral agents for T2DM.

Site of action	Drug class	Mechanism of action
Pancreas	Sulfonylureas	Enhances insulin secretion
	Nonsulfonylurea secretagogues	Enhances insulin secretion
	GLP-1 agonists	Enhances insulin secretion and suppresses glucagon secretion
	Pramlintide	Suppresses glucagon secretion
Liver	Biguanide	Decreases hepatic glucose production and increases insulin sensitivity
	Thiazolidinedione	Increases insulin sensitivity
Muscle	Biguanide	Increases insulin sensitivity
	Thiazolidinedione	Increases insulin sensitivity
Adipose tissue	Thiazolidinedione	Increases insulin sensitivity
Intestines	GLP-1 agonists	Increases satiety and regulates gastric emptying
	Pramlintide	Increases satiety and regulates gastric emptying
	Dipeptidyl peptidase-4 inhibitors	Increases endogenous GLP-1
	α-Glucosidase inhibitors	Delays absorption of carbohydrates
Kidney	SGLT2 inhibitors	Inhibits glucose reabsorption in the kidney's proximal tubule

GLP-1, glucagon-like peptide-1; SGLT2, sodium-dependent glucose cotransporter-2.

Table 2.
Site and mechanism of non insulin agents.

Expected A1c reduction for noninsulin antiglycemic drug classes			
Drug class	**Efficacy**	**A1c reduction(%)**	**HbA1 reduction(mmol/mol)**
Biguanides	High	1.5–2	17–22
Sulfonylureas	High	1.5–2	17–22
GLP-1 Agonists	High	0.78–1.9	8.8–20
Thiazolidinediones	High	up to 1.5	17
Dipeptidyl peptidase-4 inhibitors	Intermediate	0.7–1	8–11
SGLT2 inhibitors	Intermediate	0.5–1	5–11
Nonsulfonylurea secretagogues	Intermediate	0.3–1	3–11
α-Glucosidase inhibitors	Intermediate	0.3–1	3–11
Central-acting dopamine agonists	Low	0.3–0.6	3–7
Pramlintide	Low	0.4–0.5	4–5
Bile acid sequestrants	Low	0.40	4

HbA1c, hemoglobin A1c; GLP-1, glucagon like peptide-1; SGLT2, sodium-dependent glucose cotransporter-2.

Table 3.
Expected A1c reduction of noninsulin antiglycemic agents.

DOI: http://dx.doi.org/10.5772/intechopen.1002309

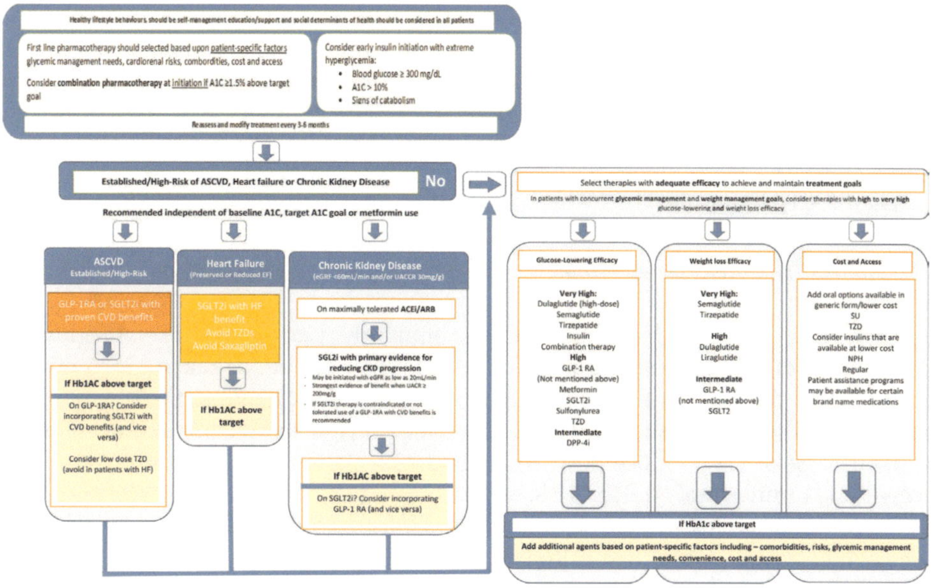

Figure 2.
Type 2 diabetes pharmacotherapy—Updated ADA 2023 treatment algorithm.

	ADA	AACE
Starting a patient on two medications	HbA1c ≥ 8.5% (69 mmol/mol)	HbA1c ≥ 7.5% (58 mmol/mol)
First-line therapy	Metformin	Six other non-insulin initial therapy options as possibilities. In patients with established or high atherosclerotic cardiovascular disease (ASCVD) risk, heart failure with reduced ejection fraction (HFrEF), and/or CKD: the preferred options are SGLT2i or GLP-1RAs

Table 4.
Key differences in ADA and AACE approach of T2DM management.

There are two generations of sulfonylureas namely first and second generation. Most commonly prescribed agents are second-generation sulfonylureas include glyburide (also known as glibenclamide), gliclazide, glipizide, and glimepiride. The ATP-sensitive potassium channels in the cell membrane of pancreatic beta cells are blocked by sulfonylureas, which lead to membrane depolarization. This allows an influx of calcium causing translocation of insulin secretory granules to the cell surface. Insulin secretion is enhanced in a non-glucose-dependent manner. Both fasting and postprandial blood glucose levels are lowered. Monotherapy produces a 1.5 (17 mmol/mol) to 2% (22 mmol/mol) decline in HbA1c and a 60–70 mg/dL (3.33–3.885 mmol/l) reduction in fasting blood glucose levels.

Maturity-onset diabetes of the young (MODY) is a type of diabetes with specific features diagnosed usually before the age of 25 years. The mutations mainly in three genes (HNF1A, HNF4A, and GCK) contribute to 95% of all individuals with MODY. Oral hypoglycemic drugs generally sulphonylureas are preferred for individuals with mutations in the HNF4A and HNFA genes. In person with mutations in GCK gene, treatment is usually not necessary [14].

Drug interactions are more likely to be associated with first-generation sulfonylureas. Cytochrome P450 2C9 pathway metabolizes most sulfonylureas. Except tolbutamide, all sulfonylureas require dosage adjustment in renal impairment [15]. Lower starting dose is necessary in elderly or individuals with compromised renal or hepatic function. Hypoglycemia and weight gain are common adverse effects. Increased risk of hemolytic anemia has been found in individuals with glucose-6 phosphate dehydrogenase deficiency [16].

5.2.2 Non-sulfonylureas secretagogues

Nateglinide and repaglinide are the two commonly used meglitinides. Meglitinides have a rapid and short duration of action. Hence, they should be taken 15–30 min before a meal three times a day. They bind to a receptor adjacent to those which sulfonylureas bind. Like sulfonylureas, they block ATP-sensitive potassium channels on the beta cells. They reduce post-meal glucose levels. A reduction of 0.3 (3 mmol/mol)–1% (11 mmol/mol) in HbA1c levels has been demonstrated [15]. Meglitinides are short-acting and associated with lower hypoglycemia risks, weight gain, and chronic hyperinsulinemia than sulfonylurea drugs [17].

Nateglinide has also been studied in individuals with maturity-onset diabetes of the young type 3(MODY3) and it has been found that a low dose of nateglinide prevents rise in acute postprandial glucose more efficiently than glibenclamide with less hypoglycemic symptoms [18]. In individuals with MODY3, improved prandial glucose control with lower risk of hypoglycemia was observed with nateglinide than glibenclamide.

5.2.3 Biguanides

In T2DM treatment, metformin is considered as a foundational therapy along with lifestyle modification. It is often used in combination with other anti-hyperglycemic agents for synergistic effects [12]. Metformin decreases hepatic glucose production and increases insulin sensitivity in both hepatic and peripheral muscle tissues. When used as monotherapy, it reduces HbA1c levels by 1.5 (17 mmol/mol)–2% (22 mmol/mol) and FPG by 60–80 mg/dL (3.33–4.44 mmol/l) [15]. The incidences of hypoglycemia are uncommon as it does not affect insulin release. The most common reported adverse effects are decreased appetite, nausea, and diarrhea. These adverse effects are often subsiding within two weeks. These adverse effects can be also minimized through use of extended release formulation and slow titration of the dose. Long-term treatment with metformin has been associated to cause vitamin B12 deficiency. Hence, periodic testing of vitamin B12 status should be done especially in individuals with macrocytic anemia or peripheral neuropathy. Lactic acidosis is one of the rare side effects reported and individuals who are at risk of lactic acidosis include those with renal impairment or elderly [16].

5.2.4 Thiazolidinedione (TZDs)

The thiazolidinediones are also known as glitazones. Pioglitazone is a TZD, which has been shown to be effective in glycemic control by lowering insulin resistance. TZDs stimulate peroxisome proliferator-activated receptor gamma which increases insulin sensitivity and decreases plasma fatty acids. As monotherapy, a decline in HbA1c is up to 1.5% (17 mmol/mol) and a reduction in FPG levels by around 60–

70 mg/dL (3.33–3.885 mmol/l) [15]. Fluid retention, weight gain, and limb fractures are known to occur with TZD therapy. An increased risk of bladder cancer has been found with pioglitazone therapy especially among men and smokers. It is contraindicated in New York Heart Association Class III and IV heart failure.

5.2.5 Alpha glucosidase inhibitors (AGIs)

Examples of AGIs are acarbose, voglibose, and miglitol. The enzymes glucoamylase, sucrase, maltase, and isomaltase that convert complex non-absorbable carbohydrates into simple absorbable carbohydrates are inhibited by AGIs. The reduction in postprandial glucose concentrations is due to delayed absorption of carbohydrates and it is up to 40–50 mg/dL (2.22–2.77 mmol/l). However only 0.3 (3 mmol/mol)–1% (11 mmol/mol) decline in HbA1c has been noted [15]. Because of high incidence of GI side effects, their use has been limited. Compared to sulfonylureas, glycemic control is inferior with AGIs [19].

5.2.6 Dipeptidyl Petidase-4 inhibitors (DPP-4i)

Sitagliptin, saxagliptin, linagliptin, and alogliptin are DPP-4 inhibitors. These drugs act through incretin hormones, which are gut hormones responsible for glucose homeostasis after oral food intake. They inhibit DPP-4, enzyme which degrades endogenous GLP-1 and hence DPP4i increases the amount of GLP-1. They lower postprandial blood glucose levels. They are approved as adjunct to diet and exercise to improve glycemic control in adults with T2DM. Typical HbA1c reductions are 0.7 (8 mmol/mol)–1% (11 mmol/mol) [15]. DPP-4 inhibitors do not seem to confer any significant cardiovascular benefit for individuals with T2DM, while they do not seem to be associated with a significant risk for any major cardiac arrhythmias [20]. Headache and nasopharyngitis are common adverse effects. Acute pancreatitis has been reported in individuals who are taking gliptins. Hence, it is contraindicated in individuals with a history of pancreatitis.

5.2.7 Sodium-dependent glucose cotransporter-2 inhibitors (SGLT2i)

Canagliflozin, dapagliflozin, empagliflozin, and ertugliflozin are SGLT2 inhibitors. They inhibit SGLT2 in the proximal tubules and lower the renal threshold for glucose reabsorption. This results in increased urinary excretion of glucose, and thus lowers plasma blood glucose concentrations. The glucose-lowering effects of SGLT2i are independent of insulin secretion or action. Typical HbA1c reductions are 0.5 (5 mmol/mol)–1% (11 mmol/mol) [15]. They may be used as monotherapy or add-on. The renal function test should be performed at baseline to guide the initial dosing and during the treatment to assess suitability of continuation of SGLT2i. Recent clinical trials have shown that SGLT2i has dramatic beneficial cardiovascular and renal outcomes, including reduced rehospitalization in subjects with heart failure, regardless of the presence of diabetes [21, 22]. In subjects with atherosclerotic cardiovascular disease or heart failure, SGLT2i is found to be effective in decreasing overall morbidity and mortality [23]. Increased incidence of urinary tract infections, genital mycotic infections are common adverse effects. Other notable adverse effects are symptomatic hypotension, euglycemic ketoacidosis, increased risk of bone fracture, newly diagnosed bladder cancer.

5.2.8 Glucagon-like peptide 1 receptor agonists (GLP-1 RA)

Exenatide, liraglutide, dulaglutide, semaglutide, and lixisenatide are glucagon-like peptide 1 receptor agonists (GLP-1 RA). They are called incretin mimetics, or GLP-1 analogs (**Table 5**) [11, 24, 25]. Blood glucose-lowering effect of GLP-1 RAs is mediated by (a) glucose-dependent insulin secretion; (b) reducing post-meal glucagon secretion; (c) increasing satiety which decreases food intake; (d) regulation of gastric emptying, which allows smooth absorption of nutrients into the circulation. These agents have been shown to reduce HbA1c (by ~0.8–1.6%), body mass (by ~1–3 kg), blood pressure, and lipids. Cardiovascular outcome trials have demonstrated that GLP1RA reduces the rates of major adverse cardiovascular events in patients with T2DM [26]. This class of drugs is associated with a low risk of hypoglycemia, and the most common adverse effects are gastrointestinal such as nausea, vomiting, and diarrhea [27]. They are contraindicated in individuals with acute pancreatitis.

5.2.9 Dual GIP/GLP-1 receptor agonists

Tirzepatide, the most advanced unimolecular dual glucose-dependent insulinotropic polypeptides (GIP/GLP-1) agonist has been recently approved. It is administered as once weekly through subcutaneous route. It stimulates release of insulin from the pancreas leading to reduction of hyperglycemia. The level of adinopectin is also increased. In comparison to GLP-1 RA, the dual agonistic action leads to a significant reduction in hyperglycemia along with reduced appetite, energy intake, and body mass. In the phase III studies, it decreased HbA1c levels upto −2.58% along with loss in body mass by −12.9 kg because of the complementarity of action of the two incretins. The cardiovascular protective effect is also being studied. It is prescribed as a second-line medications in management of T2DM. Except for higher incidence of diarrhea, gastrointestinal tolerance is comparable to that of GLP-1 analogs [28, 29]. The clinical trial evidences suggest that tirzepatide offers a new treatment option for the effective lowering of blood glucose and body mass in adults with T2DM [30].

5.2.10 Central-acting dopamine agonist

Bromocriptine is a central-acting dopamine agonist. A quick release formulation is approved for treatment of T2DM. The mechanism of action of bromocriptine is unknown. The data indicate that it improved insulin sensitivity, likely a result of its effect on dopamine oscillations [15]. It should be considered a last-line option due to the modest effect on blood sugar levels and HbA1c [8]. Rhinitis, dizziness, asthenia, headache, sinusitis, constipation, and nausea are the main side effects. It is contraindicated in syncopal migraine and women who are nursing [16].

It is an attractive treatment option for the treatment of T2DM because of its novel mechanism of action, acceptable side effect profile, and its effects to reduce cardiovascular event rates [31].

5.2.11 Bile acid sequestrants

Colesevelam is bile acid sequestrant. It is approved as adjunctive therapy to improve glycemic control in conjunction with diet, exercise, and insulin or oral agents for treatment of T2DM. It showed significant effects on glycemic control when added on to antidiabetic agents. There is insufficient data on long-term effects particularly in

Generic name	Dosage strengths	Starting dosage	Dosage interval	Titration interval	Maximum dose	Time to effect (min)	Comments and cautions
Pramlintide	2.7 mL for 60, 120 mcg doses	60 mcg	Three times a day with meals	3–7 days	120 mcg	20	Side effects: hypoglycemia, nausea, vomiting, Available in SymliPen 60 and 120
Exenatide	Immediate release 5 mcg, 10 mcg	Immediate release 5 mcg	Immediate release twice daily	Immediate release 1 month	Immediate release 10 mcg twice daily	Immediate release 15–30	Inject immediate release formulation 15–20 min before two meals of the day with 6 h separating the meals; prefilled disposable pen; may delay absorption of oral drugs; separate doses by 1 h Side effects: nausea, vomiting, diarrhea, increased hypoglycemia with sulfonylureas
	Extended release 2 mg	Extended release 2 mg	Extended release once weekly	Extended release NA	Extended release 2 mg	NA	Extended release formulation can be administered regardless of meals
Lixisenatide	10 mcg and 20 mcg pen-injector starter kit; 20 mcg pen-injector	10 mcg	Once daily	14 days	20 mcg	N/A	If missed dose, administer within 1 h of next meal
Liraglutide	18 mg/3 mL pen	0.6 mg	Once daily	1 week	1.8 mg	N/A	Can be dosed at any time of day regardless of meals; may delay absorption of oral drugs; separate doses by 1 h Side effects: nausea, vomiting, increased hypoglycemia with sulfonylureas
Dulaglutide	0.75 mg single dose pen; 1.5-mg single dose pen, 3.0 mg single dose pen; 4.5 mg single dose pen	0.75 mg	Once weekly	4–8 weeks	4.5 mg	N/A	If missed dose occurs within 3 days of regularly scheduled dose, dose should be administered at that time. If missed dose occurs more than 3 days past scheduled dose, wait until next regularly scheduled dose to administer next dose Side effects: nausea, diarrhea, vomiting, abdominal pain, decreased appetite,dyspepsia, fatigue
Semaglutide	2 mg/1.5 mL pen injector for 0.25 or 0.5 mg/dose pen; 4 mg/3 mL pen-injector for 1 mg/dose pen	0.25 mg	Once weekly	4 weeks	1 mg	N/A	If missed dose occurs within 5 days, administer the dose as soon as possible. If >5 days, do not administer until the next scheduled weekly dose Side effects: nausea, vomiting, diarrhea, abdominal pain, risk of hypoglycemia, tachycardia

Table 5.
Injectable noninsulin agents for diabetes.

cardiovascular risk management and reduction of micro- and macrovascular complications. It is rarely used [32].

5.2.12 Amylin mimetic

Pramlintide acetate is a synthetic analog of human amylin. Amylin secretion is lower than normal in individuals with T2DM who require insulin. Pramlintide is given subcutaneously before meals to lower postprandial blood glucose elevations. Hypoglycemia, nausea, and vomiting are the most common side effects. Pramlintide slows gastric emptying, suppresses glucagon secretion, and increases satiety. By slowing gastric emptying, the normal initial post-meal spike in blood glucose is reduced [16].

5.2.13 Insulin

In 1921, Banting and Best discovered insulin. They prepared an extract of pancreas after degeneration of the exocrine part and demonstrated its hypoglycemic action. The molecular weight of insulin is 6000 and it has two polypeptide chains having 51 amino acids. The A and B chain has 21 and 30 amino acids respectively. Insulin is synthesized as a single polypeptide chain containing 110 aminoacid called preproinsulin. This is processed to proinsulin and then to insulin and C-peptide. The disposal of meal-derived glucose, amino acids, fatty acids is the overall effect of insulin and promotes fuel storage. Because of its anabolic action, it promotes synthesis of glycogen, lipids, and protein [33–35].

The mainstay for treatment of virtually all type 1 and type 2 diabetes is insulin. There is no specific maximum dose of insulin and can be titrated as per the need of individual. It can be administered subcutaneously, intramuscularly, or through intravenous route. Currently, the recombinant DNA technology is being used to prepare all insulin formulations. One international unit of insulin is equal to 34.7 mcg of crystalline insulin [33]. The preparations of insulin consist of the amino acid sequence of human insulin and their variations (insulin analogs).

In addition to the combination of insulin plus insulin, insulin plus GLP1RA combinations have also been approved. Furthermore, basal insulin therapy combinations with other drugs or adjunctive therapies are also prescribed [17].

The properties of available insulins are summarized in **Table 6** [11, 16, 36]. The time of onset of action, peak effect, and duration of action of insulin greatly varies among individuals and even in the same individual with repeated doses. This depends on the dose size, the injection site, the exercise, and the desire of circulating anti-insulin antibodies.

The potential benefits of complementary pre-prandial short-acting insulin therapy in T2DM have also been studied. Insulin treatment led to improvement in Hb1Ac, mean blood glucose, body mass, and self-reported quality of life. The improved blood glucose control was evident from fourth day of treatment. Furthermore, complimentary insulin therapy was more beneficial to individuals in whom insulin was newly introduced compared to individually previously treated with insulin [37].

6. Choice of glucose-lowering therapy

The choice of pharmacologic therapy is guided by treatment goals and person-centered treatment factors including comorbidities. A person-centered approach such as

Generic name (insulin)	Strength	Onset	Peak (h)	Duration (h)	Administration options
Ultra rapid acting insulin					
Aspart with niacinamide	U-100	15–20 min	1.5–2	5–7	CSII, IV, SC; 10-mL vial; 3-mL cartridge and Flex Touch Disposable Pen
Recombinant human insulin regular	Not applicable	12–15 min	1	1.5–3	Ihh; Technosphere insulin particles for oral inhalation; 4,8, and 12 U as cartridges
Rapid acting insulin					
Lispro	U-100, U-200	15–30 min	0.5–1.5	3–4	CSII, IV, SC; 3-mL and 10 mL vial, 3-mL cartridge, KwikPen disposable pen
	U-100				CSII, IV, SC; 3-mL and 10-mL vial; 3-mL SoloStar disposable pen
Lispro aabc	U-100, U-200	15–30 min	0.5–1.5	4–7	IV, SC; 10-mL vial; 3-mL cartridge and Kwik disposable pen
Aspart	U-100	15–30 min	0.5–1.5	3–5	CSII, IV, SC; 10-mL vial; 3-mL cartridge, FlexPen disposable pen
Glulisine	U-100	15–30 min	1–2	3–4	CSII, IV, SC; 10-mL vial; 3-mL SoloStar disposable pen
Short acting insulin					
Regular	U-100, U-500	30–60 min	2–4	5–8	CSII, IV, SC; U-100 10-mL vial; U-500 20-mL vial and 3-mL KwikPen disposable pen
	U-100				CSII, IV, SC; 10-mL vial, 3-mL cartridge, 3-mL Innolet
Intermediate-acting insulin					
Neutral protamine Hagedorn	U-100	2–4 h	4–10	10–24	SC; 10-mL vial, 3-mL cartridge
	U-100				SC; 10-mL vial, 3-mL cartridge, 3-mL InnoLet
Long-acting insulin					
Glargine	U-100	2–4 h	Flat	20–24	SC; 10-mL vial, 3-mL SoloSTAR disposable pen
	U-300	6 h	Flat	36	SC;1.5-mL SoloStar disposable pen
	U-300				SC; 3-mL SoloStar disposable pen
	U-100	2–4 h	Flat	20–24	SC; 3-mL KwikPen disposable pen
	U-100	1–3 h	Flat	≥ 24	SC; 10-mLvial, 3-mL disposable pen
Detemir	U-100	1.5–4 h	6–14	16–20	SC; 10-mL vial, 3-mL FlexTouch disposable pen
Degludec	U-100, U-200	1 h	Flat	42	SC; 3-mL disposable FlexTouch pen
Combination insulin products					
Neutral protamine Hagedorn and regular	U-100	30–60 min	1.5–16	10–16	SC: 10-mL vial, 3-mL KwikPen disposable pen
	U-100	30–60 min	2–12	10–16	SC; 10-mL vial, 3-mL FlexPen disposable pen

Generic name (insulin)	Strength	Onset	Peak (h)	Duration (h)	Administration options
Neutral protamine lispro and lispro	U-100	15–30 min	1–6.5	15–18	SC; 10-mL vial, 3-mL KwikPen disposable pen
	U-100				SC; 10-mL vial, 3-mL KwikPen disposable pen
Neutral protamine aspart and aspart	U-100	15–30 min	1–4	Up to 24	SC; 10-mL vial, 3-mL cartridge, 3-mL FlexPen disposable pen
Combination insulin GLP-1 agonist products					
Degludec and liraglutide	U-100 degludec/ 3.6 mg/mL liraglutide	N/A	N/A	N/A	SC; 3-mL pen-injector
Glargine and lixisenatide	U-100 glargine/33 mcg/mL liraglutide	N/A	N/A	N/A	SC; 3-mL pen-injector

CSII, continuous subcutaneous insulin infusion; GLP-1, glucagon like peptide; Inh, inhalation; IV, intravenous; N/A, not applicable; SC, subcutaneous.

Table 6.
Insulin agents for diabetes.

the effects on cardiovascular and renal comorbidities, efficacy, hypoglycemia risk, impact on weight, cost, and access, risk for side effects and individual preferences are considered for appropriate selection of pharmacologic agents. To reduce cardiorenal risk is the ultimate goal of treatment in adults with type 2 diabetes and established/high risk of atherosclerotic cardiovascular disease, heart failure, and/or chronic kidney disease. The usual pharmacologic approaches to achieve and maintain treatment goals are treatment with metformin and other agents including combination therapy. In T2DM management, the approaches that support weight management goals are preferred. A SGLT2i and/or GLP1RA is recommended as part of glucose-lowering regimen in individuals with type 2 diabetes who have established cardiovascular disease or indicators of high cardiovascular risk, established kidney disease or heart failure. Every 3–6 months, medication regimen and medication taking behavior should be evaluated and if needed, treatment should be adjusted to incorporate specific factors that impact choice of treatment. **Table** 7 summarizes choice of glucose-lowering therapy in T2DM [3, 38].

7. Trends and newer developments in T2DM management

7.1 Trends in T2DM management

There has been substantial progress in T2DM management with promising results using various treatment regimens. The therapeutic options to treat T2DM are increasing and now there are nearly 60 FDA-approved drugs available. There is an increase in preference for newer drugs such as DPP4i and SGLT2i as per available prescription data [17, 39].

Drugs/class	Efficacy	Hypoglycemia	Impact on body weight	CV effects		Renal effects		Oral/SC	Clinical considerations
				Effect on MACE	HF	Progression of DKD	Dosing/use considerations*		
Metformin	High	No	Neutral (potential for moderate loss)	Potential benefit	Neutral	Neutral	Contraindicated with eGFR < 30 mL/min/1.73 m^2	Oral	GI side effects common: to mitigate GI side effects, consider slow dose titration, extended release formulations, and administration with food
SGLT2-Inhibitors	Intermediate to high	No	Loss (Intermediate)	Benefit: canagliflozin, empagliflozin	Benefit: canagliflozin, dapagliflozin, empagliflozin, ertugliflozin	Benefit: canagliflozin, dapagliflozin, empagliflozin	See labels for renal dose considerations of individual agents Glucose-lowering effect is lower for SGLT2 inhibitors at lower eGFR	Oral	DKA risk, rare in T2DM: discontinue, evaluate, and treat promptly if suspected; be aware of predisposing risk factors and clinical presentation (including euglycemic DKA); discontinue before scheduled surgery (e.g., 3–4 days), during critical illness or during prolonged fasting mitigate potential risk Increased risk of genitourinary tract infections Necrotizing fasciitis of perineum (Fournier gangrene), rare reports; prompt treatment recommended if suspected Attention to volume status, blood pressure, adjust other volume-contracting agents as applicable
GLP1-RAs	High to very high	No	Loss (intermediate to very high)	Benefit: dulaglutide, liraglutide, semaglutide (SQ) neutral: exenatide once weekly, lixisenatide	Neutral	Benefit for renal endpoints in CVOTs, driven by albuminuria outcomes: dulaglutide, liraglutide, semaglutide (SQ)	See labels for renal dose considerations of individual agents No dose adjustment for dulaglutide, liraglutide, semaglutide Monitor renal function when initiating or	SC; oral (semaglutide)	Risk of thyroid C-cell tumors in rodents: human relevance not determined (liraglutide, dulaglutide, exenatide extended release, semaglutide) Counsel patients on potential for GI side effects and their typically natural guidance on dietary modifications to mitigate GI side effects (reduction in meal size, eating practices (stop eating once full), decreasing intake of high-fat or spicy food) consider slower dose titration for patients experiencing GI

Drugs/class	Efficacy	Hypoglycemia	Impact on body weight	CV effects		Renal effects		Oral/SC	Clinical considerations
				Effect on MACE	HF	Progression of DKD	Dosing/use considerations*		
							escalating doses in patients with renal impairment reporting severe adverse GI reactions		challenges Pancreatitis has been reported but causality has not been established. Discontinue if pancreatitis is suspected Evaluate for gall bladder disease if cholelithiasis or cholecystitis is suspected
GIP and GLP-1RA	Very high	No	Loss (very high)	Under investigation	Under investigation	Under investigation	See labels for renal dose considerations of individual agents No dose adjustment Monitor renal function when initiating or escalating doses in patients with renal impairment reporting severe adverse GI reactions	SC	Risk of thyroid C-cell tumors in rodents: human relevance not determined Counsel patients on potential for GI side effects and their typically temporary nature; provide guidance on dietary modifications to mitigate GI side effects (reduction in meal size, eating practices (stop eating once full), decreasing intake of high-fat or spicy food) consider slower dose titration for patients experiencing GI challenges
DPP-4 inhibitors	Intermediate	No	Neutral	Neutral	Neutral (potential risk, saxagliptin)	Neutral	Renal dose adjustment required (sitagliptin, saxagliptin, alogliptin); can be used in renal impairment No dose adjustment required for linagliptin	Oral	Pancreatitis has been reported in clinical trials but causality has not been established, Discontinue if pancreatitis is suspected Joint pain Bullous pemphigoid (post-marketing): discontinue if suspected

Drugs/class	Efficacy	Hypoglycemia	Impact on body weight	CV effects		Renal effects		Oral/SC	Clinical considerations
				Effect on MACE	HF	Progression of DKD	Dosing/use considerations*		
Thiazolidinediones	High	No	Gain	Potential benefit: Pioglitazone	Increased risk	Neutral	No dose adjustment required Generally not recommended in renal impairment due to potential for fluid retention	Oral	Congestive HF (pioglitazone, rosiglitazone) Fluid retention (edema; heart failure) Benefit in NASH Risk of bone fractures Weight gain: consider lower doses to mitigate weight gain and edema
Sulfonylureas	High	Yes	Gain	Neutral	Neutral	Neutral	Glyburide: generally not recommended in chronic kidney disease Glipizide and glimepiride: initiate conservatively to avoid hypoglycemia	Oral	FDA special warning on increased risk of CV mortality based on studies of an older sulfonylurea (tolbutamide); glimepiride shown to be safe Use with caution in persons at risk for hypoglycemia
Insulin — Human	High to very high	Yes	Gain	Neutral	Neutral	Neutral	Lower insulin doses required with a decrease in eGFR; titrate per clinical response	Human: SC; inhaled	Injection site reactions Higher risk of hypoglycemia with human insulin (NPH or premixed formulations) vs. analogs.
Insulin — Analogs								Analogs: SC	

*CV, cardiovascular; CVOT, cardiovascular outcomes trial; DKA, diabetic ketoacidosis; DKD, diabetic kidney disease; DPP-4, dipeptidyl peptidase 4; eGFR, estimated glomerular filtration rate; FDA, U.S. Food and Drug Administration; GI, gastrointestinal; GIP, gastric inhibitory polypeptide; GLP-1 RA, glucagon-like peptide 1 receptor agonist; HF, heart failure; NASH, non-alcoholic steatohepatitis; MACE, major adverse cardiovascular events; SGLT2, sodium–glucose cotransporter 2; SC, subcutaneous; T2DM, type 2 diabetes mellitus. *For agent-specific dosing recommendations, please refer to manufacturers' prescribing information.*

Table 7.
Choice of glucose-lowering therapy.

In clinical trials, nearly 100 additional antidiabetic agents are being currently studied. This list includes 19 more GLP1-RA, 10 DPP4i, and 12 SGLT2i. More drugs from these newer classes will be available soon in the pharmaceutical market. They are highly effective but due to their high cost, they are more commonly prescribed to patients in economically developed countries. Metformin is the most preferred first-line drug prescribed in both China and India [40, 41]. The increased use of metformin has influenced a decrease in the prescription trends of SUs and TZDs in economically developed countries [42]. Similar trends have been observed in developing countries [43]. In India, after metformin, DPP4 inhibitors and SUs are being used as second-line treatment and SGLT2 inhibitors are being used as third- or fourth-line antidiabetic agents.

7.2 Newer developments—drugs in the pipeline

7.2.1 LY3502970

Orforglipron is an oral non-peptide GLP-1RA. It is highly potent and selective against other B G-protein-coupled receptors. It has favorable pharmacokinetic profile for oral administration. It is a partial agonist, biased toward G-protein activation over beta-arrestin recruitment at the GLP-1 receptor. The results of Phase II trial have been published and have shown −2.1% HbA1c reduction at 26 weeks and weight loss upto −14.7% at 36 weeks. Currently it is in Phase III and is being developed by Eli Lilly [44–46].

7.2.2 SCO-094

A drug candidate which has a dual target of the receptors on GIP and GLP-1 has been identified by SCOHIA Company [47].

7.2.3 PF-06882961

Pfizer is developing a small-molecule GLP 1 receptor agonist called danuglipron. The oral formulation of this molecule is being investigated for diabetes mellitus. At 16 weeks, −1.16% HbA1c reduction along with −4.17 kg weight loss has been reported in Phase II trial. To confirm this results, Phase III trial is being conducted. The Phase II trial in obese non-diabetic patient is ongoing and is expected to complete by the end of year 2023. It is a twice a day formulation, work is being done to modify this formulation to once a day formulation [48, 49].

7.2.4 CagriSema

Semaglutide 2.4 mg co-administered with the long-acting amylin analog cagrilintide is known together as CagriSema. This investigational medicine is being developed by Novo Nordisk. It is given subcutaneously once in a week. At the end of 32 weeks, −2.2% HbA1c reduction along with −15.6% weight loss has been reported in Phase II trial. This gut hormone analog has potential to treat obesity and prevent diabesity [50, 51].

7.2.5 Multi-receptor drugs

Dr. Matthias Tschöp, the recipient of 2023 Banting Medal for the scientific achievement from American Diabetes Association (ADA) suggests that discovery of novel classes of dual and triple gut hormone drugs will continue to transform the fight against diabetes and obesity [52].

7.2.6 LY3437943

Retatrutide also known as GGG tri-agonist is a GIP, GLP-1, and glucagon receptor agonist. Eli Lilly is developing it for management of T2DM and obesity. It is administered subcutaneously once in a week. At 24 weeks, upto −2.02% HbA1c reduction along with −16.94% weight loss has been reported in T2DM phase II trial. In obesity phase II trial, weight loss upto −24.2% has been observed. One of the reasons for greater weight reduction with retatrutide may be combining glucagon receptor agonist with GIP and GLP-1 receptor agonism. It is as safe as incretin-based therapies [53–55].

8. Conclusions

The availability of newer class of drugs in recent years has changed the pharmacotherapeutic approach of management of T2DM. Understanding of underlying pathophysiology of T2DM, treatment strategies can be individualized to address the specific mechanisms contributing to the disease. The effectiveness of medications such as metformin, sulfonylureas, thiazolidinediones, DPP-4 inhibitors, SGLT2 inhibitors, GLP-1 receptor agonists has been extensively studied and proven to enhance glycemic control. The results of completed trials conducted on newer molecules having distinct mechanism of action are promising. These newer potential treatment options will change the management approach of T2DM in future. This chapter has provided a comparative overview of all options available for the management of T2DM highlighting key concepts and current practices.

Author details

Pankaj Kumar Jha*, Heta Shukla, Altaf Makwana and Ashutosh Kakkad
Department of Medical Services, Torrent Pharmaceuticals Ltd., India

*Address all correspondence to: pankajjha@torrentpharma.com

References

[1] International Diabetes Federation. IDF Diabetes Atlas. 10th ed. Brussels, Belgium: International Diabetes Federation; 2021

[2] Anjana RM, Unnikrishnan R, Deepa M, et al. Metabolic non-communicable disease health report of India: The ICMR-INDIAB national cross-sectional study (ICMR-INDIAB-17). The Lancet Diabetes and Endocrinology. 2023;**11**(7):474-489

[3] American Diabetes Association. 2. Classification and diagnosis of diabetes: Standards of medical care in diabetes-2020. Diabetes Care. 2020;**43**(Suppl 1): S14-S31

[4] DeFronzo RA. From the triumvirate to the ominous octet: A new paradigm for the treatment of type 2 diabetes mellitus. Diabetes. 2009;**58**(4):773-795

[5] DeFronzo RA, Ferrannini E, Groop L, et al. Type 2 diabetes mellitus. Nature Reviews. Disease Primers. 2015;**1**:15019

[6] Diabetes Control and Complications Trial Research Group, Nathan DM, Genuth S, Lachin J, et al. The effect of intensive treatment of diabetes on the development and progression of long-term complications in insulin-dependent diabetes mellitus. The New England Journal of Medicine. 1993;**329**(14):977-986

[7] Intensive blood-glucose control with sulphonylureas or insulin compared with conventional treatment and risk of complications in patients with type 2 diabetes (UKPDS 33). UK Prospective Diabetes Study (UKPDS) Group. Lancet. 1998;**352**(9131):837-853 Erratum in: Lancet 1999 Aug 14;354(9178):602

[8] Garber AJ, Handelsman Y, Grunberger G, et al. Consensus statement by the American Association of Clinical Endocrinologists and American College of Endocrinology on the comprehensive type 2 diabetes management algorithm—2020 executive summary. Endocrine Practice. 2020;**26**:107-129

[9] Handelsman Y, Bloomgarden ZT, Grunberger G, et al. American Association of Clinical Endocrinology-Clinical practice guidelines for developing diabetes mellitus comprehensive care plan-2015. Endocrine Practice. 2015;**21** (suppl 1):1-87

[10] Davies MJ, DA D'A, Fradkin J, et al. Management of hyperglycaemia in type 2 diabetes, 2018. A consensus report by the American Diabetes Association (ADA) and the European Association for the Study of Diabetes (EASD). Diabetologia. 2019;**62**(5):873

[11] Facts & Comparisons eAnswers. Hudson, OH: Wolters Kluwer Clinical Drug Information, Inc.; 2020

[12] American Diabetes Association. 9. Pharmacologic approaches to glycemic treatment: Standards of medical care in diabetes-2020. Diabetes Care. 2020;**43** (Suppl 1):S98-S110

[13] Sola D, Rossi L, Schianca GP, Maffioli P, Bigliocca M, Mella R, et al. Sulfonylureas and their use in clinical practice. Archives of Medical Science. 2015;**11**(4):840-848

[14] Delvecchio M, Pastore C, Giordano P. Treatment options for MODY patients: A systematic review of literature. Diabetes Therapy. 2020;**11**(8): 1667-1685

[15] Trujillo J, Haines S. Diabetes Mellitus. In: JT DP, Yee GC, Posey L,

Haines ST, Nolin TD, Ellingrod V, editors. Pharmacotherapy: A Pathophysiologic Approach, 11e. McGraw Hill; 2020. Available from: https://accesspharmacy.mhmedical.com/content.aspx?bookid=2577&sectionid=228901946 [Accessed: July 01, 2023]

[16] Lexicomp Online. Hudson, OH: Wolters Kluwer Clinical Drug Information, Inc.; 2020

[17] Dahlén AD, Dashi G, Maslov I, et al. Trends in antidiabetic drug discovery: FDA approved drugs, new drugs in clinical trials and global sales. Frontiers in Pharmacology. 2022;**12**:807548

[18] Tuomi T, Honkanen EH, Isomaa B, Sarelin L, Groop LC. Improved prandial glucose control with lower risk of hypoglycemia with nateglinide than with glibenclamide in patients with maturity-onset diabetes of the young type 3. Diabetes Care. 2006;**29**(2): 189-194

[19] Van de Laar FA, Lucassen PL, Akkermans RP, Van de Lisdonk EH, Rutten GE, Van Weel C. Alpha-glucosidase inhibitors for type 2 diabetes mellitus. Cochrane Database of Systematic Reviews. 2005;**2005**(2): CD003639

[20] Patoulias DI, Boulmpou A, Teperikidis E, et al. Cardiovascular efficacy and safety of dipeptidyl peptidase-4 inhibitors: A meta-analysis of cardiovascular outcome trials. World Journal of Cardiology. 2021;**13**(10): 585-592

[21] Lopaschuk GD, Verma S. Mechanisms of cardiovascular benefits of sodium glucose co-transporter 2 (SGLT2) inhibitors: A state-of-the-art review. JACC: Basic to Translational Science. 2020;**5**(6):632-644

[22] Kubota Y, Shimizu W, et al. Clinical benefits of sodium–glucose cotransporter 2 inhibitors and the mechanisms underlying their cardiovascular effects. JACC: Asia. 2022; **2**(3_Part_2):287-293. DOI: 10.1016/j.jacasi.2022.03.009

[23] Sieracki L, Sordi C, Ostroff ML, et al. Investigating cardiovascular benefits of SGLT2 inhibitors. US Pharmacist. 2022; **47**(11):17-22

[24] Trujillo JM, Nuffer W, Ellis SL. GLP-1 receptor agonists: A review of head-to-head clinical studies. Therapeutic Advances in Endocrinology and Metabolism. 2015;**6**:19-28

[25] Nauck MA, Meier JJ. Management of endocrine disease: Are all GLP-1 agonists equal in the treatment of type 2 diabetes? European Journal of Endocrinology. 2019;**181**(6):R211-R234

[26] Hinnen D. Glucagon-like peptide 1 receptor agonists for type 2 diabetes. Diabetes Spectrum: A Publication of the American Diabetes Association. 2017; **30**(3):202-210

[27] Ussher JR, Drucker DJ. Glucagon-like peptide 1 receptor agonists: Cardiovascular benefits and mechanisms of action. Nature Reviews. Cardiology. 2023;**20**(7):463-474

[28] Ludvik B, Giorgino F, Jódar E, et al. Once-weekly tirzepatide versus once-daily insulin degludec as add-on to metformin with or without SGLT2 inhibitors in patients with type 2 diabetes (SURPASS-3): A randomised, open-label, parallel-group, phase 3 trial. Lancet. 2021;**398**(10300):583-598

[29] Dutta P, Kumar Y, Babu AT, Giri Ravindran S, Salam A, Rai B, et al. Tirzepatide: A promising drug for type 2

diabetes and beyond. Cureus. 2023;**15**(5): e38379

[30] De Block C, Bailey C, Wysham C, Hemmingway A, Allen SE, Peleshok J. Tirzepatide for the treatment of adults with type 2 diabetes: An endocrine perspective. Diabetes, Obesity & Metabolism. 2023;**25**(1):3-17

[31] Shivaprasad C, Kalra S. Bromocriptine in type 2 diabetes mellitus. Indian Journal of Endocrinology and Metabolism. 2011;**15** (Suppl 1):S17-S24

[32] Ooi CP, Loke SC. Colesevelam for type 2 diabetes mellitus. Cochrane Database of Systematic Reviews. 2012; **12**(12):CD009361

[33] Brunton LL, Hilal-Dandan R, Knollmann BC, editors. Goodman & Gilman's: The Pharmacological Basis of Therapeutics,13e. McGraw Hill; 2017. Available from: https://accessmedicine.mhmedical.com/content.aspx?bookid=2189&sectionid=165936845

[34] Tripathi KD. Essentials of Medical Pharmacology. 8th ed. New Delhi, India: Jaypee Brothers Medical; 2018

[35] Jacob S, Morsy MA, Nair A. An overview on the insulin preparations and devices. Indian Journal of Pharmaceutical Education and Research. 2018;**52**(4):550-557

[36] Humulin R. U-500 KwikPen [package insert]. Indianapolis, IN: Eli Lilly and Company; 2019

[37] Chlup R, Vaverková H, Bartek J. Complementary insulin therapy improves blood glucose and serum lipids parameters in type 2 (non-insulin-dependent) diabetic patients. I. Effects on blood glucose control. Experimental and Clinical Endocrinology & Diabetes. 1997;**105**(Suppl 2):70-73

[38] ElSayed NA, Aleppo G, Aroda VR, et al. 9. Pharmacologic approaches to glycemic treatment: Standards of care in diabetes-2023. Diabetes Care. 2023;**46** (Suppl 1):S140-S157

[39] Aloke C, Egwu CO, Aja PM, Obasi NA, Chukwu J, Akumadu BO, et al. Current advances in the management of diabetes mellitus. Biomedicine. 2022;**10**(10):2436

[40] Hu C, Jia W. Diabetes in China: Epidemiology and genetic risk factors and their clinical utility in personalized medication. Diabetes. 2018;**67**(1):3-11

[41] Singla R, Bindra J, Singla A, et al. Drug prescription patterns and cost analysis of diabetes therapy in India: Audit of an endocrine practice. Indian Journal of Endocrinology and Metabolism. 2019;**23**(1):40-45

[42] Srinivasan S, Yee SW, Giacomini KM. Pharmacogenetics of antidiabetic drugs. Advances in Pharmacology. 2018;**83**:361-389

[43] Mohan V, Khunti K, Chan SP, et al. Management of Type 2 diabetes in developing countries: Balancing optimal glycaemic control and outcomes with affordability and accessibility to treatment. Diabetes Therapy. 2020; **11**(1):15-35

[44] Kawai T, Sun B, Yoshino H, et al. Structural basis for GLP-1 receptor activation by LY3502970, an orally active nonpeptide agonist. Proceedings of the National Academy of Sciences of the United States of America. 2020; **117**(47):29959-29967

[45] Wharton S, Blevins T, Connery L, et al. Daily Oral GLP-1 receptor agonist

orforglipron for adults with obesity. The New England Journal of Medicine. 2023. DOI: 10.1056/NEJMoa2302392. Epub ahead of print

[46] Frias JP, Hsia S, Eyde S, et al. Efficacy and safety of oral orforglipron in patients with type 2 diabetes: A multicentre, randomised, dose-response, phase 2 study. Lancet. 2023:S0140-6736 (23)01302-8. DOI: 10.1016/S0140-6736 (23)01302-8. Epub ahead of print

[47] SCO-094 by Scohia Pharma for Type 2 Diabetes: Likelihood of Approval. Available from: https://www.pharmaceutical-technology.com/data-insights/sco-094-scohia-pharma-type-2-diabetes-likelihood-of-approval/ [Accessed: June 20, 2023]

[48] Saxena AR, Frias JP, Brown LS, et al. Efficacy and safety of oral small molecule glucagon-like peptide 1 receptor agonist danuglipron for glycemic control among patients with type 2 diabetes: A randomized clinical trial. JAMA Network Open. 2023;**6**(5): e2314493

[49] Available from: https://www.pfizer.com/news/press-release/press-release-detail/pfizer-provides-update-glp-1-ra-clinical-development [Accessed: July 03, 2023]

[50] Frias JP, Deenadayalan S, Erichsen L, et al. Efficacy and safety of co-administered once-weekly cagrilintide 2·4 mg with once-weekly semaglutide 2·4 mg in type 2 diabetes: A multicentre, randomised, double-blind, active-controlled, phase 2 trial. Lancet. 2023:S0140-6736(23)01163-7. DOI: 10.1016/S0140-6736(23)01163-7. Epub ahead of print

[51] Maja Clasen. Semaglutide Plus Cagrilintide Reduced Blood Sugar, Weight in T2D. Available from: https://www.medpagetoday.com/meetingcoverage/ada/105213 [Accessed: July 03, 2023]

[52] ADA. Banting Medal Recipient Discusses Emerging Promise of Pharmacologic Treatment for Obesity and Diabetes. 2023. Available from: https://www.adameetingnews.org/live-updates/session-coverage/banting-medal-recipient-discusses-emerging-promise-of-pharmacologic-treatment-for-obesity-and-diabetes/ [Accessed: July 06, 2023]

[53] Rosenstock J, Frias J, Jastreboff AM, et al. Retatrutide, a GIP, GLP-1 and glucagon receptor agonist, for people with type 2 diabetes: A randomised, double-blind, placebo and active-controlled, parallel-group, phase 2 trial conducted in the USA. Lancet. 2023: S0140-6736(23)01053-X. DOI: 10.1016/S0140-6736(23)01053-X. Epub ahead of print

[54] Jastreboff AM, Kaplan LM, Frías JP, Wu Q, Du Y, Gurbuz S, et al. Retatrutide phase 2 obesity trial investigators. Triple-hormone-receptor agonist retatrutide for obesity-A phase 2 trial. The New England Journal of Medicine. 2023. DOI: 10.1056/NEJMoa2301972. Epub ahead of print

[55] Lilly's phase 2 retatrutide results published in The New England Journal of Medicine show the investigational molecule achieved up to 17.5% mean weight reduction at 24 weeks in adults with obesity and overweight. Eli Lilly and Company. Jun 26 2023. Available from: https://investor.lilly.com/news-releases/news-release-details/lillys-phase-2-retatrutide-results-published-new-england-journal [Accessed: July 03, 2023]

Chapter 13

Perspective Chapter: Exploring the Potential of Vagus Nerve Neuromodulation as a Personalized and Enhanced Therapeutic Experience for Type 2 Diabetics

Jonathan Waataja, Sayeed Ikramuddin, Dov Gal and Charles Billington

Abstract

Glucagon-like peptide-1 (GLP-1) receptor agonists have become the gold standard for the treatment of type 2 diabetes mellitus (T2D). The therapeutic benefits of GLP-1 are marred by compliance, cost, and side effects. Vagus nerve modulation (VNM) holds great potential for current and future neuromodulation therapies in a range of medical conditions. Treatment for T2D using VNM is a potential new area of research. Most VNM studies investigating glycemic control utilize glucose tolerance tests. There are few long-term chronic studies examining both fasting plasma glucose and plasma glucose in the absorptive state. This chapter explores literature involving the use of VNM to enhance glycemic control. Also, results of a novel method of multi-site, multi-frequency sub-diaphragmatic vagal neuromodulation will be reviewed as well as a discussion of mechanisms associated with this VNM technique. This modality holds promise in enhancing glycemic control in the fasting and postprandial states. Multi-site multi-frequency neuromodulation offers a multitude of different therapy parameters for personalized medicine.

Keywords: type 2 diabetes, diabetes, glucose intolerance, vagus nerve, vagal nerve, sub-diaphragmatic vagus, vagus nerve stimulation, VNS, bioelectronics, neuromodulation

1. Introduction

Despite advances in diabetic medications, the use of bariatric surgery and lifestyle modification, there is still an unmet need for novel treatments for type 2 diabetes mellitus (T2D). For example, outside of clinical trials, discontinuation rates of glucagon like peptide 1 (GLP)-1 Receptor Agonist (GLP-1 RA) therapy has been reported to be approximately 45% at 1 year [1, 2] due to unwanted side effects [3], high cost [4], and unwillingness to follow physician's treatment advice [5]. There are questions regarding the long-term durability of bariatric surgery to treat T2D [6] and as many as 75% of diabetics fail at lifestyle modification [7]. This chapter will explore current treatment options and the advances, and potential advantages, of new non-pharmacological methods in development as treatment options for T2D. These include insulin pump technology, duodenal mucosal resurfacing, gene therapy, external electrical stimulation, peripheral focused ultrasound, direct stimulation to visceral organs, and vagus nerve modulation (VNM) technologies. Benefits of many of these therapies include a decreased need for compliance, decreased long term costs, and decreased unwanted side effects. Finally, this chapter will highlight a novel technique comprising of multi-site, multi-frequency electrical modulation of the sub-diaphragmatic vagus nerve for the treatment of T2D.

1.1 Limitations of current T2D treatment options

According to the American Academy of Clinical Endocrinologist (AACE) Treatment Guidelines, T2D therapeutic options follow an algorithm of three escalating scales of intervention starting with lifestyle modification (LSM), and escalating to monotherapy with pharmacological agents, concurrent dual therapy, triple therapy, and eventually medical and surgical weight loss [8]. These pharmacologic treatments begin with Metformin, and then are combined with other drugs such as sulfonylureas, thiazolidinedione, DPP-4 & SGLT2 inhibitors and GLP-1 RAs. The medications are not without side effects, potentially inducing hypoglycemia, heart failure, ketoacidosis, diarrhea, nausea, abdominal pain, orthopedic fracture and weight gain [9].

As an adjunct to pharmacotherapy, insulin therapy is an effective tool to increase glycemic control, however, there is a risk of hypoglycemia and a large portion of diabetics fears insulin injections [10–15]. A study by Stotland et al. [16] found that 45% of diabetic subjects avoided injections because of anxiety, phobia and fear. Injection anxiety has been related to poorer treatment adherence, greater psychological distress, a greater incidence of diabetes-related hospitalization and a higher risk of retinopathy and neuropathy [10].

Weight-loss surgery for T2D has demonstrated efficacy as a non-pharmacological treatment for T2D. However, it is not without challenges and potential complications. T2D has shown to be recurrent in 58% of bariatric surgical patients, albeit with sustained reductions in medications and insulin [17]. While a safe option, with mortality rates below 1%, the side effects of some bariatric surgeries still carry the risks of bowel obstructions, staple line dehiscence, sepsis, gallstones, GERD, Barret's Esophagus, hernia, and dumping syndrome [18]. Non-anatomical sparing bariatric surgeries such as the Roux-Y-Gastric Bypass (RYGB) and its variants, Vertical Sleeve Gastrectomy (VSG) and the Biliopancreatic Diversion with Duodenal Switch (BPD-DS) can cause a number of nutritional complications secondary to these malabsorptive procedures, such as anemias, metabolic bone disease, calcium deficiencies, sarcopenic obesity, and neurologic disorders if a patient is non-compliant with their post-operative nutritional protocols [19].

GLP-1 receptor agonists have gained much recent popularity and have shown promise for the treatment of T2D. In clinical trials HbA1c reduction ranges from −14.8 to −2.7 mmol/mol [20] and weight loss up to 12% from baseline [21]. However, real-world studies have demonstrated lower positive outcomes with this class of drugs. In a retrospective cohort study by Weiss et al. [2], weight and adherence were

Study	Study duration	GLP-1 agonist	Adherence (%)
Divino et al. (2019) [22]	1 year	Dulaglutide	36.8–67.2
		Exenatide twice daily	5.9–44.4
		Exenatide once weekly	24.7–44.2
		Liraglutide	22.2–57.5
		Lixisenatide	15.5–40.0
Johnston et al. (2014) [23]	1 year	Exenatide once weekly	78.3
		Exenatide twice daily	50
		Liraglutide once daily	72.2
Uzoigwe et al. (2021) [24]	1 year	Semaglutide once weekly	67.0
		Dulaglutide	56.0
		Liraglutide	40.4
		Exenatide one weekly	35.5
Weiss et al. (2020) [1]	1 year	Once daily GLP-1RA	43.8
		Once Weekly GLP-1 RA	64.2
Weiss et al. (2022) [2]	1 year	Once daily GLP-1RA	59.8
		Once Weekly GLP-1 RA	82.1
	2 years	Once daily GLP-1RA	55.3
		Once Weekly GLP-1 RA	74.1

Table 1.
Multiple studies demonstrate issues with adherence to taking GLP-1 RAs. This is observed in once daily and once week injections. A major problem for lack of adherence is forgetfulness to take medications.

analyzed at 12 and 24 months in 589 subjects that were prescribed GLP-1 RAs. At 12 months only 33% of patients achieved weight loss of ≥5%, adherence was 65% and the discontinuation rate was 45%. At 24 months 44% of type 2 diabetics achieved weight loss of ≥5%, adherence was 59% and 65% of patients discontinued GLP-1 RAs. Non-adherence to GLP-1 RAs has been observed in multiple other studies (**Table 1**). Low adherence to new oral forms of GLP-1 RAs is predicted, with only 50% of type 2 diabetics adhering to oral medications as prescribed [25] mainly due to forgetfulness [26]. Approximately 5–10% of type 2 diabetics cannot tolerate GLP-1 RAs [20] due to nausea, vomiting and diarrhea [3].

2. Non-pharmacological technologies under development

There are multiple non-pharmacological T2D treatment methodologies in various stages of development. Clinical trials have included next generation closed loop insulin pumps, duodenal mucosal resurfacing, external electrical stimulation, direct stimulation of visceral organs and transcutaneous auricular vagus nerve stimulation. Preclinical tests have involved gene therapies, peripheral focused ultrasound, direct visceral organ stimulation and various approaches to vagus nerve stimulation. The following is a summary of these emerging technologies.

2.1 Next generation closed-loop insulin pumps

For many type-1 diabetics insulin pumps have demonstrated efficacy in increasing targeted glycemic outcomes, decreasing glucose variability and increasing quality of life. Studies have indicated that this technology may be beneficial for insulin delivery for therapy for type 2 diabetics on insulin therapy [27]. However, there are many drawbacks of using pump technology. Hypoglycemic events still remain an issue for both diabetic populations using this technology [27, 28]. Continuous glucose monitoring (CGM) sensor-augmented insulin pump therapy reduces the incidence of hypoglycemia [29],though these systems cannot actively raise plasma glucose (PG). To compensate for unidirectional glycemic control, CGM sensor-augmented pump algorithms incorporate a significant safety floor margin when defining target blood glucose range. This results in average HbA1c levels greater than the recommended <53 mmol/mol [30], at which point diabetes-associated complications develop [31, 32]. Alternatively, bidirectional glycemic control systems have been explored to increase time-in-range. Dual-hormone pumps using both insulin and glucagon enable tighter glycemic control, including reducing the number of hypoglycemia episodes. Challenges associated with the stability of glucagon at room-temperature have prevented widespread acceptance of dual-hormone therapies [33]. A significant drawback for the use of insulin pump technology for type 2 diabetics is the considerably greater amount of daily insulin required for T2D insulin therapy versus that required to treat T1DM (approximately 100 Units for T2D vs. 10 units for T1DM [27]). This would require frequent daily refills of the pump revisor. For these reasons, insulin pump therapy has not been well adopted by type 2 diabetics.

2.2 Duodenal mucosal resurfacing

Duodenal mucosal resurfacing (DMR) is a potential new method of increasing glycemic control for T2D. It has demonstrated positive results in early single-arm, open-label clinical trials [34]. The procedure involves thermal energy ablation of duodenal mucosa using an endoscopic procedure [35]. Two-year results demonstrated a HbA1c level reduction from 69.4 ± -15.8 to 58.5 ± -11.5 mmol/mol [34]. Despite promising early results, the endoscopic DMR procedure carries potential risks of perforation of the intestine and intestinal leaks [36]. Further research is required to establish the long-term safety and effectiveness of DMR.

2.3 Gene therapies

Gene therapy for type 2 diabetes is an emerging field of research and there are several promising approaches that are being investigated. One approach is to use gene therapy to increase the production of insulin in the pancreas [37]. Another approach is to modify genes that regulate blood glucose levels outside of pancreatic function. This involves using gene editing tools such as CRISPR-Cas9 to modify genes associated with insulin resistance or glucose metabolism [38]. These approaches are still in the early stages of research and many further studies are needed to ensure safety and efficacy in type 2 diabetics.

Evidence is accumulating that obesity-associated and/or adipose tissue-derived circulating miRNAs are promising new therapeutic targets for the treatment of obesity and T2D [39]. The development of novel therapeutics, such as miRNA mimetics, anti-miRNA oligonucleotides and exosomes loaded with miRNAs, might allow the clinical application of miRNA-based therapeutics for T2D.

Another exciting branch of gene therapy for the treatment of T2D utilizes opto- and chemogenetic neuromodulation. Optogenetics involves two components, genetic modulation, and optics. The genetic component comprises cellular expression of light sensitive ion channels, or opsins, that are typically isolated from sensory photoreceptors from green algae. There are two major classes of opsins: channelrhodopsins which conduct cations that induce neuronal excitation and anion-conducting channelrhodopsins which induce neuronal inhibition. A cell specific promoter actuator gene is fused to the opsin for expression to specific neuronal populations, allowing for cell type specific excitation or inhibition. Genes coding for opsins are delivered to the cell by generating lines of transgenic animals, transfection, or viral transduction.

A study by Fontaine et al. [40] utilized a non-diabetic transgenic mouse line that employed an acetyltransferase promoter to express Channelrhodopsin-2 (ChR2) in vagal pre-ganglionic afferent nerves innervating the pancreas. When optically stimulating the pancreas, they observed a decrease in blood glucose by 2.8 mmol/l which recovered to baseline following cessation of stimulation. Insulin was increased by 84% but did not reach significance and there was no change in glucagon. Optogenetic stimulation enhanced performance on glucose tolerance tests and there was an observed increase in insulin in these experiments. One drawback was that isoflurane was used in these acute experiments which may have confounded the results.

Studies employing chemogenetic stimulation have exhibited effects on glycemic control. Chemogenetic stimulation has similarities to optogenetic stimulation which requires genetic modification and cell specific stimulation, or inhibition, by utilizing cell specific promoters to express desired genes. However, in contrast to optogenetics, pharmacologically inert compounds are used to active transfected designed mutated receptors. The most common receptors are genetically altered G protein-coupled receptors [41] with GqD and GiD used to activate or silence neurons, respectively. Chemogenetic stimulation has advantages over optogenetic modulation in that it does not require the complexity of introducing a light source inside the animal.

Many chemogenetic-targeted-tissues include extra-neuronal cells such as alpha and beta-cells, L-cells, adipocytes, hepatocytes and skeletal muscle [42–47]. Effects of chemogenetic stimulation on these tissues involve an enhanced glucose uptake in skeletal muscle, reduced glucagon secretion, increased insulin secretion and beta cell proliferation [42–47]. Chemogenetic neuronal targets have focused on AgRP and POMC neurons [47, 48]. Modulation of activity in these neuronal populations may increase glycose homeostasis primarily through modulating food intake [47, 48].

Despite promising experimental results using gene therapy, there are many obstacles to overcome for this methodology to be utilized for a treatment of T2D. The use of adeno-associated viruses (AAVs) is a common method to deliver genes in vivo and the most reasonable method to be used clinically for delivery of genes for gene therapy. However, there are inherent risks involved with AAV-mediated gene delivery and many barriers for acceptance for a treatment of T2D. The type of diseases that have been accepted for gene therapy are sever, rare and debilitating [49]; and not metabolic disorders.

Serious adverse events are associated with the delivery of genes using AAVs which are associated with complement immune system activation [50, 51]. Due to this immunosuppressant therapy is required which is a clinical risk. Hepatotoxicity, kidney damage and dorsal root ganglia toxicity have been observed with use of AAVs [52].

2.4 External electrical stimulation

Studies have tested the effects of electrical stimulation delivered to the surface of the skin on increasing glycemic control. A study by Lee et al. [53] examined stimulation in 12 subjects using applications microcurrents at an ultra-low frequency of 0.0007 Hz delivered to the surface of the skin for 3.5 hours per day, 5 days per week for 2–4 months. Results were reported for 6 subjects at the conclusion of the trial. HbA1c decreased in these subjects from 55.2 ± -13.7 to 44.3 ± -15.8 mmol/mol (average $\pm$ stdev). Limitations of this study include a lack of a control group, a small sample size, and no statistical analysis.

Catalogna et al. [54] studied peripheral electrical stimulation (PES) in 12 T2D subjects in an interventional, open label, randomized, crossover trial. Two adhesive electrodes were placed bilaterally, one on the anterior aspect of the legs, below the kneecap, and lateral to the anterior crest of the tibia in proximity to the common peroneal and tibial branches of the sciatic nerve. Electrical current was applied for 5 minutes every morning before breakfast for 14 days. They found a significant decrease in average nocturnal PG (from 7.4 $\pm$ 0.6 mmol/l at baseline to 6.5 $\pm$ 0.5 mmol/l) and FPG decreased from 7.6 $\pm$ 0.4 to 6.7 $\pm$ 0.4 mmol/l following treatment. There was no change in insulin. A controlled experiment with a larger sample is needed to draw conclusions regarding the use of this technique as a treatment for T2D.

2.5 Peripheral focused ultrasound

Peripheral focused ultrasound (pFUS) has been tested as a novel approach to externally modulate neuronal activity [55]. Cotero et al. [56] evaluated the effects of daily pFUS on restoring glycemic control in rat and mouse models of T2D. Ultrasound was focused on the hepatoportal nerve plexus, known to contain glucose metabolism sensory neurons. The study demonstrated that pFUS increased glycemic control by reversing the onset of LPS-induced hyperglycemia and improved performance on glucose tolerance tests. Interestingly, they found that pFUS modulated firing rates in the hypothalamus at areas that are innervated by vagal projects and altered levels of neurotransmitters regulated to metabolism. In non-diabetic swine they demonstrated increased insulin sensitivity by using hyperinsulinemic-euglycmic clamps. The authors note that there are barriers to the practicality of this system. At home use of this methodology requires large technological advancements. Currently pFUS systems require physicians and technicians to operate the system. Hand-held ultrasound devices with flexible body-conformal ultrasound patches are under development [57], which may help bridge this technical gab. However, the focal depth of these systems is 10–20 mm and would not reach the hepatoportal nerve plexus in humans. Also, daily use of an external device may have problems with adoption in the T2D population.

2.6 Direct stimulation to visceral organs

Stimulation of the duodenum has demonstrated increased glycemic control in rodents [58] as well as in T2D subjects. In an open-labeled, prospective, single-arm study by Aberle et al. [59] electrodes were implanted into the subserosal layer of the anterior duodenal wall in 12 obese type 2 diabetic subjects with a mean HbA1c of 63.9 mmol/mol at baseline. After 12 months of duodenal stimulation there was a $-$ 15.8 mmol/mol decrease in HbA1c and a drop in FPG of 1.8 mmol/l from

9.6 mmol/l at baseline. There was no change in c-peptide at 12 months. Further investigation with adequately powered blinded clinical trials is required to determine the effects of this approach.

Direct hepatic electrical stimulation has demonstrated increased glycemic control in rodents. Chen et al. [60] placed cardiac pacing electrodes on two lopes of the livers in the Zucker obese (fatty) rat (ZDF fa/fa) T2D animal model. The locations of the electrodes on the liver were described as at the "the top and middle lobe". The rat's FPG decreased from 17.1 ± 2.2 to 15.9 ± 2.1 mmol/l with 3 hours of stimulation. There was also a slight increase in performance during an oral glucose tolerance test (OGTT) with hepatic stimulation. Limitations to this technique are the possibility of perforation to the liver at the site of the implanted electrodes as well as stimulation induced hypoglycemia.

Carotid sinus nerve (CSN) stimulation has been assessed as an approach of increasing glycemic control. In a study by Sacramento et al. [61] a 50 kHz signal was applied to the CSN in a diet induced model of type 2 diabetes in rat. Stimulation increased performance on OGTTs as well as potentiating insulin sensitivity. However, there was no change in FPG. A limitation to this procedure is possible adverse effects on ventilatory control and chemoreflexes during stimulation [62].

2.7 Vagus nerve modulation

Studies investigating the therapeutic potential of using vagus nerve modulation (VNM) have involved both external and implanted electrodes. Locations of internal stimulation have included cervical and abdominal vagus nerve segments. The auricular segment of the vagus nerve has been widely evaluated as a site for external vagus stimulation.

Transcutaneous auricular vagus nerve stimulation (taVNS) has shown mixed results to increase glycemic control. The physiological concept behind taVNS is excitation of the auricular branch of the vagus nerve (ABVN) which runs close to the external ear [63, 64]. Supportive evidence that transcutaneous auricular stimulation effects vagal function is demonstrated through changes in heart rate variability [65, 66], known to be affected by many vagus nerve stimulation approaches, and fMRI evidence showing increased central nervous system (CNS) activity in central vagal projections areas [67, 68] during taVNS.

Preclinical and clinical studies have evaluated the effects of taVNS on glycemic control. A study by Li et al. [69] examined if taVNS prevents the development of hyperglycemia in the Zucker rats. taVNS was delivered for 30 minutes a day for 34 days. Zucker rats that received taVNS did not develop hyperglycemia and had a lower HbA1c compared to control after 34 days. Insulin receptors were upregulated in hypothalamus, liver, and skeletal muscle.

Clinical studies evaluating taVNS have had mixed results. A study by Kozorosky et al. [70] measured blood glucose, C-peptide, insulin, leptin, glucagon, ghrelin, baroreceptor-heart rate reflex sensitivity and heart rate variability in non-diabetic subjects following a glucose tolerance test involving ingestion of a beverage containing: 9 g protein, 33 g total carbohydrates (10 g glucose), and 9 g fat. The results were confounding. The sham group demonstrated a decrease in blood glucose similar to the taVNS group. In the glucose tolerance experiments taVNS did not affect blood glucose, glucagon, insulin and C-peptide. There was no change in heart rate variability or baroreceptor-heart rate reflex sensitivity (as would be expected with vagus nerve excitation). However, taVNS decreased postprandial plasma ghrelin levels.

In a single blind randomized controlled trial [71] involving 72 subjects with impaired glucose tolerance (baseline HbA1c = 45.4 mmol/mol) taVNS was applied for 12 weeks twice per day. Fasting plasma glucose (FPG), 2-hour plasma glucose (2hPG, during OGTTs) and HbA1c were evaluated. There was a modest decrease in FPG from 6.2 to 5.7 mmol/l after 12 months with taVNS and a decrease in 2hPG from 9.7 to 7.5 mmol/l. However, the sham groups also saw a decrease in FPG from 9.1 to 8.0 mmol/l. There was a very modest, clinically insignificant, decrease in HbA1c from 45.4 to 43.2 mmol/l with taVNS, however, the sham group experienced a drop from 44.3 to 42.1 mmol/mol. Taken together this study demonstrated no (or at least very modest) improvement in glycemic control and the subjects were not diabetic.

Another clinical study [72] demonstrated no effect of taVNS on glycemic control. In this study OGTTs were carried out on fifteen non-diabetic male subjects and demonstrated no increase in glycemic control. Application of taVNS did not affect serum catecholamine levels or a change in heart rate as would be expected during vagus nerve stimulation.

Overall, taVNS studies have either shown a very modest increase in glycemic control or none. Internal stimulation may be required to increase the effectiveness of vagus nerve stimulation for modulation of PG. Indeed, cervical, and sub-diaphragmatic vagus nerve stimulation approaches have repeatedly demonstrated efficacy to modify glycemic control.

The effects of efferent and/or afferent cervical vagus nerve stimulation on glycemia has been evaluated in preclinical studies. In a study by Meyers et al. [73] stimulation was applied to the cervical vagus nerve non-diabetic rats. Experimental conditions involved ligation of the vagus nerve and stimulation at either the cranial or distal segments, as well as stimulation to an intact nerve. When the uncut nerve was stimulated there was an increase in PG 30 minutes following the initiation of stimulation as well as an increase in plasma glucagon but not insulin. When the cranial side was stimulated there was also an increase in PG but no change in insulin or glucagon. Interestingly, when the distal side of the cut vagus nerve was stimulated there was an increase in PG at 30 minutes as well as an increase in glucagon, however, following 120 minutes of stimulation PG decreased with a corresponding increase in insulin and a decrease in glucagon. Despite these intriguing findings, cervical vagus nerve ligation was required, making it unrealistic for human use.

The results of the Mayer et al. study were replicated by stimulation of intact cervical vagus nerve [74]. In addition to experiments in the Mayer et al. study, researchers also accessed glycemic control with an intraperitoneal glucose tolerance test (IPGTT). Results from glucose tolerance test demonstrated decreased glycemic control with a corresponding decrease in insulin. Interestingly, both right and left cervical vagus stimulation caused a decrease in blood insulin. This suggests that stimulation of *either* celiac branch or accessory celiac branch vagal pathways may affect pancreatic function (anatomical vagal branch depiction can be found on **Figure 1**).

Payne et al. [75] also found similar results as Meyers et al. [73] which was demonstrated by increased glycemic control in a rat model of T2D by selective stimulation of efferent vagal fibers of the anterior sub-diaphragmatic vagal trunk. The Payne et al. methodology is clinically practical compared to the one tested by Meyers et al. in that selective efferent stimulation was achieved by the combination of an electrical nerve blockade signal (stimulation at 26 kHz), in lieu of vagotomy, and stimulation distal to the site of nerve blockade. Also, the modulation was below the level of the heart, decreasing possible cardiac effects. The procedure induced an increase in glycemic

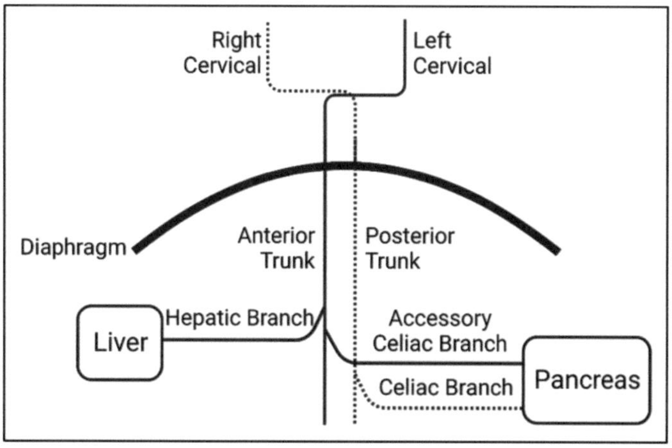

Figure 1.
Various sub-diaphragmatic vagus nerve branches innervate the liver and the pancreas. The pancreas is innervated by the celiac and accessory celiac vagal branches. The celiac branch stems from the posterior sub-diaphragmatic vagal trunk and the accessory celiac branch bifurcates from the anterior sub-diaphragmatic vagal trunk. The hepatic branch, innervating the liver, stems from the anterior sub-diaphragmatic vagal trunk. Note: Crossing of axon projects between right/posterior and left/anterior vagal trunks also occurs. Image created by biorender.com.

control as assessed by OGTTs. Pancreatic function was *possibly* affected with a trend ($p = 0.057$) in decreased glucagon during neuromodulation. This may have occurred through modulating accessory celiac branch activity. The group did not report changes in FPG.

In a study by Yin et al. [76] the dorsal sub-diaphragmatic vagus was stimulated in a rat model of T2D. The group applied various frequencies (5, 14, 40, 5000 Hz as well as intermittent stimulation with 10 seconds on and 90 seconds off at 5 Hz) and determined that 14 Hz with a 0.3 ms pulse width, 5000 Hz and intermittent stimulation significantly increase glycemic control. They also found an increase in insulin sensitivity with stimulation at 5 Hz. They did not report changes in FPG.

Radio frequency applied to the walls of hepatic vessels has been studied to induce a sub-diaphragmatic hepatic vagotomy with the goal to decrease sympathetic nervous system tone to increase glycemic control [77]. Experiments using this technique have demonstrated increased glycemic control by enhanced performance on OGTTs. Also, plasma insulin and c-peptide were shown to increase during the OGTT experiments. Despite the positive findings hepatic vagotomy may be problematic. Hepatic vagotomy has been shown to cause negative changes in feeding behavior, increased hypoglycemic episodes, negative effects on liver regeneration, and cause increased metastasis during liver cancer [78–81].

Methods to increase glycemic control through VNM may not be entirely dependent on modulation of pancreatic or hepatic function. Vagal neuromodulation-induced decreases in systemic inflammation and weight may facilitate controlling glycemic dysfunction. Many studies have shown that inflammation dysregulation is prevalent in T2D [82–85]. VNS decreases pro-inflammatory cytokines [86–88] and reduces effects of inflammatory diseases such as rheumatoid arthritis [89]. Utilizing VNS strategies that decrease inflammation may be a target for T2D treatments [90], but further study is required.

Neuromodulation involving electrical-induced conduction block of the anterior and posterior vagal trunks has demonstrated weight loss and increased glycemic control in human subjects. In a study by Herrera et al. [91] HbA1c decreased by −16.9 mmol/mol, from a baseline of 61.7 mmol/mol, and FPG decline by 1.0 mmol/l, from a baseline of 8.4 mmol/l, following 3 years of vagal blockade. This coincided with a 21% loss of excess weight from baseline.

In summary, multiple studies have demonstrated the ability to increase glycemic control by utilization of VNM. The translation of many of the above preclinical studies to human application requires ongoing research, including studies by our research group. Below highlights recent results from our work utilizing a new approach to VNM. This involves a novel method of electrically modulating multiple sites along the vagus nerve to treat glucose dysregulation.

3. Exploring a targeted multisite/multifrequency vagal neuromodulation approach as a treatment for type 2 diabetes mellitus

Since multiple organ systems involved in blood glucose regulation are influenced by different vagus nerve branches, there may be necessity for electrical modulation of multiple vagus nerve branches to achieve optimal effects on plasma glucose (PG) regulation. This idea has led our team to investigate a new dual neuromodulation concept involving combined stimulation of celiac fibers of the vagus nerve innervating the pancreas along with reversible electrical blockade of neuronal hepatic fibers of the vagus nerve innervating the liver (sites of neuromodulation are depicted in **Figure 2**). This technique is termed Diabetic Block Stimulation Neuromodulation (DBSN) and has shown efficacy of increasing glycemic control in animal models of T2D. The following highlights key findings of DBSN experimental results in rodent and swine models of T2D [92].

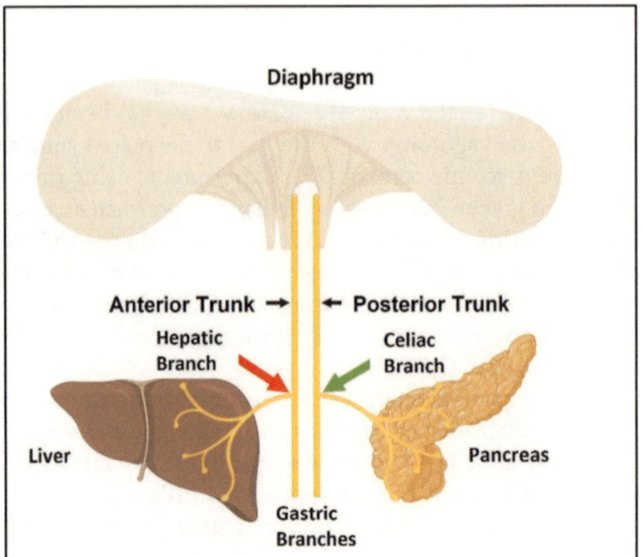

Figure 2.
The sites of dual neuromodulation involve the hepatic can celiac sub-diaphragmatic vagus nerve branches. The red arrow indicates the site of electrical neuronal blockade, and the green arrow indicates the cite of stimulation. Image adapted from Waataja (2022) [92]. Image originally created by biorender.com.

The Zucker obese (fatty) male rats (ZDF fa/fa) rat is a well-established rodent model of T2D [93–97]. Zucker rats are homozygous for a non-functional leptin receptor which causes obesity and insulin resistance [98]. Pancreatic ß-cells have also been shown to fail to respond to glucose in these rats [98]. This model was used to test our hypothesis that DBSN will reversibly increase glycemic control in an animal model of T2D.

Various VNM techniques were tested in Zucker rats. Since hepatic vagotomy has demonstrated a decrease in insulin resistance and celiac stimulation has demonstrated increased insulin release, both VNM techniques were tested during intravenous glucose tolerance tests (IVGTTs). These methods failed to increase glycemic control (**Figure 3a**).

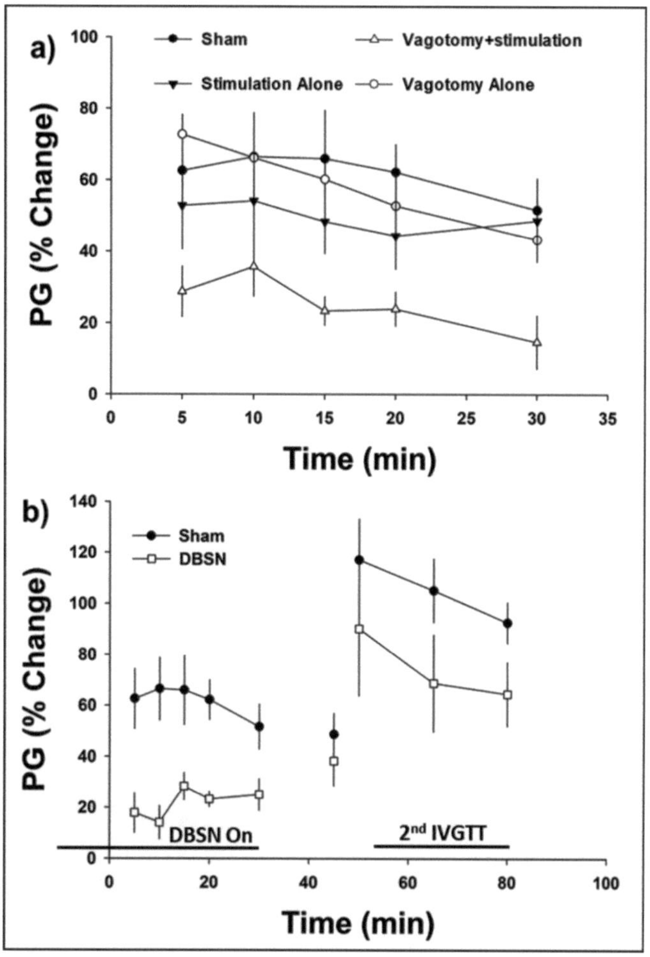

Figure 3.
As assessed by IVGTT experiments, HFAC+stimulation and DBSN increased glycemic control in the Zucker rat model of T2D compared to controls (a) Application of HFAC+stimulation increased performance on IVGTTs compared to sham, celiac branch stimulation alone or hepatic vagotomy alone. The various neuromodulation techniques were applied 1 hour before the IVGTT and during the 30 minutes course of blood sampling during the IVGTT, (b) DBSN demonstrated improved performance on IVGTTs compared to sham. DBSN was applied 15 minutes prior to the IVGTT and during 30 minutes of blood sapling after the glucose injection. As part of the DBSN experiments, a subsequent IVGTT was performed with the devices turning off to demonstrate reversibility of glucose tolerance following termination of the electrical signals. Also, to note, the IVGTT results from the HFAC +stimulation (DBSN) experiments mimicked the results from the vagotomy+stimulation suggesting that HFAC mimicked a vagotomy.

However, their coadministration (vagotomy+stimulation) demonstrated improved performance on the IVGTT compared to sham (**Figure 3a**). Despite the increased glycemic control observed with vagotomy+stimulation, the procedure would be undesirable clinically in that hepatic vagotomy is non-reversible, the body may adapt to hepatic vagotomy over time and significant unwanted side effects may be associated with hepatic vagotomy [78–81]. Therefore, in lieu of a hepatic vagotomy, a high frequency alternating current (HFAC at 5 kHz) blocking signal was applied to the hepatic branch which has shown to reversibly block conduction through the sub-diaphragmatic vagus nerve [99]. Application of HFAC to the hepatic branch with concurrent celiac branch stimulation (the DBSN procedure) reversibly increased glycemic control during IVGTTs (**Figure 3b**).

We next tested DBSN in Alloxan treated swine, a common model used in the study of diabetes [100–104]. In our preparation a titrated amount of Alloxan was delivered to the swine that partially ablated β-cells. This procedure decreased glycemic control but did not induce an insulin dependent state [92]; indicative of a T2D animal model.

DBSN was delivered to swine by an implantable ReShape Lifesciences Viking DBSN™ system (**Figure 4**) which increased glycemic control compared to sham by assessment of OGTTs (**Figure 5**). Interestingly, following the cessation of DBSN signals, a sustained decrease in FPG was observed. Over 3 OGTTs, with 2 days rest between experiments, sham conditions demonstrated a consistent FPG of 6.7 ± 0.8 mmol/l. When DBSN was first applied during an OGTT experiment blood glucose declined to 3.7 ± 0.3 mmol/l. Surprisingly, at the initiation of the subsequent DBSN experiment, FPG remained decreased at 3.8 ± 0.2 mmol/l. Following 16 days of

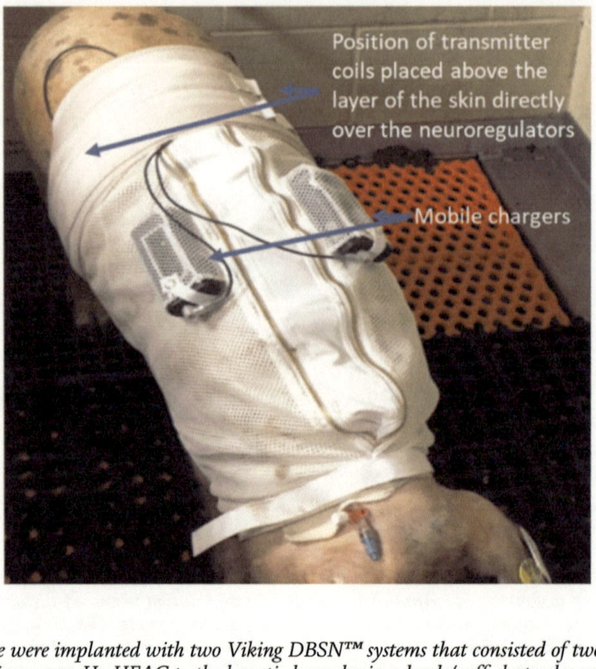

Figure 4.
Alloxan treated swine were implanted with two Viking DBSN™ systems that consisted of two implanted pulse generators, one to deliver 5000 Hz HFAC to the hepatic branch via 2 leads/cuff electrodes and the other to deliver 1 Hz stimulation to the celiac branch via a second pair of leads/cuff electrodes. Above is an implanted swine during a recharging session between glucose tolerance experiments. Two external mobile chargers were connected to two transmitter coils placed superficial to the skin and above the implanted pulse generators. The mobile chargers transmitted energy through the transmitter coils as well as stimulation parameter to be used in subsequent experiments.

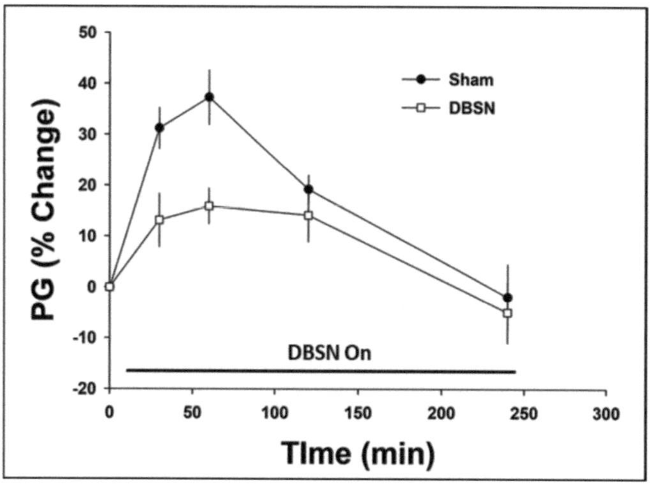

Figure 5.
Alloxan treated swine demonstrated increased glycemic control with DBSN as assessed by OGTTs. DBSN signals were applied 5 minutes after the swine consumed glucose and continued for the course of the OGTT experiment.

DBSN experiments FPG remained depressed at 3.9 ± 0.2 mmol/l and there were no signs of hypoglycemia.

We also tested if HFAC applied to the hepatic branch alone would decrease glucose following an OGTT and found that there was no effect of the single modality modulation on glycemic control.

4. Discussion

These experiments demonstrated that DBSN is an effective method of increasing glycemic control in animal models of T2D. The necessity of the addition of concurrent celiac stimulation to hepatic block was demonstrated. Possible DBSN mechanisms are discussed below.

The rational to induce a hepatic branch conduction block to increase glycemic control is fourfold: decreasing the liver's sensitivity to glucagon with increased hepatic sensitivity to insulin, increasing serum levels of GLP-1, increasing tonic release of pancreatic insulin, and decreasing insulin resistance.

It has been demonstrated that hepatic cholinergic denervation decreases the liver's sensitivity to glucagon. This was shown though a decrease in glucagon-induced hepatic glucose production following hepatic vagotomy [105]. Sub-diaphragmatic vagotomy has also demonstrated an increase in hepatic insulin sensitivity through an upregulation of hepatic insulin receptors and a stronger insulin-induced activation of AKT following vagotomy [106]. Vagotomized mice in this study also demonstrated elevated levels of GLP-1.

Hepatic vagotomy may enhance tonic pancreatic insulin release. In a study by Lee and Miller [107], ligation of the vagus hepatic branch induced increases in both arterial and portal plasma insulin concentrations. Stimulation of the cranial end of the sectioned hepatic branch suppressed this effect. Interestingly, ligation of the celiac branch abolished the hormonal changes due to the vagotomy and the stimulation. These physiological results support the hypothesis that hepatic afferents emit tonic inhibition of celiac preganglionic vagal efferents. Literature suggests a likely mechanism of this flip in activity which involves a glycemic reflexive arc with central nervous system (CNS) processes mainly located in the brain stem [108]. DBSN's effects on this reflex arc are as follows.

Many studies indicate involvement of hepatic afferent and celiac efferent activity [108] in a glycemic reflex arc with much CNS activity localized to dorsal medullary neural circuits [109]. Similar reflex arcs have been proposed in various vago-vagal loops such as those involved in cardiovascular/respiratory processes [110–116], digestive processes [117–120] and the regulation of inflammation [86]. The glycemic reflex arc is initiated with activation of glucose receptors in the portal vein leading to decreased hepatic branch axonal discharge rates [121]. Hepatic branch fibers project to the nucleus tractus solitarius (NST) in the dorsal medulla and form a glutamatergic synapse with their first order neuronal targets [116, 122]. Many of these target neurons involve the multitude of inhibitory GABAergic cells found in metabolic NTS pathways [108, 123]. These neurons project to sites of preganglionic celiac vagal efferents [109] and exert tonic inhibition [108, 124]. Decreased NTS GABAergic activity leads to a release of tonic inhibition of DMV neurons, leading to increased excitatory vagal efferent celiac tone [108]. This neural circuitry can be appreciated though increased discharge rates of celiac efferent fibers resulting from decreased hepatic afferent discharge rates during delivery of glucose to the hepatic portal vein [121, 125]. Blockade of hepatic afferent activity during delivery of DBSN would lead to high celiac discharge rates, increasing tonic pancreatic insulin release. A graphical depiction of this metabolic reflex arc is demonstrated in **Figure 6**.

It should be noted that communication between the NTS and DMV is not limited to GABAergic projections. Glutamatergic projections from the NTS to the DMV have also been described [109] and there are hypothalamic projections to the DMV [126] that may modify the reflex (**Figure 6**). However, the vast number of projects from NTS to DMV are GABAergic [108, 123, 127, 128] and localization of the majority of reflex neuronal circuitry located in the brainstem is supported by electrophysiology experiments [108, 109]. This indicates a simple reflexive GABAergic-induced activity flip between the NTS and DMV. Concurrent electrical block, or ligation, with celiac nerve stimulation was required to improve glycemic control in the Zucker rat experiments and demonstrated efficacy in Alloxan treated swine studies.

The final rational for including hepatic block in the DBSN signal is evidence that it may improve insulin resistance. Hepatic nerve ligation has been shown to decrease insulin resistance through attenuation of hepatic PPARα [129] expression as well as to the aforementioned increase expression of hepatic insulin receptors and activation of hepatic AKT [106], a principle molecule in intracellular insulin signaling pathways.

Stimulation of the celiac branch during hepatic block has importance for induction of pancreatic insulin release in the postprandial and fasting states. One limitation of blocking conduction through the hepatic branch is the disruption of the glycemic reflex arcs in the postprandial period. Nagase et al. [125] demonstrated decreased celiac efferent activity and lower insulin release during IPGTTs following hepatic branch ligation. The addition of celiac stimulation may augment these undesired decreases by increasing celiac efferent tone and inducing insulin release (many studies have demonstrated insulin release as a result of vagus nerve stimulation [130–135] with the requirement that stimulation occurs cranial to either the celiac, or accessory celiac, branching points). In the case of DBSN, the stimulation site was chosen to occur at the celiac branching point to limit possible off target stimulation effects.

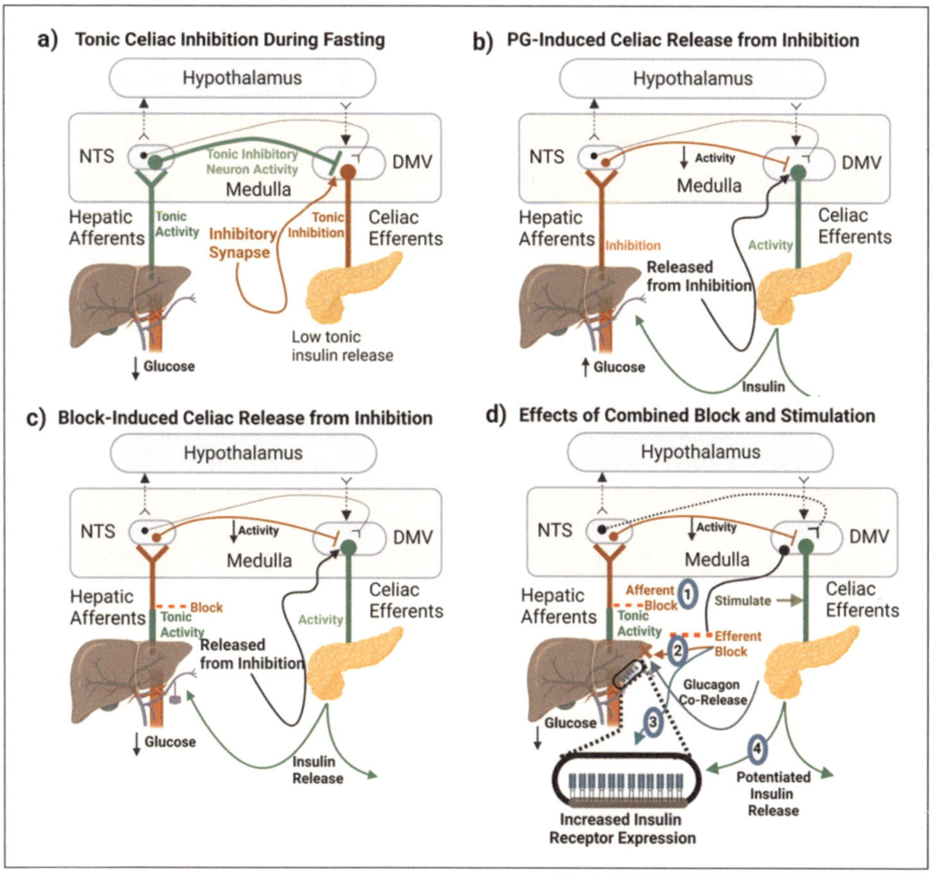

Figure 6.
Diabetes block stimulation Neuromodulation affects multiple sub-diaphragmatic vagus nerve physiological processes involved in plasma glucose regulation (a) Tonic activity of vagus nerve's hepatic branch decreases pancreatic insulin release. Research has demonstrated that increased hepatic branch activity excites inhibitory neurons in the NTS. These neurons then project to the DMV resulting in decreased celiac branch efferent activity. Decreased celiac branch activity leads to decreased tonic insulin release, (b) Increased portal vein glucose concentration induces a decrease in afferent hepatic axon activity leads to celiac axon activity upregulation. This celiac branch efferent activity has been shown to induce pancreatic insulin release, (c) Blocking conduction through the hepatic branch inhibits hepatic neuron tone and, in turn, increases celiac efferent activity, (d) the combination of celiac branch stimulation and hepatic branch blockade may influence various physiological processes leading to increased glycemic control through the following proposed mechanisms: (1) hepatic branch block decreasing hepatic tone leading to increased tonic insulin release, (2) hepatic branch block decreasing the liver's sensitivity to glucagon, (3) hepatic branch block increasing expression of hepatic insulin receptors, and (4) celiac stimulation potentiating pancreatic insulin release. Despite the greater number of proposed benefits involving block, stimulation was necessary in both our Zucker rat and alloxan treated swine experiments to achieve significantly increased glycemic control. Images created by biorender.com.

Experimental results demonstrate the necessity for adding stimulation to blocking to achieve glycemic in the Zucker rat IVGTT experiments.

In the fasting state, vagus stimulation has demonstrated increased insulin concentration in pancreatic venous and in systemic blood circulation [134]. However, a caveat to vagal stimulation-induced insulin release is the co-release of glucagon [133, 134] which can lead to increased blood glucose levels [73, 133, 134]. Decreased hepatic sensitivity to glucagon following vagus nerve hepatic branch ligation [105] suggests hepatic nerve blockade may nullify the effects of glucagon co-release. There was a decrease in FPG during our DBSN experiments.

It should be highlighted that DBSN demonstrated efficacy with signal initiation 5 minutes following the start of the OGTT. This inspires utilizing DBSN with continuous glucose monitoring (CGM) technology to deliver signals on demand, during glucose spikes. Blunting glucose spikes and decreasing blood glucose variability (GV) has positive ramifications for decreasing diabetic co-morbidities [136–141].

AI and machine learning may be utilized for DBSN parametric set optimization similar to what has been proposed in other systems such as closed-loop insulin pump technology [142]. DBSN has advantages by offering a fully implanted device and multi-site/multi-frequency modulation gives a multitude of parametric combinations to test to maximize glycemic control with AI and machine learning. CGM technology would also enable AI the to refine the timing of DBSN delivery in relation to glucose spikes by using PG prediction algorithms that are in development [143, 144].

One note of particular interest is the observation of lasting changes in FPG following cessation of DBSN signals. One possible mechanism may be due to neuronal plasticity in the glycemic reflex arc induced by applications of DBSN (**Figure 7**). Experiments demonstrate long term depression of synaptic strength between vagal afferents and their first order glutamatergic synapse in the NST [145] and DBSN signals impact activity at this synapse. Higher order plasticity is also likely to occur in hypothalamic circuits during different glycemic states [126]. Neuronal plasticity has been demonstrated in similar respiration [110–116] and digestion control neuronal circuitry [117–120].

Exploiting neuronal plasticity has importance for the design of bio-electronic VNM devices to treat T2D. As observed in synaptic long-term potentiation (LTP) and long-term depression (LTD) simulation protocols, only transient stimulation is required for long lasting changes in synaptic strength which can last for hours, days, months or greater. Utilizing neuronal plasticity may hold great importance in minimizing bio-electronic device energy expenditure aiding in the miniaturization of future devices.

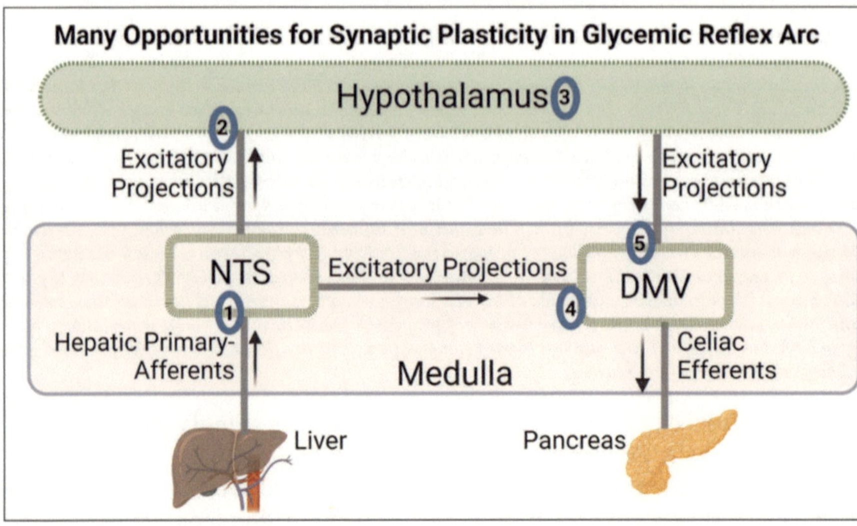

Figure 7.
Multiple plastic glutamatergic synapses in the glycemic reflex arc offers many opportunities for activity induced long lasing changes in to increase glycemic control. The above figure labels 5 of such synapses: (1) between hepatic afferents of the tractus solitarius and the NTS, (2) between projection neurons from the NTS to the hypothalamus, (3) between intra-hypothalamic nuclei, (4) between excitatory synaptic projections between the NTS and DMV, and (5) between projections from the hypothalamus to the NTS. Images created by biorender.com.

5. Conclusion

The use of vagus nerve neuromodulation to treat T2D has great potential. The localized targeting of specific organs responsible for glycemic control may decrease unwanted side effects, a one-time procedure may decrease long term costs of T2D treatments, and an implantable system decreases the need for patient compliance. A key metric to determine the effectiveness and durability of a therapy to treat T2D is the progression of diabetic medication use. First in human clinical trials involving electrical sub-diaphragmatic VNM to treat type 2 diabetics have demonstrated substantially resolved medication use [91] (results in **Table 2**). These positive results highlight the importance of continued research into VNM which holds the potential of an enhanced therapeutic experience to treat T2D.

Medication change	Percent of subjects (%)
Able to stop taking diabetes medications	22
Decrease in either the number or dosage of medications	16
No change in either the number or dosage of medications	44
Increase in either the number or dosage of medications	17
Advanced to insulin therapy	0

Table 2.
A three-year clinical trial using sub-diaphragmatic vagus nerve neuromodulation demonstrated delayed progression, and often resolution, of T2D medication requirements [91].

Author details

Jonathan Waataja[1*], Sayeed Ikramuddin[2], Dov Gal[1] and Charles Billington[3]

1 ReShape Lifesciences Inc., Irvine, CA, USA

2 Department of Surgery, University of Minnesota, Minneapolis, MN, USA

3 Minnesota Veterans' Administration Medical Center, Minneapolis, MN, USA

*Address all correspondence to: jwaataja@reshapelifesci.com; waat0006@umn.edu

References

[1] Weiss T et al. Real-world adherence and discontinuation of glucagon-like Peptide-1 receptor agonists therapy in type 2 diabetes mellitus patients in the United States. Patient Preference and Adherence. 2020; **14**:2337-2345

[2] Weiss T et al. Real-world weight change, adherence, and discontinuation among patients with type 2 diabetes initiating glucagon-like peptide-1 receptor agonists in the UK. BMJ Open Diabetes Research & Care. 2022;**10**(1)

[3] Sikirica MV et al. Reasons for discontinuation of GLP1 receptor agonists: Data from a real-world cross-sectional survey of physicians and their patients with type 2 diabetes. Diabetes, Metabolic Syndrome and Obesity: Targets and Therapy. 2017;**10**:403-412

[4] Guerci B et al. Efficacy and adherence of glucagon-like peptide-1 receptor agonist treatment in patients with type 2 diabetes mellitus in real-life settings. Diabetes & Metabolism. 2019;**45**(6): 528-535

[5] Farr AM et al. Retrospective analysis of long-term adherence to and persistence with DPP-4 inhibitors in US adults with type 2 diabetes mellitus. Advances in Therapy. 2014;**31**(12): 1287-1305

[6] Brethauer SA et al. Can diabetes be surgically cured? Long-term metabolic effects of bariatric surgery in obese patients with type 2 diabetes mellitus. Annals of Surgery. 2013;**258**(4):628-636. discussion 636-7

[7] Perez Unanua MP et al. Adherence to healthy lifestyle behaviours in patients with type 2 diabetes in Spain. Semergen. 2021;**47**(3):161-169

[8] (ACE) A.a.A.C.o.E., Clinical Practice Guidelines for Developing a Diabetes Mellitus Comprehensive Type 2 Diabetes Management Algorithm. 2020. Available from: https://www.aace.com/pdfs/diabetes/algorithm-exec-summary.pdf

[9] Chaudhury A et al. Clinical review of antidiabetic drugs: Implications for type 2 diabetes mellitus management. Frontiers in Endocrinology (Lausanne). 2017;**8**:6

[10] Brod M et al. Psychological insulin resistance: Patient beliefs and implications for diabetes management. Quality of Life Research. 2009;**18**(1): 23-32

[11] Nam S et al. Factors associated with psychological insulin resistance in individuals with type 2 diabetes. Diabetes Care. 2010;**33**(8):1747-1749

[12] Harris Interactive. Injection Impact Survey-Executive Summary. Rochester, NY, USA: Harris Interactive; 2008

[13] Peragallo-Dittko V. Removing barriers to insulin therapy. The Diabetes Educator. 2007;**33**(Suppl 3):60S-65S

[14] Rubin RR et al. Barriers to insulin injection therapy: Patient and health care provider perspectives. The Diabetes Educator. 2009;**35**(6):1014-1022

[15] Zambanini A et al. Injection related anxiety in insulin-treated diabetes. Diabetes Research and Clinical Practice. 1999;**46**(3):239-246

[16] Stotland NL. Overcoming psychological barriers in insulin therapy. Insulin. 2006;**1**:38-45

[17] Aminian A et al. Late relapse of diabetes after bariatric surgery: Not rare, but not a failure. Diabetes Care. 2020; **43**(3):534-540

[18] Eldar S et al. Bariatric surgery for treatment of obesity. International Journal of Obesity. 2011;**35**(Suppl 3): S16-S21

[19] Mahawar KK et al. Patient perspectives on adherence with micronutrient supplementation after bariatric surgery. Obesity Surgery. 2019; **29**(5):1551-1556

[20] Trujillo JM, Nuffer W, Smith BA. GLP-1 receptor agonists: An updated review of head-to-head clinical studies. Therapeutic Advances in Endocrinology and Metabolism. 2021;**12**: 2042018821997320

[21] Jensterle M et al. Efficacy of GLP-1 RA approved for weight Management in Patients with or without diabetes: A narrative review. Advances in Therapy. 2022;**39**(6):2452-2467

[22] Divino V et al. GLP-1 RA treatment and dosing patterns among type 2 diabetes patients in six countries: A retrospective analysis of pharmacy claims data. Diabetes Therapy. 2019; **10**(3):1067-1088

[23] Johnston SS et al. Retrospective study of adherence to glucagon-like peptide-1 receptor agonist therapy in patients with type 2 diabetes mellitus in the United States. Advances in Therapy. 2014;**31**(11):1119-1133

[24] Uzoigwe C et al. Semaglutide once-weekly persistence and adherence versus other GLP-1 RAs in patients with type 2 diabetes in a US real-world setting. Diabetes Therapy. 2021;**12**(5):1475-1489

[25] Nichols GA, Hillier TA, Brown JB. Progression from newly acquired impaired fasting glusose to type 2 diabetes. Diabetes Care. 2007;**30**(2): 228-233

[26] Alshehri KA et al. Type 2 diabetic patients adherence towards their medications. Cureus. 2020;**12**(2):e6932

[27] Freckmann G et al. Insulin pump therapy for patients with type 2 diabetes mellitus: Evidence, current barriers, and new technologies. Journal of Diabetes Science and Technology. 2021;**15**(4): 901-915

[28] Karges B et al. Association of Insulin Pump Therapy vs insulin injection therapy with severe hypoglycemia, ketoacidosis, and glycemic control among children, adolescents, and young adults with type 1 diabetes. JAMA. 2017; **318**(14):1358-1366

[29] Bosi E et al. Efficacy and safety of suspend-before-low insulin pump technology in hypoglycaemia-prone adults with type 1 diabetes (SMILE): An open-label randomised controlled trial. The Lancet Diabetes and Endocrinology. 2019;7(6):462-472

[30] Kanapka LG et al. Extended use of the control-IQ closed-loop control system in children with type 1 diabetes. Diabetes Care. 2021;**44**(2):473-478

[31] UK Prospective Diabetes Study (UKPDS) Group. Intensive blood-glucose control with sulphonylureas or insulin compared with conventional treatment and risk of complications in patients with type 2 diabetes (UKPDS 33). Lancet. 1998;**352**(9131):837-853

[32] Miller RG et al. Hemoglobin A1c level and cardiovascular disease incidence in persons with type 1 diabetes: An application of joint

modeling of longitudinal and time-to-event data in the Pittsburgh epidemiology of diabetes complications study. American Journal of Epidemiology. 2018;**187**(7):1520-1529

[33] El-Khatib FH et al. Home use of a bihormonal bionic pancreas versus insulin pump therapy in adults with type 1 diabetes: A multicentre randomised crossover trial. Lancet. 2017;**389**(10067): 369-380

[34] van Baar ACG et al. Durable metabolic improvements 2 years after duodenal mucosal resurfacing (DMR) in patients with type 2 diabetes (REVITA-1 study). Diabetes Research and Clinical Practice. 2022;**184**:109194

[35] Rajagopalan H et al. Endoscopic duodenal mucosal resurfacing for the treatment of type 2 diabetes: 6-month interim analysis from the first-in-human proof-of-concept study. Diabetes Care. 2016;**39**(12):2254-2261

[36] Rogalski P et al. Endoscopic management of gastrointestinal perforations, leaks and fistulas. World Journal of Gastroenterology. 2015; **21**(37):10542-10552

[37] Yue Z, Zhang L, Li C, Chen Y, Tai Y, Shen Y, et al. Advances and potential of gene therapy for type 2 diabetes mellitus. Biotechnology & Biotechnological Equipment. 2019;**33**(1):1150-1157

[38] Eksi YE et al. Genome engineering and disease modeling via programmable nucleases for insulin gene therapy; promises of CRISPR/Cas9 technology. World Journal of Stem Cells. 2021;**13**(6): 485-502

[39] Ji C, Guo X. The clinical potential of circulating microRNAs in obesity. Nature Reviews. Endocrinology. 2019; **15**(12):731-743

[40] Fontaine AK et al. Optogenetic stimulation of cholinergic fibers for the modulation of insulin and glycemia. Scientific Reports. 2021;**11**(1):3670

[41] Meister J et al. Chemogenetic approaches to identify metabolically important GPCR signaling pathways: Therapeutic implications. Journal of Neurochemistry. 2021;**158**(3):603-620

[42] Guettier JM et al. A chemical-genetic approach to study G protein regulation of beta cell function in vivo. Proceedings of the National Academy of Sciences of the United States of America. 2009; **106**(45):19197-19202

[43] Zhu L et al. Intra-islet glucagon signaling is critical for maintaining glucose homeostasis. JCI Insight. 2019;**5** (10)

[44] Lewis JE et al. Selective stimulation of colonic L cells improves metabolic outcomes in mice. Diabetologia. 2020; **63**(7):1396-1407

[45] Wang L et al. Selective activation of G(s) signaling in adipocytes causes striking metabolic improvements in mice. Molecular Metabolism. 2019;**27**: 83-91

[46] Akhmedov D et al. Gs-DREADD Knock-In mice for tissue-specific, temporal stimulation of cyclic AMP signaling. Molecular and Cellular Biology. 2017;**37**(9)

[47] Bone DBJ et al. Skeletal muscle-specific activation of G(q) signaling maintains glucose homeostasis. Diabetes. 2019;**68**(6):1341-1352

[48] Uner AG et al. Role of POMC and AgRP neuronal activities on glycaemia in mice. Scientific Reports. 2019;**9**(1): 13068

[49] Delhove J et al. Public acceptability of gene therapy and gene editing for human use: A systematic review. Human Gene Therapy. 2020;**31**(1-2):20-46

[50] Mendell JR et al. Current clinical applications of In vivo gene therapy with AAVs. Molecular Therapy. 2021;**29**(2): 464-488

[51] Chand DH et al. Thrombotic microangiopathy following onasemnogene abeparvovec for spinal muscular atrophy: A case series. The Journal of Pediatrics. 2021;**231**:265-268

[52] Ertl HCJ. Immunogenicity and toxicity of AAV gene therapy. Frontiers in Immunology. 2022;**13**:975803

[53] Lee BY et al. Ultra-low microcurrent in the management of diabetes mellitus, hypertension and chronic wounds: Report of twelve cases and discussion of mechanism of action. International Journal of Medical Sciences. 2009;**7**(1): 29-35

[54] Catalogna M et al. Effect of peripheral electrical stimulation (PES) on nocturnal blood glucose in type 2 diabetes: A randomized crossover pilot study. PLoS One. 2016;**11**(12):e0168805

[55] Bao SC et al. Peripheral focused ultrasound stimulation and its applications: From therapeutics to human-computer interaction. Frontiers in Neuroscience. 2023;**17**:1115946

[56] Cotero V et al. Stimulation of the hepatoportal nerve plexus with focused ultrasound restores glucose homoeostasis in diabetic mice, rats and swine. Nature Biomedical Engineering. 2022;**6**(6): 683-705

[57] Pashaei V et al. Flexible body-conformal ultrasound patches for image-guided neuromodulation. IEEE Transactions on Biomedical Circuits and Systems. 2020;**14**(2):305-318

[58] Khawaled R et al. Intestinal electrical stimulation decreases postprandial blood glucose levels in rats. Surgery for Obesity and Related Diseases. 2009;**5**(6):692-697

[59] Aberle J et al. Duodenal electric stimulation: Results of a first-in-man study. Obesity Surgery. 2016;**26**(2): 369-375

[60] Chen J et al. Hepatic electrical stimulation reduces blood glucose in diabetic rats. Neurogastroenterology and Motility. 2010;**22**(10):1109-e286

[61] Sacramento JF et al. Bioelectronic modulation of carotid sinus nerve activity in the rat: A potential therapeutic approach for type 2 diabetes. Diabetologia. 2018;**61**(3):700-710

[62] Mouradian GC, Forster HV, Hodges MR. Acute and chronic effects of carotid body denervation on ventilation and chemoreflexes in three rat strains. The Journal of Physiology. 2012;**590**(14): 3335-3347

[63] Bermejo P et al. Innervation of the human cavum conchae and Auditory Canal: Anatomical basis for transcutaneous auricular nerve stimulation. BioMed Research International. 2017;**2017**:7830919

[64] Redgrave J et al. Safety and tolerability of transcutaneous Vagus nerve stimulation in humans; a systematic review. Brain Stimulation. 2018;**11**(6):1225-1238

[65] Badran BW et al. Short trains of transcutaneous auricular vagus nerve stimulation (taVNS) have parameter-specific effects on heart rate. Brain Stimulation. 2018;**11**(4):699-708

[66] Forte G et al. Ear your heart: Transcutaneous auricular vagus nerve stimulation on heart rate variability in healthy young participants. PeerJ. 2022; **10**:e14447

[67] Frangos E, Ellrich J, Komisaruk BR. Non-invasive access to the Vagus nerve central projections via electrical stimulation of the external ear: fMRI evidence in humans. Brain Stimulation. 2015;**8**(3):624-636

[68] He JK et al. Transcutaneous auricular Vagus nerve stimulation modulates the prefrontal cortex in chronic insomnia patients: fMRI study in the first session. Frontiers in Neurology. 2022;**13**:827749

[69] Li S et al. Therapeutic effect of vagus nerve stimulation on depressive-like behavior, hyperglycemia and insulin receptor expression in Zucker fatty rats. PLoS One. 2014;**9**(11):e112066

[70] Kozorosky EM et al. Transcutaneous auricular vagus nerve stimulation augments postprandial inhibition of ghrelin. Physiological Reports. 2022; **10**(8):e15253

[71] Huang F et al. Effect of transcutaneous auricular vagus nerve stimulation on impaired glucose tolerance: A pilot randomized study. BMC Complementary and Alternative Medicine. 2014;**14**:203

[72] Vosseler A et al. No modulation of postprandial metabolism by transcutaneous auricular vagus nerve stimulation: A cross-over study in 15 healthy men. Scientific Reports. 2020; **10**(1):20466

[73] Meyers EE et al. Contrasting effects of afferent and efferent vagal nerve stimulation on insulin secretion and blood glucose regulation. Physiological Reports. 2016;**4**(4)

[74] Stauss HM et al. Cervical vagal nerve stimulation impairs glucose tolerance and suppresses insulin release in conscious rats. Physiological Reports. 2018;**6**(24):e13953

[75] Payne SC et al. Blood glucose modulation and safety of efferent vagus nerve stimulation in a type 2 diabetic rat model. Physiological Reports. 2022; **10**(8):e15257

[76] Yin J et al. Vagal nerve stimulation for glycemic control in a rodent model of type 2 diabetes. Obesity Surgery. 2019; **29**(9):2869-2877

[77] Kraft G et al. Sympathetic denervation of the common hepatic artery lessens glucose intolerance in the fat- and fructose-fed dog. Diabetes. 2019;**68**(6):1143-1155

[78] Hiramoto T et al. Protective role of the hepatic Vagus nerve against liver metastasis in mice. Neuroimmuno-modulation;**24**(6):341-347

[79] Donovan CM, Watts AG. Peripheral and central glucose sensing in hypoglycemic detection. Physiology (Bethesda);**29**(5):314-324

[80] Kiba T. The role of the autonomic nervous system in liver regeneration and apoptosis—Recent developments. Digestion. 2002;**66**(2): 79-88

[81] Okazaki H et al. Modulation of insulin secretion by hepatic vagotomy in cirrhotic rats. Physiology & Behavior. 1993;**53**(3):521-525

[82] Wroblewski A et al. Dysregulation of inflammation, oxidative stress, and glucose metabolism-related genes and miRNAs in visceral adipose tissue of women with type 2 diabetes mellitus.

Medical Science Monitor. 2023;**29**: e939299

[83] Dludla PV et al. Pancreatic beta-cell dysfunction in type 2 diabetes: Implications of inflammation and oxidative stress. World Journal of Diabetes. 2023;**14**(3):130-146

[84] Lempesis IG, Georgakopoulou VE. Physiopathological mechanisms related to inflammation in obesity and type 2 diabetes mellitus. World Journal of Experimental Medicine. 2023;**13**(3):7-16

[85] Tsalamandris S et al. The role of inflammation in diabetes: Current concepts and future perspectives. European Cardiology Review. 2019; **14**(1):50-59

[86] Bonaz B, Sinniger V, Pellissier S. Anti-inflammatory properties of the vagus nerve: Potential therapeutic implications of vagus nerve stimulation. The Journal of Physiology. 2016; **594**(20):5781-5790

[87] Caravaca AS et al. Vagus nerve stimulation promotes resolution of inflammation by a mechanism that involves Alox15 and requires the alpha7nAChR subunit. Proceedings of the National Academy of Sciences of the United States of America. 2022;**119**(22): e2023285119

[88] Bosmans G et al. Vagus nerve stimulation dampens intestinal inflammation in a murine model of experimental food allergy. Allergy. 2019; **74**(9):1748-1759

[89] Drewes AM et al. Short-term transcutaneous non-invasive vagus nerve stimulation may reduce disease activity and pro-inflammatory cytokines in rheumatoid arthritis: Results of a pilot study. Scandinavian Journal of Rheumatology. 2021;**50**(1):20-27

[90] Sorski L, Gidron Y. The vagal nerve, inflammation, and diabetes-a holy triangle. Cell. 2023;**12**(12)

[91] Herrera MF. Vagal nerve block for improvements in glycemic control in obese patients with type 2 diabetes mellitus: Three-year results of the VBLOC DM2 study. Journal of Diabetes and Obesity. 2017;**4**(1)

[92] Waataja JJ et al. Use of a bio-electronic device comprising of targeted dual neuromodulation of the hepatic and celiac vagal branches demonstrated enhanced glycemic control in a type 2 diabetic rat model as well as in an Alloxan treated swine model. Frontiers in Neuroscience. 2022;**16**:1005932

[93] Friedman JE et al. Altered expression of muscle glucose transporter GLUT-4 in diabetic fatty Zucker rats (ZDF/Drt-fa). The American Journal of Physiology. 1991;**261**(6 Pt 1):E782-E788

[94] Sparks JD et al. Lipoprotein alterations in 10- and 20-week-old Zucker diabetic fatty rats: Hyperinsulinemic versus insulinopenic hyperglycemia. Metabolism. 1998; **47**(11):1315-1324

[95] Corsetti JP et al. Effect of dietary fat on the development of non-insulin dependent diabetes mellitus in obese zucker diabetic fatty male and female rats. Atherosclerosis. 2000;**148**(2): 231-241

[96] Schmidt RE et al. Analysis of the zucker diabetic fatty (ZDF) type 2 diabetic rat model suggests a neurotrophic role for insulin/IGF-I in diabetic autonomic neuropathy. The American Journal of Pathology. 2003; **163**(1):21-28

[97] Reinwald S et al. Skeletal changes associated with the onset of type 2

diabetes in the ZDF and ZDSD rodent models. American Journal of Physiology. Endocrinology and Metabolism. 2009; **296**(4):E765-E774

[98] Chen D, Wang MW. Development and application of rodent models for type 2 diabetes. Diabetes, Obesity & Metabolism. 2005;7(4):307-317

[99] Waataja JJ, Tweden KS, Honda CN. Effects of high-frequency alternating current on axonal conduction through the vagus nerve. Journal of Neural Engineering. 2011;**8**(5):056013

[100] Boullion RD et al. Porcine model of diabetic dyslipidemia: Insulin and feed algorithms for mimicking diabetes mellitus in humans. Comparative Medicine. 2003;**53**(1):42-52

[101] Zhao G et al. Reduced coronary NO production in conscious dogs after the development of alloxan-induced diabetes. The American Journal of Physiology. 1999;**277**(1):H268-H278

[102] Dolkart RE, Torok EE, Wright PH. Hepatic enzyme activities in rats made diabetic with alloxan and with Guinea pig anti-insulin serum. Diabetes. 1964; **13**:78-82

[103] Lenzen S, Panten U. Alloxan: History and mechanism of action. Diabetologia. 1988;**31**(6):337-342

[104] Badin JK et al. Effect of age on diabetogenicity of alloxan in ossabaw miniature swine. Comparative Medicine. 2019;**69**(2):114-122

[105] Xue C et al. Isolated hepatic cholinergic denervation impairs glucose and glycogen metabolism. The Journal of Surgical Research. 2000;**90**(1):19-25

[106] Khound R et al. GLP-1 elicits an intrinsic gut-liver metabolic signal to ameliorate diet-induced VLDL overproduction and insulin resistance. Arteriosclerosis, Thrombosis, and Vascular Biology. 2017;**37**(12):2252-2259

[107] Lee KC, Miller RE. The hepatic vagus nerve and the neural regulation of insulin secretion. Endocrinology. 1985; **117**(1):307-314

[108] Pitra S, Smith BN. Musings on the wanderer: What's new in our understanding of vago-vagal reflexes? VI. Central vagal circuits that control glucose metabolism. American Journal of Physiology. Gastrointestinal and Liver Physiology. 2021;**320**(2):G175-G182

[109] Davis SF et al. Excitatory and inhibitory local circuit input to the rat dorsal motor nucleus of the vagus originating from the nucleus tractus solitarius. Brain Research. 2004;**1017**(1–2):208-217

[110] Andresen MC, Yang M. Dynamics of sensory afferent synaptic transmission in aortic baroreceptor regions on nucleus tractus solitarius. Journal of Neurophysiology. 1995;**74**(4):1518-1528

[111] Butcher JW, Paton JF. K+ channel blockade in the NTS alters efficacy of two cardiorespiratory reflexes in vivo. The American Journal of Physiology. 1998;**274**(3):R677-R685

[112] Chan RK, Peto CA, Sawchenko PE. Fine structure and plasticity of barosensitive neurons in the nucleus of solitary tract. The Journal of Comparative Neurology. 2000;**422**(3): 338-351

[113] Chen CY et al. Neuroplasticity in nucleus tractus solitarius neurons after episodic ozone exposure in infant primates. Journal of Applied Physiology (1985). 2003;**94**(2):819-827

[114] Chen CY et al. Extended allergen exposure in asthmatic monkeys induces neuroplasticity in nucleus tractus solitarius. The Journal of Allergy and Clinical Immunology. 2001;**108**(4): 557-562

[115] Liu Z, Chen CY, Bonham AC. Metabotropic glutamate receptors depress vagal and aortic baroreceptor signal transmission in the NTS. The American Journal of Physiology. 1998; **275**(5):H1682-H1694

[116] Mifflin SW. Short-term potentiation of carotid sinus nerve inputs to neurons in the nucleus of the solitary tract. Respiration Physiology. 1997;**110**(2–3):229-236

[117] Baptista V et al. Cholecystokinin octapeptide increases spontaneous glutamatergic synaptic transmission to neurons of the nucleus tractus solitarius centralis. Journal of Neurophysiology. 2005;**94**(4):2763-2771

[118] Appleyard SM et al. Proopiomelanocortin neurons in nucleus tractus solitarius are activated by visceral afferents: Regulation by cholecystokinin and opioids. The Journal of Neuroscience. 2005;**25**(14):3578-3585

[119] Hayes MR, Covasa M. Dorsal hindbrain 5-HT3 receptors participate in control of meal size and mediate CCK-induced satiation. Brain Research. 2006; **1103**(1):99-107

[120] Wan S et al. Presynaptic melanocortin-4 receptors on vagal afferent fibers modulate the excitability of rat nucleus tractus solitarius neurons. The Journal of Neuroscience. 2008; **28**(19):4957-4966

[121] Niijima A. Glucose-sensitive afferent nerve fibres in the hepatic branch of the vagus nerve in the Guinea-pig. The Journal of Physiology. 1982;**332**: 315-323

[122] Adachi A. Projection of the hepatic vagal nerve in the medulla oblongata. Journal of the Autonomic Nervous System. 1984;**10**(3–4):287-293

[123] Browning KN, Travagli RA. Plasticity of vagal brainstem circuits in the control of gastric function. Neurogastroenterology and Motility. 2010;**22**(11):1154-1163

[124] Gao H, Smith BN. Tonic GABAA receptor-mediated inhibition in the rat dorsal motor nucleus of the vagus. Journal of Neurophysiology. 2010; **103**(2):904-914

[125] Nagase H et al. Hepatic glucose-sensitive unit regulation of glucose-induced insulin secretion in rats. Physiology & Behavior. 1993;**53**(1): 139-143

[126] Guemes A, Georgiou P. Review of the role of the nervous system in glucose homoeostasis and future perspectives towards the management of diabetes. Bioelectronic Medicine. 2018;**4**:9

[127] Affleck VS, Coote JH, Pyner S. The projection and synaptic organisation of NTS afferent connections with presympathetic neurons, GABA and nNOS neurons in the paraventricular nucleus of the hypothalamus. Neuroscience. 2012;**219**(1–2):48-61

[128] Babic T, Browning KN, Travagli RA. Differential organization of excitatory and inhibitory synapses within the rat dorsal vagal complex. American Journal of Physiology. Gastrointestinal and Liver Physiology. 2011;**300**(1):G21-G32

[129] Bernal-Mizrachi C et al. An afferent vagal nerve pathway links hepatic

PPARalpha activation to glucocorticoid-induced insulin resistance and hypertension. Cell Metabolism. 2007; **5**(2):91-102

[130] Daniel PM, Henderson JR. The effect of vagal stimulation on plasma insulin and glucose levels in the baboon. The Journal of Physiology. 1967;**192**(2): 317-327

[131] Frohman LA, Ezdinli EZ, Javid R. Effect of vagotomy and vagal stimulation on insulin secretion. Diabetes. 1967;**16**(7):443-448

[132] Kaneto A, Kosaka K, Nakao K. Effects of stimulation of the vagus nerve on insulin secretion. Endocrinology. 1967;**80**(3):530-536

[133] Adrian TE, Bloom SR, Edwards AV. Neuroendocrine responses to stimulation of the vagus nerves in bursts in conscious calves. The Journal of Physiology. 1983; **344**:25-35

[134] Ahren B, Taborsky GJ Jr. The mechanism of vagal nerve stimulation of glucagon and insulin secretion in the dog. Endocrinology. 1986;**118**(4): 1551-1557

[135] Berthoud HR et al. Evidence for a role of the gastric, coeliac and hepatic branches in vagally stimulated insulin secretion in the rat. Journal of the Autonomic Nervous System. 1983;**7**(2):97-110

[136] Hirakawa Y et al. Impact of visit-to-visit glycemic variability on the risks of macrovascular and microvascular events and all-cause mortality in type 2 diabetes: The ADVANCE trial. Diabetes Care. 2014;**37**(8):2359-2365

[137] Zinman B et al. Day-to-day fasting glycaemic variability in DEVOTE: Associations with severe hypoglycaemia and cardiovascular outcomes (DEVOTE 2). Diabetologia. 2018;**61**(1): 48-57

[138] Takahashi H et al. Glycemic variability determined with a continuous glucose monitoring system can predict prognosis after acute coronary syndrome. Cardiovascular Diabetology. 2018;**17**(1):116

[139] Gerbaud E et al. Glycemic variability is a powerful independent predictive factor of midterm major adverse cardiac events in patients with diabetes with acute coronary syndrome. Diabetes Care. 2019;**42**(4):674-681

[140] Zhou JJ et al. Glycemic variation and cardiovascular risk in the veterans affairs diabetes trial. Diabetes Care. 2018;**41**(10):2187-2194

[141] Martinez M et al. Glycemic variability and cardiovascular disease in patients with type 2 diabetes. BMJ Open Diabetes Research & Care. 2021;**9**(1)

[142] Jin X, Cai A, Xu T, Zhang X. Artificial intelligence biosensors for continuous glucose monitoring. Interdisciplinart Materials. 2022;**2**: 209-307

[143] Marcus Y et al. Improving blood glucose level predictability using machine learning. Diabetes/Metabolism Research and Reviews. 2020;**36**(8):e3348

[144] Perez-Gandia C et al. Artificial neural network algorithm for online glucose prediction from continuous glucose monitoring. Diabetes Technology & Therapeutics. 2010;**12**(1):81-88

[145] Zhou Z, Champagnat J, Poon CS. Phasic and long-term depression in brainstem nucleus tractus solitarius neurons: Differing roles of AMPA receptor desensitization. The Journal of Neuroscience. 1997;**17**(14):5349-5356

Section 4

Case Reports and Real Global Therapeutic Effectiveness

Chapter 14

Pathophysiology-Oriented Treatment of Type 2 Diabetes: 10 Case Reports

Noemi Nováková, Martin Nezval and Viktória Molnárová

Abstract

The effects of pathophysiology-oriented treatment using metformin and/or insulin analogs and/or incretin GLP-1 receptor agonists and/or dapagliflozin and/or pioglitazone were individually evaluated in ten people with type 2 diabetes (T2D) at an urban diabetes center. Some of them had microangiopathy and/or neuropathy and/or nephropathy. The observation period ranged from 2 to 12 years. Treatment efficiency was estimated according to changes in HbA_{1c}, body mass, insulin dose per day, blood pressure, lipoproteins, albuminuria, estimated glomerular filtration rate (eGFR), and general clinical condition. The results suggest that adequate education, early implementation of self-monitoring of capillary plasma glucose (SMPG)/continuous glucose monitoring (CGM), and long-term carefully selected/combined medication (see above) appears to result in improved metabolic control and enhanced quality of life for people with T2D.

Keywords: type 2 diabetes, insulin, incretins, continuous glucose monitoring (CGM), case report, metformin, dapagliflozin

1. Introduction

Type 2 diabetes (T2D) is the predominant form of diabetes, accounting for approximately 90–95% of all diabetes cases. A distinctive feature of type 2 diabetes is that many individuals may not require insulin treatment for their survival, particularly in the early stages and often throughout their lives [1]. The establishment of therapeutic goals encompasses individual preferences, coexisting medical conditions, age, duration of diabetes, life expectancy, quality of life, psychosocial circumstances, and the individual's capabilities [2, 3].

The rising prevalence of T2D has led to the emergence of numerous novel approaches aimed at safely managing hyperglycemia. Nevertheless, individual responses to treatment modalities may vary due to the diverse and complex pathophysiology underlying T2D. Correct understanding and addressing this heterogeneity may influence the choice of therapeutic approach [4]. As per the guidelines provided by the ADA/EASD, older adults who are in good health with minimal coexisting chronic conditions and intact cognitive and functional abilities should aim for lower glycemic targets, typically with an HbA_{1c} level of <53–58 mmol/mol. For older adults facing multiple chronic illnesses, cognitive impairment, or functional dependence, goals with HbA_{1c} < 64 mmol/mol are recommended [5–7].

Prompt initiation of pharmacotherapy is recommended at the time when T2D is diagnosed unless contraindications exist. Metformin or other agents, including combination therapy, should be considered. Agents that reduce cardiorenal risk should be included in the treatment regimen for adults with a high risk of atherosclerotic cardiovascular disease (ASCVD), heart failure (HF), and/or chronic kidney disease (CKD). These involve consideration of agents such as dulaglutide, semaglutide (SEMA), insulin, and gliflozins should be considered [3, 8].

In people with T2D and obesity, the medication's impact on body mass should be considered [9, 10].

In addition to pharmacological therapy, people with T2D should adopt their physical activity and well-balanced diet [2].

In this chapter, we present ten case reports that demonstrate the application of pathophysiology-oriented treatment strategies in individuals with T2D [11]. These case reports were created at an urban diabetes center. The observation period ranged from 2 to 12 years. The effectiveness of the pathophysiology-oriented treatment was evaluated based on various parameters, including changes in HbA_{1c}, body mass, amount of insulin per day, and general clinical condition. Additionally, the importance of adequate education and early implementation of self-monitoring of capillary plasma glucose (SMPG) or continuous glucose monitoring (CGM) is plays a significant role [12].

2. Case reports

This collection of case reports aims to demonstrate the diverse challenges and various aspects of T2D treatment. We have selected six men and four women. Their age varies between 52 and 78 years, and the duration of diabetes from 2 years to 27 years. Case reports were ordered according to the duration of T2D. The overview of these ten cases is in **Table 1**.

Each case report serves a specific focus, presenting the unique reason for its inclusion in this collection. They offer a glimpse into the medical history and pharmacological background of each individual, shedding light on their specific challenges and treatment journeys, and future plans marked as looking ahead. The case reports are complemented by graphical representations of absolute values, illustrating the progress of HbA_{1c} (glycated hemoglobin), BMI (body mass index), and INS/d (insulin dosage) over time.

Relative values are depicted in a graph where 100% corresponds to the highest physiological range for HbA_{1c}, BMI, and INS/d. This allows for a better understanding of each individual's progress in relation to the optimal target range.

No	Name	Age (years)	T2D (years)	Study period (years)	BM start (kg)	BM end (kg)	HbA_{1c} start (mmol/mol)	HbA_{1c} end (mmol/mol)
1	Amy	78	27	9	82	79	84	53
2	Benjamin	60	25	11	123	103	81	59
3	Connor	72	24	12	113	99	76	85

No	Name	Age (years)	T2D (years)	Study period (years)	BM start (kg)	BM end (kg)	HbA_{1c} start (mmol/mol)	HbA_{1c} end (mmol/mol)
4	David	72	24	3	116	98	60	51
5	Emma	65	23	12	108	90	88	83
6	Fatima	73	16	11	83	79	65	52
7	Gerry	71	16	5	106	107	82	45
8	Henry	52	5	5	111	102	66	48
9	Irene	65	2	2	112	105	110	58
10	Jacob	52	2	2	130	112	129	37

Table 1.
Overview of the individual case reports, ordered according to the duration of T2D.

2.1 Case report Amy

Focus: Crucial role of the family in ensuring medication intake adherence of IDegLira and DAPA by the subject with T2D and progressing cognitive impairment [13].

History: Amy, a 78-year-old woman, was diagnosed with T2D in 1995 when she was 51 years of age. Despite attempts to control her diabetes with an MDI regimen, her HbA_{1c} remained persistently high, around 80 mmol/mol, coupled with fluctuating BM, and polyneuropathy.

In 2014, Amy was referred to our center. MDI was replaced with CSII and introduced to the fixed combination of dapagliflozin and metformin (DAPA/MET) in 2016. This was followed by the replacement of her insulin pump with a combination of degludec and liraglutide (IDegLira) in June 2018. However, the unrecognized progression of the cognitive impairment led to difficulties in keeping up with the new treatment, resulting in worsening glycemic control.

To further investigate the issue, Amy was hospitalized (H1), which led to a decrease in HbA_{1c} from 90 to 70. Her GP refused home care service due to Amy's ability to administer medication herself; therefore, family members were asked to ensure Amy adheres to her medication schedule, and they agreed.

Despite these precautions, Amy's glycemic control rapidly deteriorated during outpatient care. As Amy lives alone and was usually only supervised remotely through phone calls from her family, her intellectual dysfunction interfered with her ability to accurately report her medication adherence, leading to an alarming HbA_{1c} of 131 mmol/mol by December 2020.

Addressing this, the healthcare team implemented a more comprehensive approach. Amy was admitted to the hospital for rehabilitation including diabetes control (H2, H3, and H4), see **Figure 1**. During her hospital stay, her family members were educated about her condition and the importance of their active involvement in her care. A home care service was also arranged to ensure regular monitoring and assistance. With these interventions, Amy's HbA_{1c} dropped to 51 mmol/mol in May 2023; see **Figures 2** and **3** for data values.

Looking ahead: Regular check-ups at in-home care senior house.

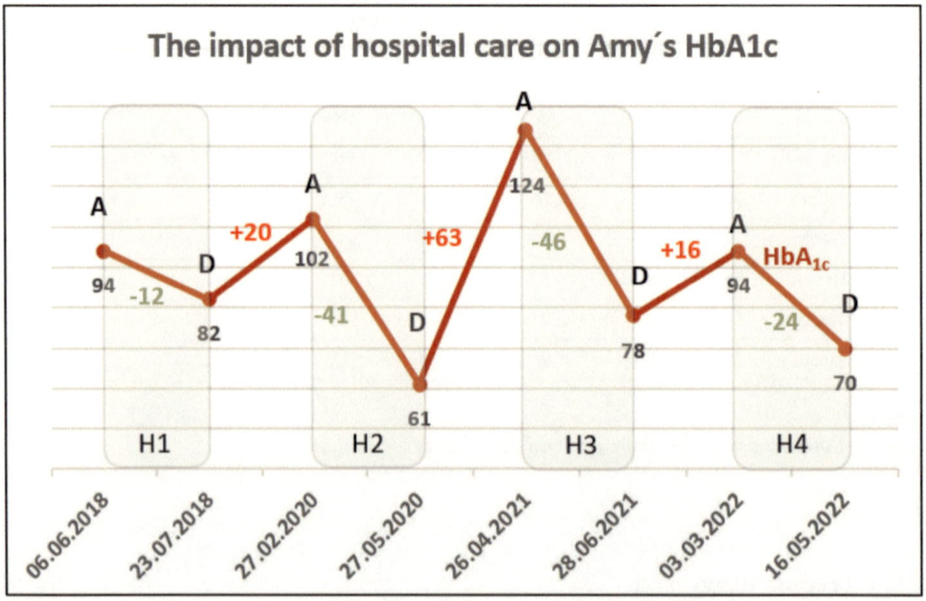

Figure 1.
Four hospitalizations (H1-H4) marked as four green boxes, with marked admission (A) values of HbA1c and dismission (D) values of HbA1c. Green and red numbers indicate the change between each measurement.

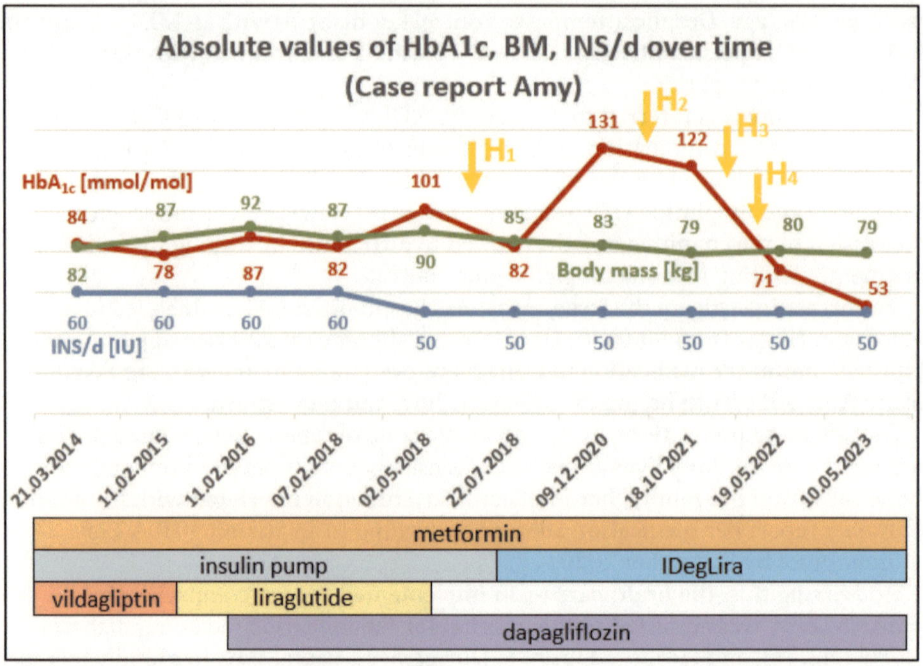

Figure 2.
*Absolute values of HbA_{1c}, BM, and INS/d over 9 years period showing that the first hospitalization (H1) led to a decrease in HbA_{1c}, yet due to poorly managed self-care and inability to adhere to the prescribed medication, the HbA_{1c} value escalated to 131 mmol/mol. Following further hospitalizations, coupled with family support and home care, a noticeable decrease in HbA_{1c} was achieved (see also **Figure 1**). Insulin usage was constant, with 60 IU/d, and then, decreased to 50 IU/d.*

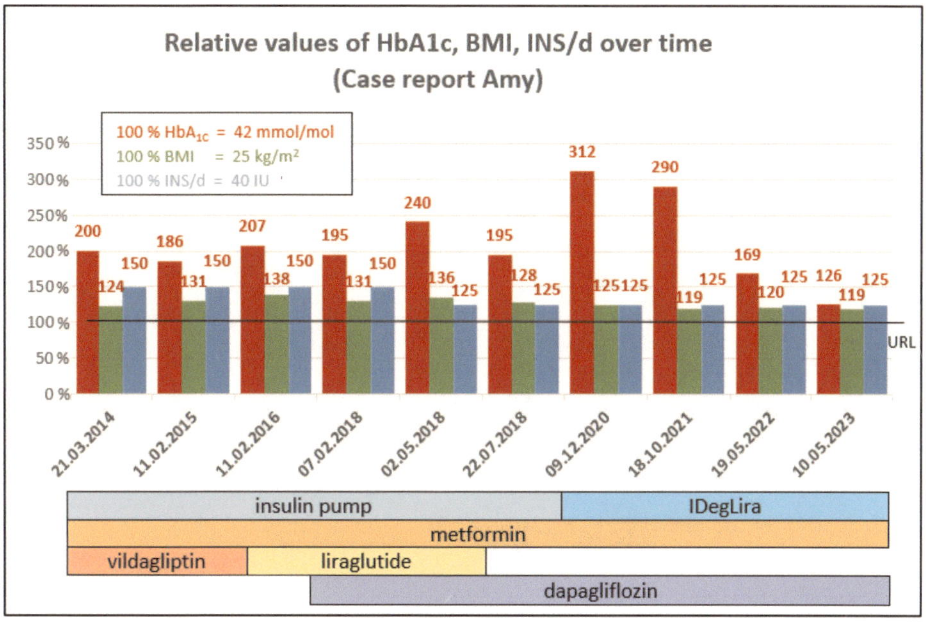

Figure 3.
Relative values of HbA_{1c}, BMI, and INS/d over the last 9 years show that none of the observed parameters reached under the upper limit of the reference range (URL), depicted as a line on 100% level.

2.2 Case report Benjamin

Focus: remarkable influence of CGM/hybrid insulin pump, DAPA, and SEMA on reduction of BM and HbA_{1c} and on improving overall metabolic health.

History: Benjamin, 60 years-old-man, was first diagnosed with DM2 in 1998. A subsequent diagnosis of polyneuropathy in 2007 suggests that his diabetes was most likely not optimally controlled.

Benjamin began our regimen of care in August 2012, presenting with an HbA_{1c} of 81 mmol/mol and a daily insulin requirement of 80 IU. The introduction of an insulin pump in early 2013 led to a commendable decrease in his HbA_{1c} to 71 mmol/mol and a reduction in his daily insulin requirement to 70 IU by the beginning of 2014 [14]. Nevertheless, Benjamin grappled with personal challenges in controlling his eating habits, which he found particularly difficult to overcome.

In an effort to curb his overeating, we strategically reduced Benjamin's daily insulin intake. Despite this, his glycated HbA_{1c} remained around 80 mmol/mol from 2017 to 2019. To address this, we introduced a combination of dapagliflozin/metformin (DAPA/MET) into his treatment plan in 2019, which successfully brought down his HbA_{1c}. (**Figures 4** and 5).

In early 2021, SEMA s.c. (once weekly) was added to his regimen. This led to a notable improvement in his glycemic control, with HbA_{1c} dropping to a promising 56 mmol/mol. However, Benjamin's struggle with overeating resurfaced. Later in the same year (November 2021), flash glucose monitoring started. In 2022, a hybrid insulin pump MiniMed 780G, replaced the previous pump Paradigm Veo [15]. CareLink statistics can be seen in **Figure 6**.

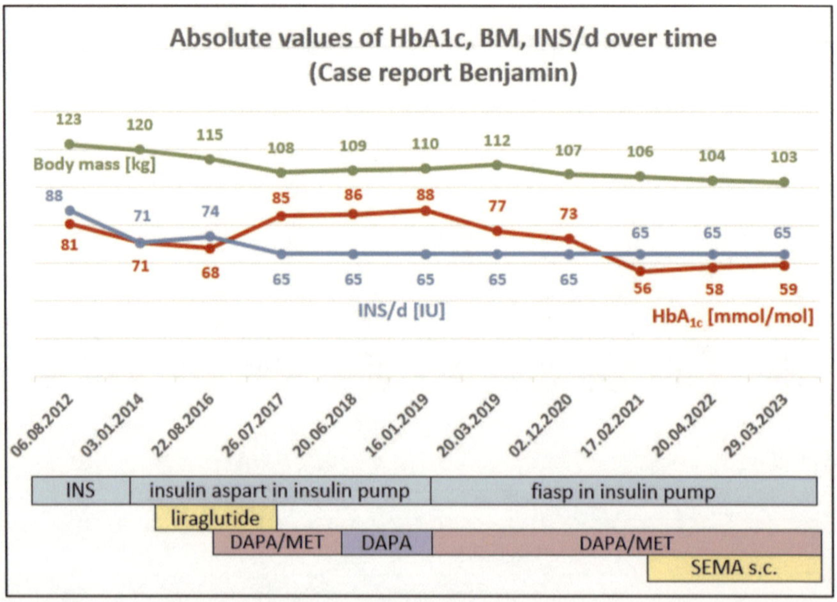

Figure 4.
CareLink Statistics: A comparison between the date range of 1 month A (blue) and B (orange). Progress between both date ranges, time in range (TIR), blood glucose (BG), insulin usage, and saccharides consumed.

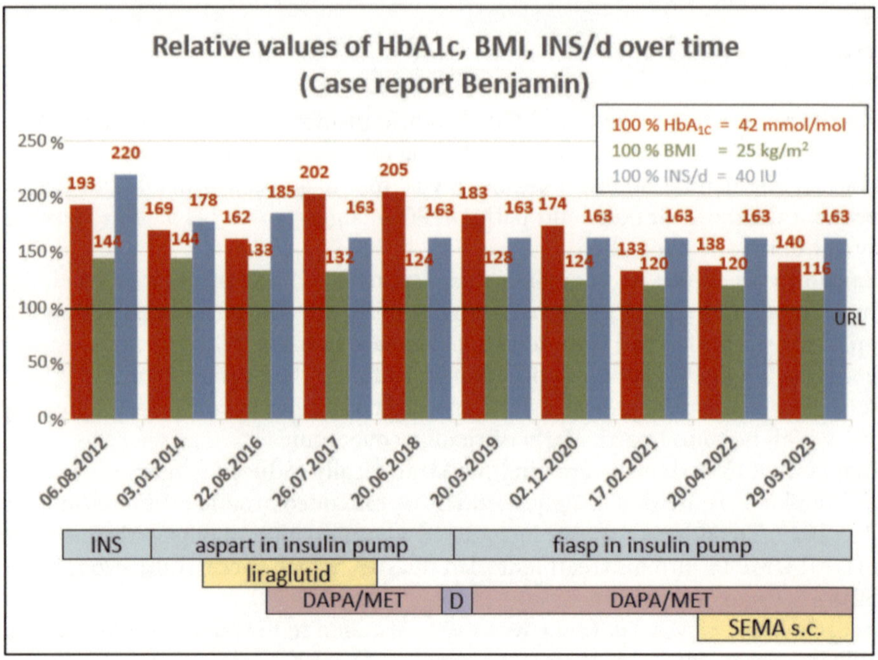

Figure 5.
Absolute values of HbA_{1c}, BM, INS, since Benjamin has been in our care. The daily dose of insulin has been reduced from 88 to 71 IU by the implementation of an insulin pump. After lowering the INS/d and adding liraglutide to the treatment plan, HbA_{1c} increased, but body mass decreased by 7 kg. There is an apparent body mass decreasing trend, with a further decrease after SEMA was added to the treatment plan.

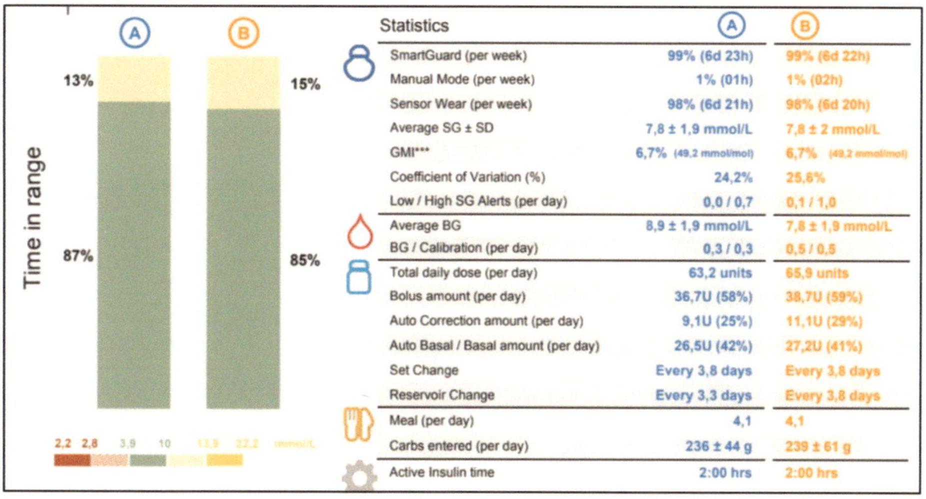

Figure 6.
Relative values of HbA_{1c}*, BMI, INS/d over the last 11 years showing that all the parameters are above the upper reference limit (URL). The BMI values show a decreasing trend.*

Despite this setback, Benjamin's glycemic control has remained commendably stable over the last 3 years, with HbA_{1c} maintaining below 60 mmol/mol. Moreover, his Body Mass Index (BMI) has also been reduced to below 30.

Looking Ahead: Reducing insulin intake and BM while maintaining/improving his glycemic control (HbA_{1c}). Improvement in his overall health and well-being.

2.3 Case report Connor

Focus: Unfortunate case with the focus on BM and HbA_{1c} reduction with no sustainable effect of CSII, exenatide, liraglutide, DAPA, >MET, SEMA.

History: A 72-year-old man, diagnosed with T2D in 1999 and on insulin therapy since 2007, was registered in our diabetes center on May 30, 2011. Upon admission, Connor's treatment plan comprised insulin lispro (86 ID/d), insulin glargine (48 IU/d) (LIS + GLA in **Figure** 7), and MET (1700 mg daily). Soon after, insulin adjustments were made: insulin lispro was replaced with insulin aspart and insulin glargine with insulin detemir. This case will be further described using **Figures 8–11**.

September 30, 2011, the INS/d was reduced from 134 to 81 IU. April 13, 2012, in line with the special study, Connor was given an insulin pump, with 81 IU/d of insulin aspart; also MET increased to 3 g/day [14]. The outcome of the special study, which ended on October 12, 2012: despite reducing INS/d by 12 IU, HbA_{1c} decreased from 92 to 69 mmol/mol, and his body mass remained unchanged. Connor continues to use CSII [15].

January 21, 2013, liraglutide (LIRA) 6 mg/ml was prescribed, but on November 18, 2013, LIRA was replaced with exenatide (EX) (10–0-10 mg s.c./d) (as shown on **Figure 9**). March 3, 2014, exenatide was discontinued, but after a month exenatide QW (EX QW) was prescribed again. As the body mass was 111 kg, he was advised on the need for physical activity and a healthy lifestyle. Treatment with exenatide, metformin, and insulin delivery via the insulin pump led to improvement of HbA_{1c}, but its value still did not drop 60 mmol/mol below, so on November 23, 2015, dapagliflozin was added to the therapeutic plan. Exenatide and dapagliflozin were discontinued on February 29, 2016, due to gastric issues. June 27, 2016, exenatide

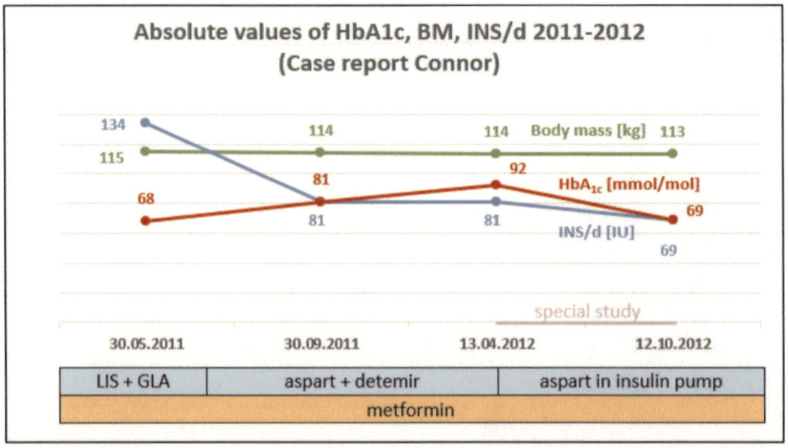

Figure 7.
Absolute values of HbA$_{1c}$, BM, INS, in 2011–2013.

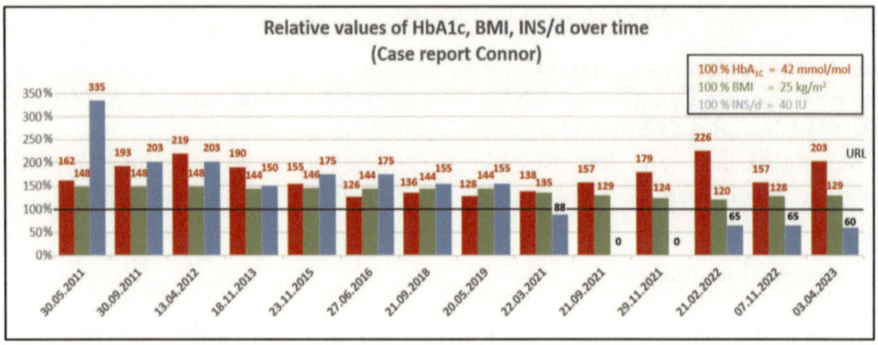

Figure 8.
Overview of Connor's relative values from 2011 until 2023.

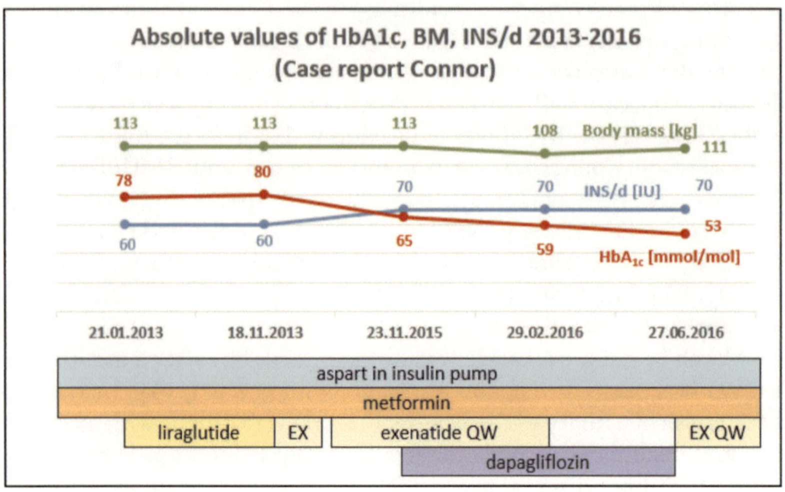

Figure 9.
Absolute values of HbA$_{1c}$, BM, INS/d over time.

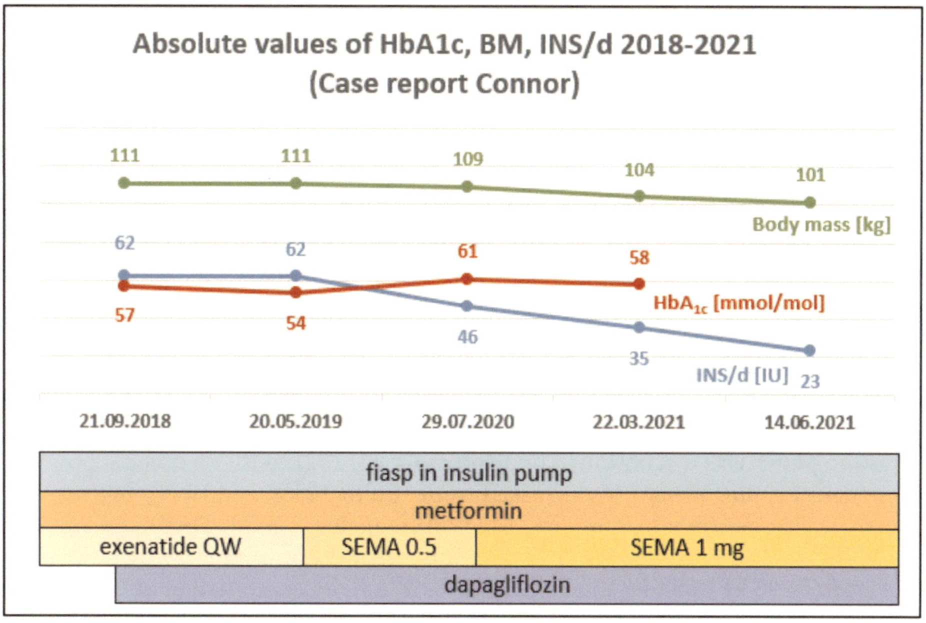

Figure 10.
Absolute values of HbA_{1c}, BM, INS/d in 2018–2021.

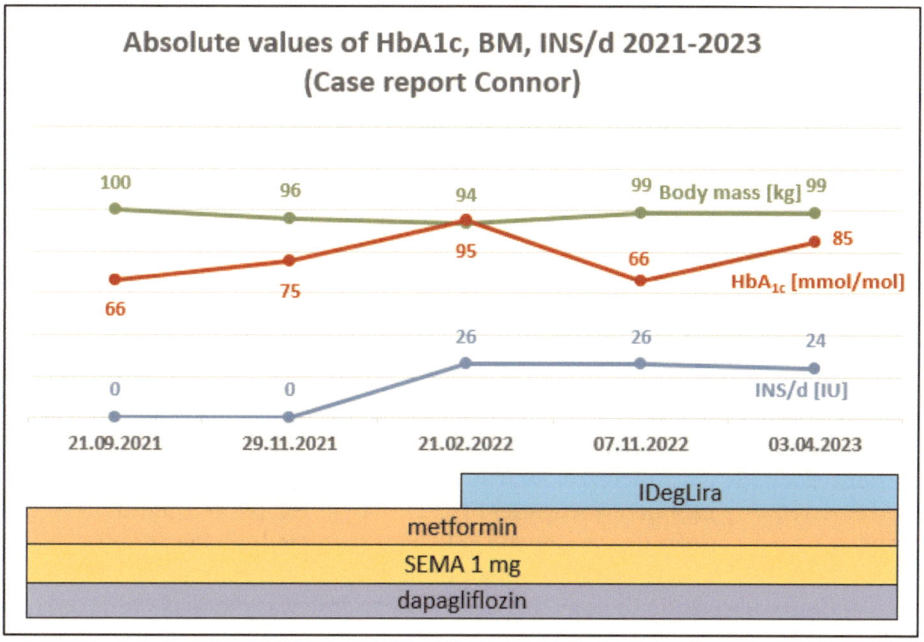

Figure 11.
Absolute values of HbA_{1c}, BM, INS/d in 2021–2023.

therapy was restarted, which was interrupted due to surgery on the biliary tract, resulting in HbA_{1c} dropping below 50 mmol/mol after 6 months.

In 2017, the basal insulin dose was gradually reduced. April 22, 2018, insulin Fiasp was prescribed for the insulin pump. Due to persistently elevated blood pressure (157/

80) and HbA_{1c} (57 mmol/mol) despite insulin pump, exenatide, and metformin treatment, dapagliflozin was added again on September 21, 2018. This treatment combination led to a slight improvement in HbA_{1c} to 55 mmol/mol. HbA_{1c} value shows a slight decrease, but as no change in body mass occurs, exenatide was replaced with s.c. SEMA on May 20, 2019. On July 29, 2020, HbA_{1c} values increased from 54 to 61 mmol/mol, and body mass remained unchanged; thus, SEMA dose was increased from 0.5–1 mg.

BM remained unchanged, HbA_{1c} decreased to 59 mmol/mol (by 2 mmol/mol). Therefore, the basal rate is reduced from 27 to 16.5 IU per day. With concurrent DAPA and SEMA, BM decreased by 2.5 kg in 3 months, and treatment continues.

March 22, 2021: With this treatment, where the total daily insulin dose was 34 IU/day, there was a slight decrease in HbA_{1c} to 58 mmol/mol, and body mass decreased by 5.5 kg – now 104.5 kg. After another 3 months, June 14, 2021, there is a BM reduction of 4 kg (i.e., to 100.7 kg). Due to favorable body mass development, the basal insulin dose was reduced by 0.1 IU every hour to 14.1 IU per day – INS/d is 25 IU.

Insulin pump was discontinued on September 21, 2021, with no other supply of endogenous insulin. Then, BM decreased from 100 to 96 kg, and HbA_{1c} increased from 66 to 75 mmol/mol in 3 months. Medication includes MET, DAPA, and SEMA.

Due to an increase in HbA_{1c} from 75 mmol/mol to 95 mmol/mol, with body mass reduced from 96 kg to 94 kg since the last check, a fixed combination of IDegLira at a dose of 22 units was initiated on February 21, 2022.

Since the last check-up, while on IDegLira treatment of 22 units, dapagliflozin, and metformin 1-0-1, HbA_{1c} decreased from 95 to 80 mmol/mol, but body mass increased to 96 kg. IDegLira dose increased to 26 units on May 16, 2022.

After 6 months (November 7, 2022) with this treatment combination, HbA_{1c} decreased from 80 mmol/mol to 66 mmol/mol but also led to an increase in body mass (now 99 kg).

Looking Ahead: Adequate algorithm for DAPA, MET, incretin, and insulin administration resulting in HbA_{1c} decrease without BM increase should be sought. Bariatric surgery should be discussed.

2.4 Case report David

Focus: Effective replacement of insulin with IDegLira followed by DAPA and SEMA: challenging reduction of both BM and HbA_{1c}, higher satisfaction, no insulin.

History: David, a 72-year-old man, sought medical care at our clinic after relocating to a new area. At the time of his visit, he was facing challenges with his diabetes management. His daily insulin requirement exceeded 100 units, and he experienced a body mass increase, with an elevated HbA_{1c} of around 60 mmol/mol. David had a history of mononeuropathy of the left peroneal nerve and had developed advanced axonal sensory-motor diabetic polyneuropathy in both lower limbs since 2019. Additionally, he was already taking fibrates for hyperlipidemia.

To optimize his insulin therapy, his daily insulin dose was gradually reduced from 102 IU to 76 IU.

During a subsequent follow-up, adjustments were made to his insulin regimen. Insulin glargine at a dose of 40 IU was replaced with insulin degludec at a dose of 30 IU, while maintaining insulin aspart at a dose of 30 IU. This modification resulted in a total daily insulin dose of 60 IU. Despite 6 months of intensive insulin therapy, there were no notable improvements in HbA_{1c} or body mass.

In light of the unsatisfactory outcomes, both insulin aspart (30 IU) and degludec (30 IU) were substituted with a fixed combination of insulin degludec and the incretin liraglutide (IDegLira), totaling 16 units. David was educated on the need for titration and diligently adjusted his daily dose to stabilize it at 50 units. Unfortunately, even with this medication change, the desired reduction in clinical and laboratory parameters was not achieved (see **Figures 12** and **13**).

Considering David's intolerance to MET, DAPA 10 mg was introduced as an additional treatment option. However, after a year of this regimen, David began experiencing fatigue during daily activities, which resulted in a decrease in his physical activity level. Consequently, his HbA_{1c} once again reached 63 mmol/mol, while his body mass remained around 110 kg. At this point, David received further education on the importance of energy intake restriction and increasing physical activity.

During a subsequent check-up, his body mass increased by 3 kg, and his HbA_{1c} rose to 71 mmol/mol. To address these concerns, treatment with 0.5 mg of SEMA was initiated for David, with his explicit preference for the injectable form. After 3 months of SEMA 0.5 mg treatment (once weekly), his body mass decreased by 9 kg. Since there was no simultaneous decrease in HbA_{1c}, the SEMA dose was increased to 1 mg, subcutaneously.

Following 6 months of treatment with SEMA 1 mg subcutaneously (s.c.), pioglitazone 15 mg, and dapagliflozin 10 mg, David's body mass decreased from 103 kg to 97 kg, and his HbA_{1c} dropped from 72 mmol/mol to 55 mmol/mol. As his TAG exceeded 4 mmol/L, David was advised to pay closer attention to his fat intake.

Additionally, he was encouraged to further increase his physical activity. Treatment with this medication combination continues to be ongoing for David, and regular monitoring and follow-up are being conducted.

Looking ahead: Identifying a treatment approach that can lead to relative values below 100% for both HbA_{1c} and body mass.

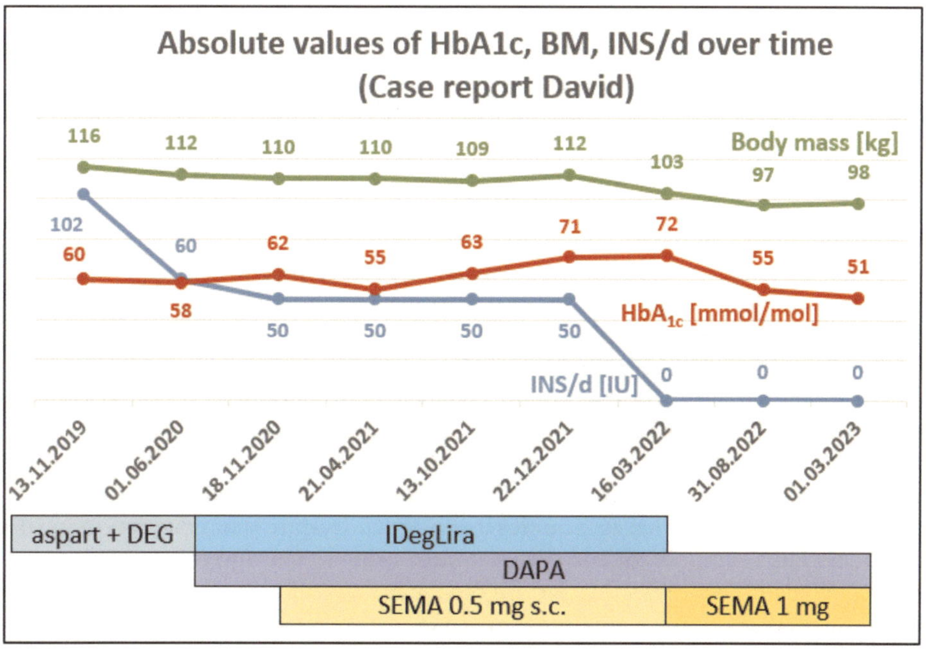

Figure 12.
Absolute values of HbA_{1c}, BM, INS/d over time. By the admission, David's daily use of insulin was 102 IU. Insulin usage was reduced, and eventually, IDegLira was prescribed with a starting dose of 16 units with a final titration of 50 units per day. During this period, his body mass remained relatively stable. After exogenous insulin intake was stopped and the SEMA dose was increased to 1 mg, HbA_{1c} started to drop along with his body mass.

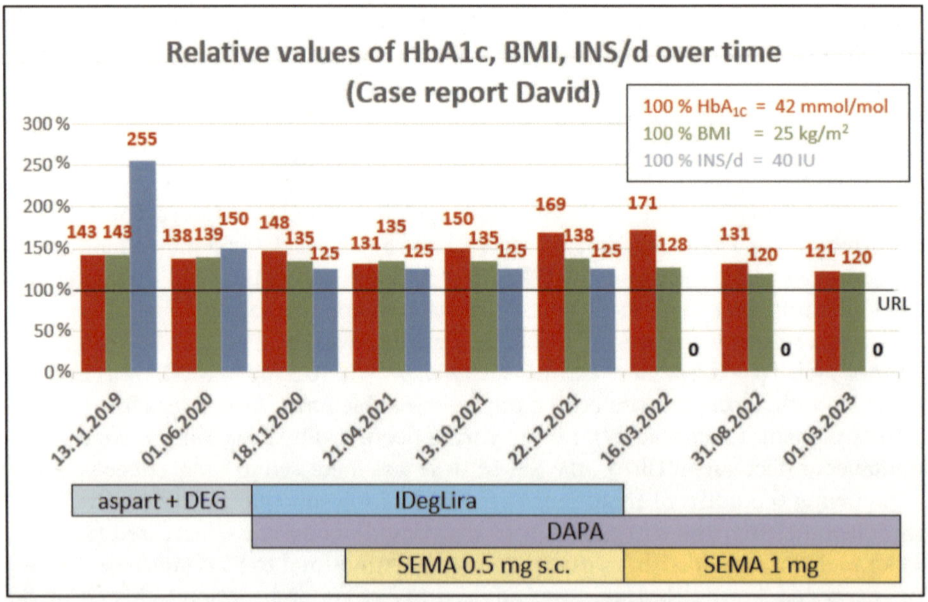

Figure 13.
Relative values of HbA_{1c}, BMI, INS/d over time showing red values of given parameters that represent being above the upper reference limit (URL). After exogenous insulin doses were decreased to 0, a treatment consisting of dapagliflozin (DAPA) and semaglutide 1 mg (SEMA 1 mg) and increased physical activity, the values of HbA_{1c} and BMI are getting closer to the URL line, indicating an improvement.

2.5 Case report Emma

Focus: A person with a long history of T2D with multiple pharmacologic approaches including DAPA, pioglitazone, saxagliptin, liraglutide, exenatide QW, SEMA IDegLira, MET, and insulin delivery through an insulin pump and its effect on body mass and HbA_{1c}.

History: Emma, born in 1958, was diagnosed with type 2 diabetes (T2D) in 2000 and has been on insulin therapy since 2005. In 2011, she was referred to our care due to her inability to adequately compensate for her diabetes.

Emma presented with multiple comorbidities, including obesity, hyperlipoproteinemia, retinopathy, and a history of postsurgical complications following ovarian cyst removal. At the time of referral, her HbA_{1c} was around 88 mmol/mol and prandial glycemia fluctuated between 10 and 15 mmol/L. The complexity of this case, notably attributed to the diverse pharmacological interventions, is depicted and emphasized with accompanied visual representations in **Figures 14–16**.

Not long after enrolling at our diabetes center, Emma became a participant in a specialized study [14]. During this study, the Paradigm Veo insulin pump was introduced, initially reducing her insulin dosage to 37 IU. Despite the reduction in insulin dosage, her HbA_{1c} improved, and she continued using the insulin pump even after the study concluded. Eventually, her insulin dosage increased to 68 IU (and remained this high until February 2016). On January 21, 2013, she was prescribed liraglutide 0.6 mg, and after 3 months, the dosage was escalated to 1.2 mg. Unfortunately, due to gastrointestinal issues, liraglutide was discontinued from her treatment plan on November 18, 2013. During this period, there were also adjustments to MET doses, since after an increase to a maximum dose of 3000 mg, Emma did not feel well. **Figure 17** shows an overview of relative values since admission.

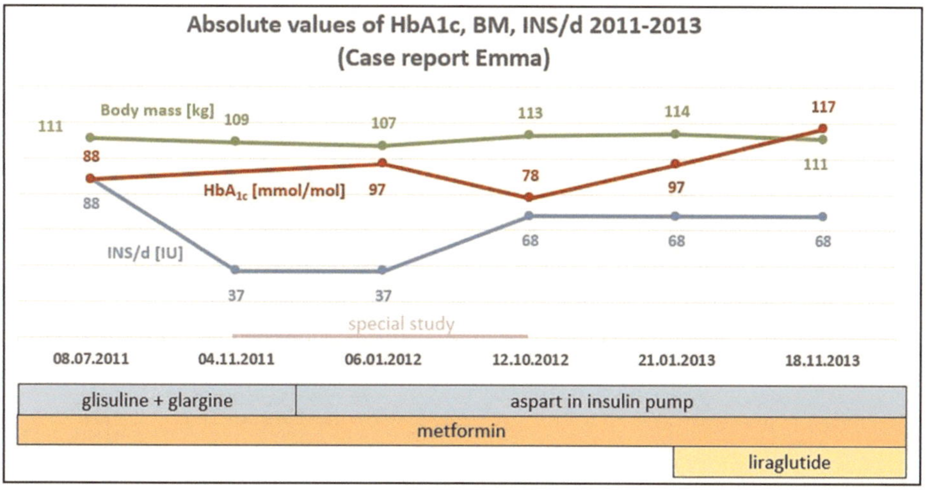

Figure 14.
Absolute values of Emma's HbA_{1c}, BM, INS/d since her registration in our center until the year 2013. The purple line special study demarcates its duration period.

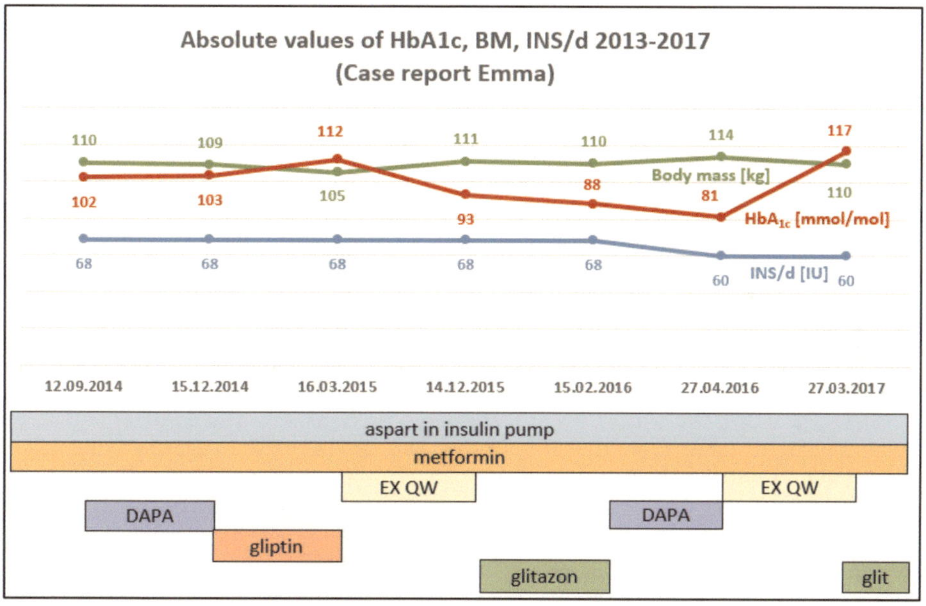

Figure 15.
Absolute values of HbA_{1c}, BM, INS/d in years 2014–2017.

There is an overview of Ema's medication in **Table 2**.

Emma's persistent struggle with exceedingly high HbA_{1c} levels, surpassing 100 mmol/mol, prompted the addition of DAPA to her treatment regimen on September 12, 2014. Nevertheless, owing to discomfort and gynecological inflammations, DAPA was discontinued on December 15, 2014, and saxagliptin was introduced as an alternative. With her HbA_{1c} level escalating to 112 mmol/mol, saxagliptin was subsequently halted and replaced with exenatide QW (EX QW). For her next visit on December 14, 2012, Emma's body mass increased to 111 kg, despite a decline in her

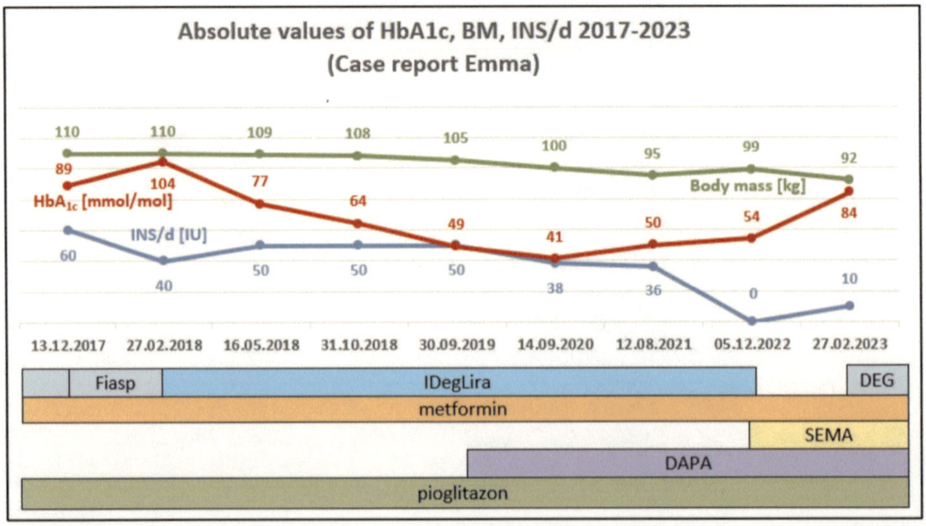

Figure 16.
Absolute values of HbA_{1c}, BM, INS/d in years 2017–2023.

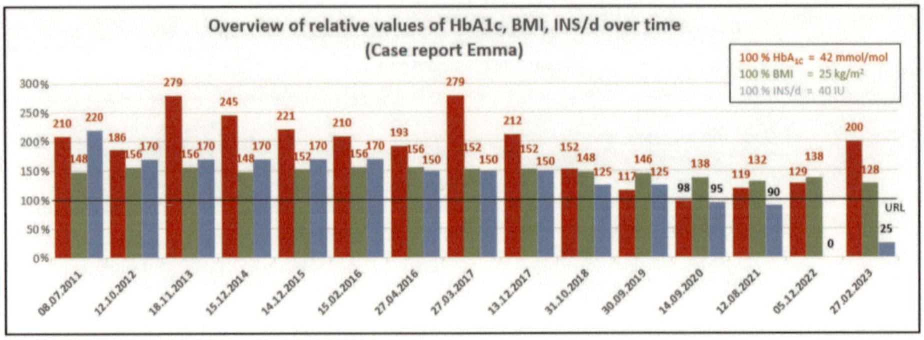

Figure 17.
Overview of Ema's relative values from 2011 until 2023.

Medication	From	Up to
Metformin	Beginning	Present
Aspart insulin pump	04.11.2011	13.12.2017
Liraglutide	21.01.2013	18.11.2013
Dapagliflozin	12.09.2014	15.12.2014
Saxagliptine	15.12.2014	16.03.2015
Exenatide QX	16.03.2015	14.12.2015
Pioglitazone	14.12.2015	15.02.2016
Dapagliflozin	15.02.2016	27.04.2016
Exenatide QX	27.04.2016	27.03.2017
Pioglitazone	27.03.2017	Present
FIASP for insulin pump	13.12.2017	27.02.2018

Medication	From	Up to
IDegLira	27.02.2018	05.12.2022
Dapagliflozin	30.09.2019	Present
Semaglutide 1 mg	05.12.2022	Present
Insulin degludec	27.02.2023	Present

Table 2.
Overview of Emma's medication.

HbA_{1c} levels. As her treatment journey unfolded, exenatide QW was eventually phased out, and pioglitazone was prescribed. Over the following year, a therapeutic sequence involving DAPA, exenatide, and pioglitazone was established. Presently, Emma remains on pioglitazone as part of her ongoing treatment regimen.

On December 13, 2017, the insulin aspart was changed to the faster-acting insulin aspart within the insulin pump. Despite this adjustment, HbA_{1c} levels persisted in their ascent, peaking at 104 mmol/mol. In response, following a deliberation with Emma, the decision was made to discontinue CSII on February 27, 2018. As a substitution, IDegLira was introduced (initially at 40 units). The titration of IDegLira to 50 units, in conjunction with a combination of DAPA, MET, and pioglitazone, yielded a remarkable improvement, driving HbA_{1c} levels to 41 mmol/mol. This success led to the gradual reduction of IDegLira dosages—first to 38 units, then to 36 units. This adjustment in insulin degludec dosage influenced liraglutide levels as well, contributing to a rise in appetite, HbA_{1c}, and body mass. In light of these developments, a novel treatment approach was devised, involving the cessation of IDegLira and the initiation of SEMA on December 5, 2022. Despite the holiday season, this shift resulted in a reduction in body mass from 99 kg to 92 kg. Unfortunately, there was an increase in HbA_{1c} to 84 mmol/mol. This rise serves as a clear indication that Emma's optimal glycemic control necessitates exogenous insulin supplementation, leading to the prescription of insulin degludec [16].

Looking ahead: Determining the lowest effective dosage of insulin to achieve optimal HbA_{1c} control, all the while carefully managing body mass.

2.6 Case report Fatima

Focus: Impact of oral SEMA on INS/d, BM, HbA_{1c}, and lifestyle modifications in a lady with T2D treated by means of CSII and DAPA.

History: Fatima, a 73-year-old woman, visited our diabetes center in 2011 for therapy adjustment and a transition to an insulin pump [14]. Prior to that, she had been treated with 68 IU of insulin aspart and 32 IU of insulin detemir, along with 1000 mg of metformin twice a day, for 3 years. Fatima was provided with the Paradigm 754 Veo pump equipped with insulin aspart in our clinic. Through gradual use of the pump, her average daily insulin dose stabilized at around 60 IU. She quickly adapted to using the pump and handled it very well.

After nearly 3 years of treatment with the pump and metformin (3x1000 mg/day), Fatima started experiencing higher PG during the day. She also developed moderate diabetic retinopathy. As a result, she was prescribed saxagliptin 5 mg once daily. During a follow-up after 4 months, her HbA_{1c} decreased from 64 mmol/mol to 57 mmol/mol.

After 10 months, her HbA_{1c} increased to 61 mmol/mol without any increase in body mass. Consequently, saxagliptin 5 mg was replaced with dapagliflozin 10 mg/

day. As the desired effect was still not achieved, dapagliflozin treatment was supplemented with metformin in a fixed combination of dapagliflozin 5 mg and metformin 1000 mg (DAPA/MET), with a dosage of twice daily.

In 2017, the insulin aspart, that Fatima was taking, was switched to the same type but with a faster onset of action. Her daily insulin usage remained unchanged. Despite repeated education, dietary adjustments, and efforts to increase physical activity, her diabetes compensation was not satisfactory. In January 2018, she received a recommendation for comprehensive balneotherapy in Luhačovice spa.

Fatima continued taking her diabetes medication without changes for almost three more years. During this period, she was monitored for hypertension in our internal clinic. Fatima repeatedly reported frequent dizziness, nausea, and occasional unexplained falls. Consequently, she underwent several examinations by relevant physicians, but the findings were repeatedly negative. In August 2020, Fatima was scheduled for a planned hospitalization to address these problems. During her stay, attention was also focused on improving her diabetes compensation.

Due to the outbreak of the COVID-19 pandemic, Fatima did not return for further check-ups and blood tests until a year after her hospitalization. During this period, her HbA_{1c} increased by 8 mmol/mol, while her body mass remained unchanged. As part of her current treatment, she was prescribed oral SEMA at a starting dose of 3 mg daily, gradually increasing to 7 mg and eventually 14 mg, with increments every month.

The first follow-up after 3 months of using oral SEMA, DAPA/MET, and the insulin pump showed a decrease in HbA_{1c} from 60 mmol/mol to 43 mmol/mol with minimal body mass change. Fatima felt well and experienced no adverse effects from SEMA. Hypoglycemia did not occur. Her daily insulin dose gradually decreased to 55 IU and then to 36 IU per day. After a year of treatment combination consisting of oral SEMA, the insulin pump, and DAPA/MET, she lost 5 kg and her HbA_{1c} decreased by 23 mmol/mol (**Figures 18** and **19**).

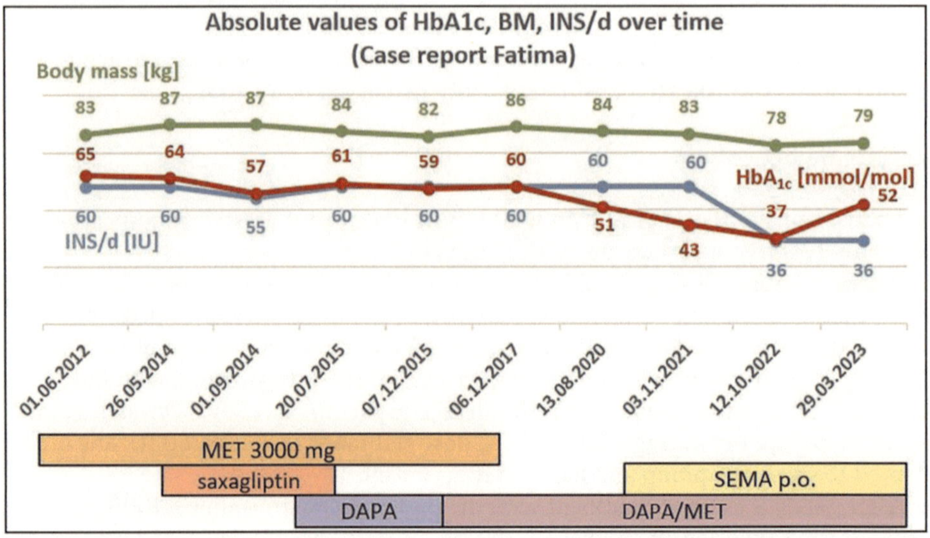

Figure 18.
Absolute values of parameters from 2012 showing relatively constant body mass that slightly decreased after oral SEMA (SEMA p.o.) was added to the treatment plan, and insulin dosage was lowered to nearly half – from 60 IU to 36 IU. After adding dapagliflozin/metformin (DAPA/MET) in combination with SEMA p.o., the HbA_{1c} level lowered from 60 mmol/mol to 37 mmol/mol. A recent check-up in March 2023 showed an increase in HbA_{1c}.

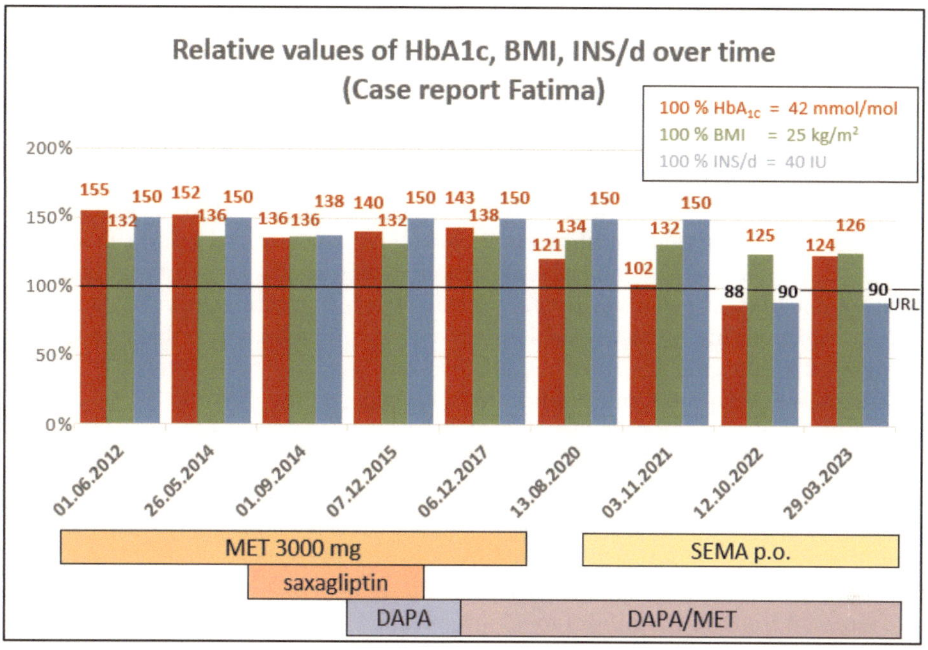

Figure 19.
Relative values of HbA_{1c}, BMI, INS/d over time showing the values of given parameters being written in red, above URL. In 2022, her HbA1c improved and got under 100%, showing sufficient glycemic control. This led to an insulin dosage decrease, 90% of the upper reference limit (36 IU). This resulted in an HbA_{1c} increase.

Fatima continues with her established treatment, although her most recent check-up in March 2023 showed an increase in HbA_{1c}. Fatima was once again educated about the importance of adhering to proper lifestyle principles.

Looking ahead: Continue to adjust Fatima's medication regimen based on her response to treatment and her glycemic control. Consider alternating or combining different classes of antidiabetic medication to achieve HbA_{1c} lower than 42 mmol/mol and body mass reduction (BMI under 28).

2.7 Case report Gerry

Focus: Effect of INS, IDegLira, and consequent complementation with DAPA/MET on BM, HbA_{1c}, cardiovascular complications, and lifestyle modifications.

History: Gerry, a 71-year-old man, arrives at our diabetes center due to the recommendation of his cardiologist. He is currently being monitored for heart failure with a left ventricular ejection fraction of 45% and falls under NYHA class I-II. Gerry has been managing diabetes since 2007 and has been receiving treatment with insulin detemir (18 IU) and gliclazide (a sulfonylurea derivative) at a dosage of 60 mg once a day. Under this treatment regimen, his HbA_{1c} level was recorded at 82 mmol/mol, and his body mass stood at 106 kg. It became evident that a change in medication was necessary.

As part of the revised treatment plan, insulin detemir was substituted with 16 IU of insulin degludec in a fixed combination with liraglutide, and gliclazide was discontinued. Unfortunately, Gerry faced challenges in the initial 2 months of this new treatment regimen. He struggled with proper insulin administration, often missing several daily doses. To address this issue, Gerry received repeated guidance on sticking to a dietary regimen and was motivated to avoid consuming foods high in fat content.

After 4 months of gradual titration, he successfully reached a stable daily insulin dose of 30 IU. Furthermore, after 3 months of treatment, there was a notable decrease in his HbA_{1c} level by 19 mmol/mol, accompanied by a body mass increase of 2 kg. Encouraged by these positive results, Gerry remained committed to the gradual titration of his medication and continued to make adjustments to his lifestyle. One of his dietary habits involved a high intake of carbohydrates, such as white bread, potatoes, and sweetened beverages. Over time, he made efforts to modify the composition of his diet, incorporating more vegetables. Gerry diligently adhered to this treatment regimen for nearly a year.

Given the development of ischemic heart disease and the ongoing insufficient control of his diabetes, a fixed combination of dapagliflozin and metformin (DAPA/MET) was added to his medication (as depicted in **Figures 20** and **21**).

Over the course of 4 years, during which Gerry has been taking DAPA/MET (5/1000 mg) alongside 50 IU of insulin degludec, his blood pressure readings at our clinic have predominantly demonstrated normal values. Additionally, his HbA_{1c} level has decreased from 60 mmol/mol to 45 mmol/mol. His body mass has remained relatively stable, consistently above 100 kg.

Despite Gerry's consistent efforts and adherence to dietary modifications, he has faced challenges in achieving body mass below 100 kg and maintaining HbA_{1c} within the physiological range. Over a period of 7 years under our monitoring, Gerry's left ventricular ejection fraction (LVEF) has declined to 30%. The inclusion of SEMA in

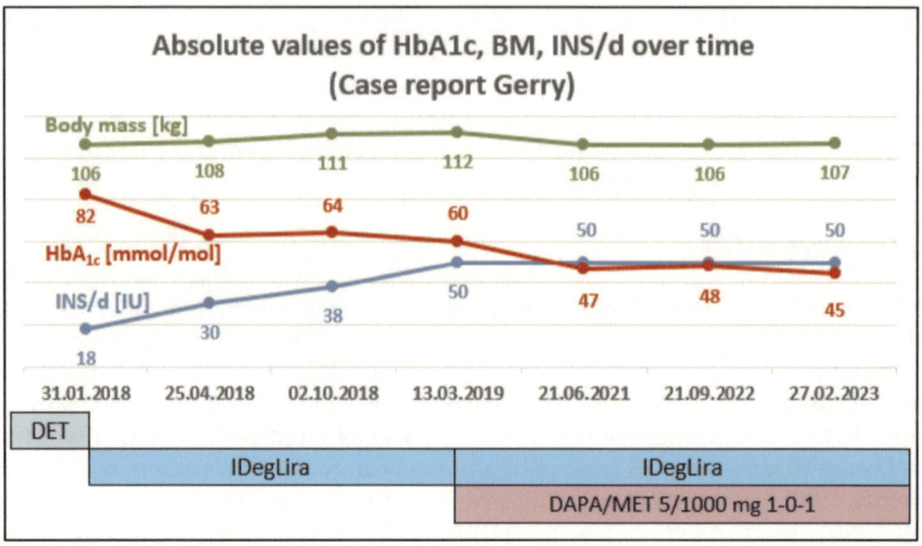

Figure 20.
The absolute values of HbA_{1c}, BM, INS/d over 5 years period. Values of HbA_{1c} recorded a decrease from 82 to 63 mmol/mol during the first 3 months of using IDegLira. Through gradual titration, Gerry's dose was stabilized at 50 units of IDegLira. When using this dose, HbA_{1c} values decreased to 47 mmol/mol. Body mass gradually increased from the beginning of IDegLira treatment, leading to the addition of a combination of DAPA/MET 5/1000 mg to the dose of 50 units IDegLira. This change resulted in a body mass decrease from 112 kg to 106 kg, which has been maintained.

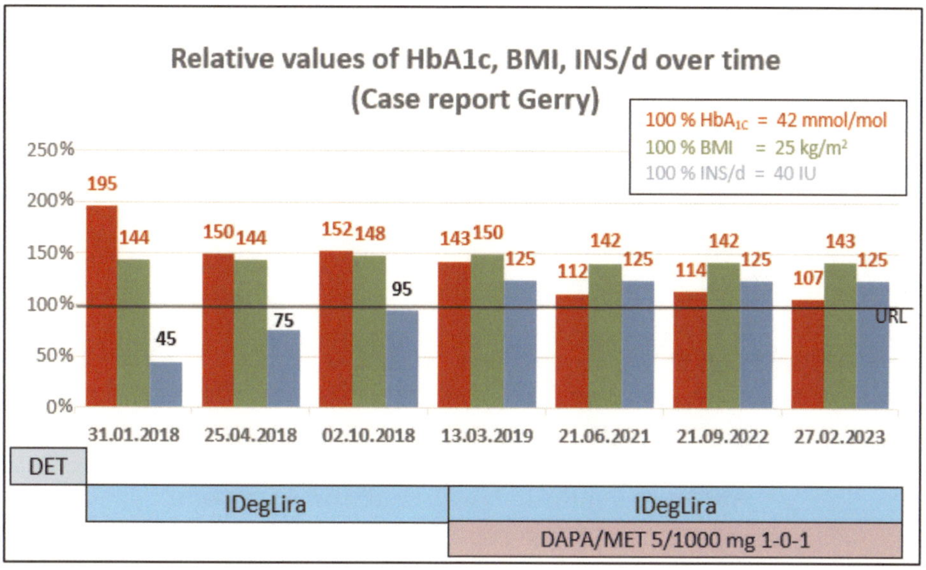

Figure 21.
Relative values of HbA_{1c}, BMI, INS/d over time. Values over the upper reference limit (URL) are depicted in red. There is an apparent decreasing trend in the HbA_{1c} level, which started almost at 200% and got nearly to 100% of the reference range, signing a sufficient glycemic control.

his medication regimen is being contemplated due to its potential cardioprotective effects [17].

Gerry continues to prioritize the improvement of his dietary choices and lifestyle habits with ongoing support from his healthcare team.

Looking ahead: A potential switch from IDegLira to SEMA is being considered in the future.

2.8 Case report Henry

Focus: Impact of SEMA p.o. on BM and HbA_{1c} in a man treated with metformin and DAPA without insulin.

History: Henry came to the clinic on the recommendation of his general practitioner due to the detection of hyperglycemia of 10.8 mmol/L and 13.1 mmol/L in June 2018. The general practitioner prescribed MET, which Henry tolerates well without any gastrointestinal issues. In addition to type 2 diabetes mellitus, Henry has also been diagnosed with hypertension and dyslipidemia. He was advised to quit smoking, and the dose of MET was increased to 1500 mg per day. Due to elevated TAG reaching 5.9 mmol/L, fenofibrate 200 mg once daily was also prescribed (**Table 3**). Henry received counseling and was recommended to reduce caloric intake and achieve a reduction of body mass of at least 5 kg.

After 3 months of this treatment regimen, Henry returned for a follow-up visit. However, the HbA_{1c} remained at 65 mmol/mol (**Figures 22** and **23**). Considering the risk of his wife's suicide and the potential misuse of insulin, a combination of DAPA/MET 5/1000 mg twice daily was initiated. He tolerates this medication well but has noticed increased urination.

After 3 months, HbA_{1c} decreased from 65 mmol/mol to 56 mmol/mol, and metformin 1000 mg was added, resulting in a total daily MET dose of 3000 mg.

Medication	From	Up to	Dosage
metformin 1000 mg	June 2018	21.09.2018	1/2-1/2-1/2
metformin 1000 mg	10.12.2018	present	0-1-0
oral SEMA 3-7-14 mg	13.12.2021	present	1-0-0
dapagliflozin/metformin 5/1000 mg	21.09.2018	present	1-0-1
fenofibrate 200 mg	June 2018	present	1-0-0
atorvastatin 20 mg		present	0-0-1

Table 3.
Overview of Henry's medication.

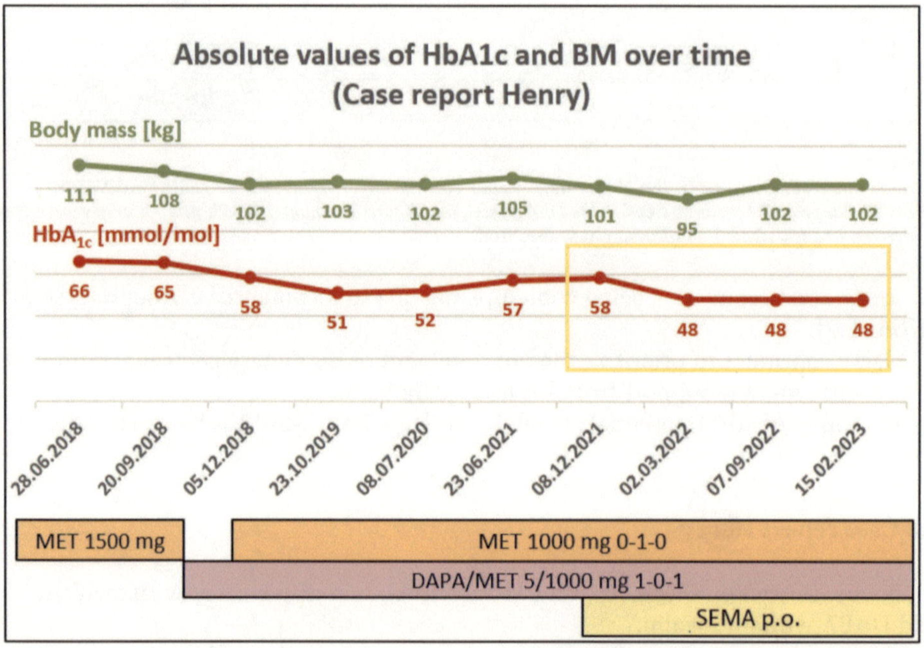

Figure 22.
Absolute values showing the progression of parameters over 5 years. His treatment initially involved metformin (MET) with a dosage of 500 mg three times a day. Subsequently, dapagliflozin/metformin (DAPA/MET) was introduced, resulting in a decrease in HbA_{1c}. Further improvement in HbA_{1c} was observed upon adding oral SEMA (SEMA p.o.), demonstrating its effectiveness in reducing HbA_{1c} (yellow box).

Since starting the combination of DAPA/MET 5/1000 mg twice daily with metformin 1000 mg, Henry's body mass has remained nearly the same, but there has been a gradual increase in HbA_{1c}. Therefore, oral SEMA is added. In the first month, Henry is instructed to take 3 mg of SEMA daily. In the second month, the dose is increased to 7 mg, and in the third month, it is further increased to 14 mg.

After 3 months of treatment with oral SEMA, no adverse effects have been reported, and Henry experienced a decrease in appetite. His body mass decreased from 100 kg to 94 kg, and his HbA_{1c} dropped from 58 mmol/mol to 48 mmol/mol.

During the subsequent 6-month follow-up, it was noted that Henry had gained 7 kg, with HbA_{1c} remaining the same. Henry was once again advised to increase

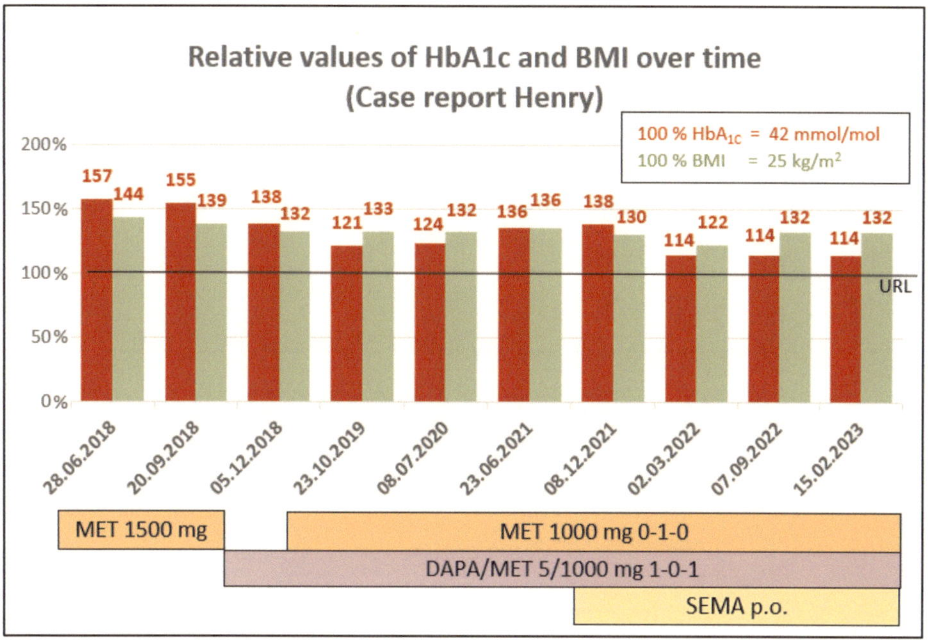

Figure 23.
Over the course of 5 years, Henry's HbA_{1c} and BMI values were consistently elevated, surpassing the highest reference values, as indicated by the red color.

physical activity and limit caloric intake. He is aware that his physical activity level is minimal and his dietary habits are not optimal.

Looking ahead: Both body mass and HbA_{1c} reductions are required by increasing his physical activity and improving his diet.

2.9 Case report Irene

Focus: Influence of the INS replacement with SEMA s.c., DAPA, and MET on BM, HbA_{1c} in a lady with recent T2D and heart failure.

History: Irene, a 65-year-old woman, was diagnosed with type 2 diabetes (T2D) in 2015 and initiated oral antidiabetic medication. Insulin was added to her treatment regimen in 2018.

In 2021, Irene experienced cardiopulmonary failure, leading to hospitalization in the intensive care unit of a local hospital. She was prescribed 46 IU of insulin (insulin aspart 36 IU and insulin glargine 10 IU) per day during her hospital stay. Following her discharge, Irene was referred to a diabetologist for ongoing management.

During her initial assessment at our diabetes center, Irene's HbA_{1c} was measured at 110 mmol/mol, and her body mass was recorded as 112 kg. Based on these results, insulin therapy was temporarily discontinued, and Irene was prescribed a subcutaneous dose of 0.25 mg of SEMA. Irene's medication is summed up in **Table 4**.

After 1 month of treatment, the dosage was increased to 0.5 mg. Over the course of 3 months, Irene experienced a 4 kg body mass loss, accompanied by a 32 mmol/mol reduction in HbA_{1c}. Consequently, the SEMA dosage was further increased to 1 mg (as depicted in **Figures 24** and **25**).

Medication	From	Up to	Dosage
Insulin aspart	Diagnosis of T2D	30.08.2021	14-14-8
Insulin glargin	Diagnosis of T2D	30.08.2021	0-0-0-10
Semaglutide	30.08.2021	Present	Once a week
DAPA/MET	07.02.2022	Present	1-0-1

Table 4.
Overview of Irene's medication.

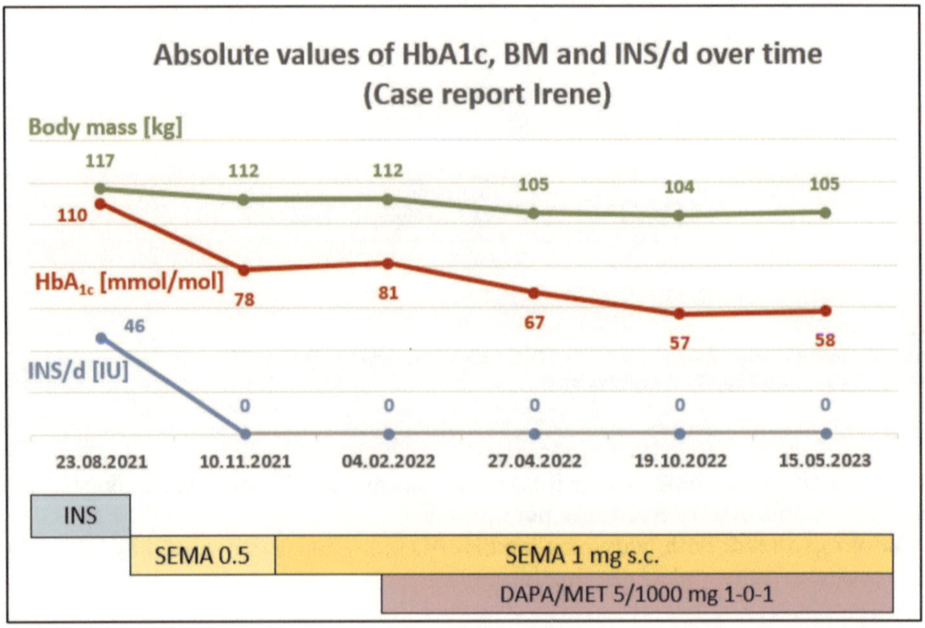

Figure 24.
The HbA_{1c} values of Irene, recorded since her registration at our diabetes center, demonstrate a notable reduction from 110 mmol/mol to 78 mmol/mol over a 3-month period after discontinuation of insulin therapy and initiation of semaglutide (SEMA) treatment following standard titration starting at a dose of 0.25 mg and gradually increasing to 1 mg subcutaneously once a week. Additionally, there is a clear and consistent downward trend observed in body mass and HbA_{1c} throughout the course of treatment.

During the subsequent 3-month follow-up, no significant improvement was observed with SEMA treatment. Considering Irene's cardiovascular comorbidities, a combination medication containing dapagliflozin 5 mg and metformin 1000 mg (DAPA/MET) was introduced. This combination therapy resulted in continued improvements in HbA_{1c} and body mass reduction. Irene occasionally experienced diarrhea after consuming fatty meals.

During a subsequent check-up, Irene reported frequent morning nausea and feelings of weakness, which subsided after breakfast.

Consequently, Irene's treatment was adjusted to semaglutide and a fixed combination of dapagliflozin and metformin (DAPA/MET), with insulin being discontinued. This modification led to a decrease in HbA_{1c} from 110 mmol/mol to 57 mmol/mol, as well as a reduction in body mass from 117 kg to 104 kg. Irene continued with this combination therapy.

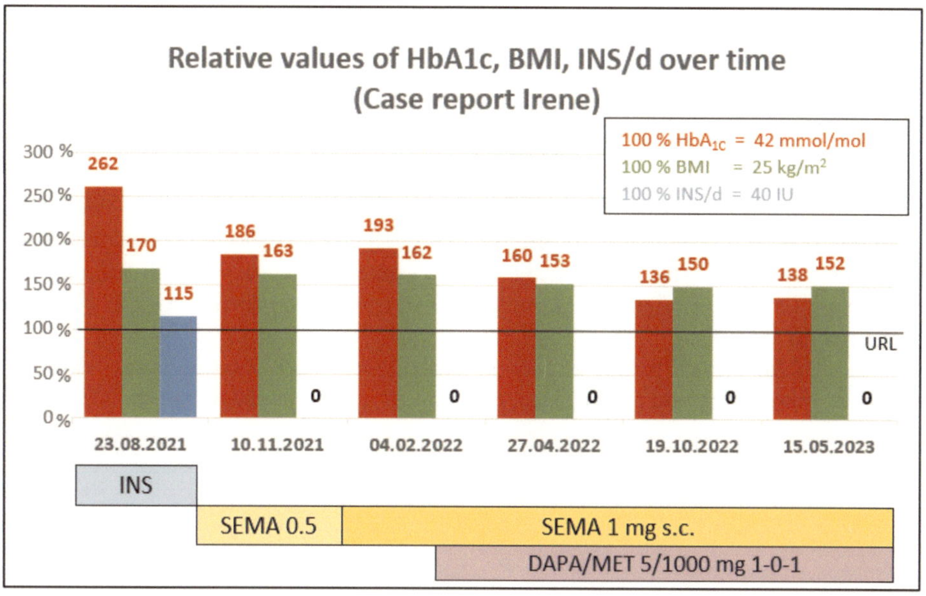

Figure 25.
Despite the decreasing trend in HbA_{1c} levels and BMI following the discontinuation of insulin and implementation of a new treatment plan, it is important to note that the relative values still exceed the upper limit of the physiological range (depicted as red).

Given the gradual deterioration of Irene's vision over the past year, an ophthalmic examination was indicated. The examination ruled out diabetic retinopathy and confirmed a diagnosis of senile cataract (cataracta senilis).

Due to the unavailability of the subcutaneous form of SEMA, Irene's medication was switched to the tablet form in May 2023.

Looking ahead: The tolerance and the effect of oral SEMA will be observed, and further medication adjustments will be made if needed. Body mass reduction is needed.

2.10 Case report Jacob

Focus: Impact of slow insulin replacement with SEMA and MET on BM and HbA_{1c} in a man with recent T2D diagnosis.

History: Jacob, a 52-year-old man, presented to his general practitioner with a hyperglycemia reading of 24.1 mmol/L during a routine check-up. Further laboratory tests, including measurements of C-peptide and autoantibodies, confirmed the diagnosis of type 2 diabetes mellitus. Jacob's medical history revealed that his father and cousin also have type 2 diabetes.

Upon diagnosis, Jacob's treatment plan was initiated by his general practitioner, who prescribed the following medication: Insulin aspart at a dosage of 40 IU per day and insulin detemir at a dosage of 30 IU per day.

Upon referral to our diabetes center, Jacob's treatment plan was reevaluated and modified. The new treatment regimen comprised several medications. Insulin degludec was prescribed at a dosage of 20 IU per day to address his glycemic control. SEMA was initiated at a starting dosage of 0.25 mg in the first month, which was subsequently increased to 0.5 mg from the second month onwards to further enhance glucose management. MET was prescribed at a dosage of 850 mg twice daily, providing additional support in glycemic control. In addition to these diabetes-specific medications (**Table 5**), Jacob continued his treatment with atorvastatin for cholesterol management and perindopril/amlodipine for hypertension management.

Over a span of 6 months, Jacob showed a notable improvement in his condition. His body mass decreased from an initial 130 kg to 112 kg, demonstrating successful body mass management. Moreover, his HbA_{1c} decreased from 130 to 37 mmol/mol, indicating effective blood glucose control and an improved metabolic state. (Depicted in **Figures 26** and 27).

In June 2022, a modification to Jacob's treatment regimen was necessary due to a noticeable increase in body mass. He had gained 7 kg in the previous 6 months,

Medication	From	Up to	Dosage
Semaglutide 1 mg s.c.	21.06.2021	Present	Once weekly
Metformin 850 mg	21.06.2021	Present	1-0-1
Atorvastatin 20 mg		Present	0-0-1/2
Indacaterol/glycopyrronium 85/43 MCG		Present	1-0-0
Insulin degludec	22.06.2021	22.07.2022	20-0-0 IU

Table 5.
Overview of all Jacob's medication.

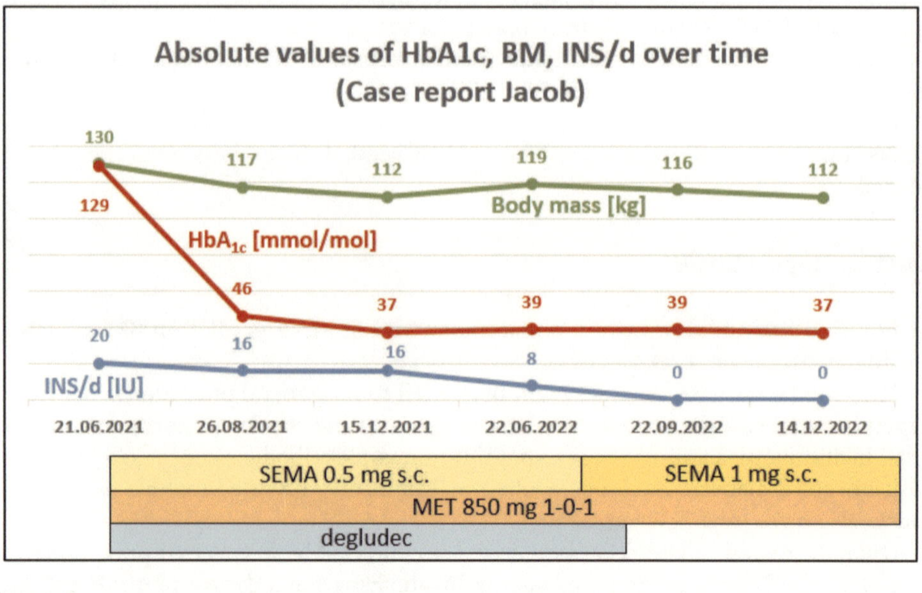

Figure 26.
The absolute values of HbA_{1c} demonstrate a consistent downward trend despite the gradual reduction and eventual discontinuation of insulin degludec usage. Jacob's body mass initially decreased and remained relatively stable, with a slight increase observed in June 2022. Following the adjustment of semaglutide (SEMA) to 1 mg and the discontinuation of insulin, his body mass started decreasing again. These findings suggest that the combination of medication adjustments, including increased SEMA dosage and insulin discontinuation, contributed to improved glycemic control and body mass management.

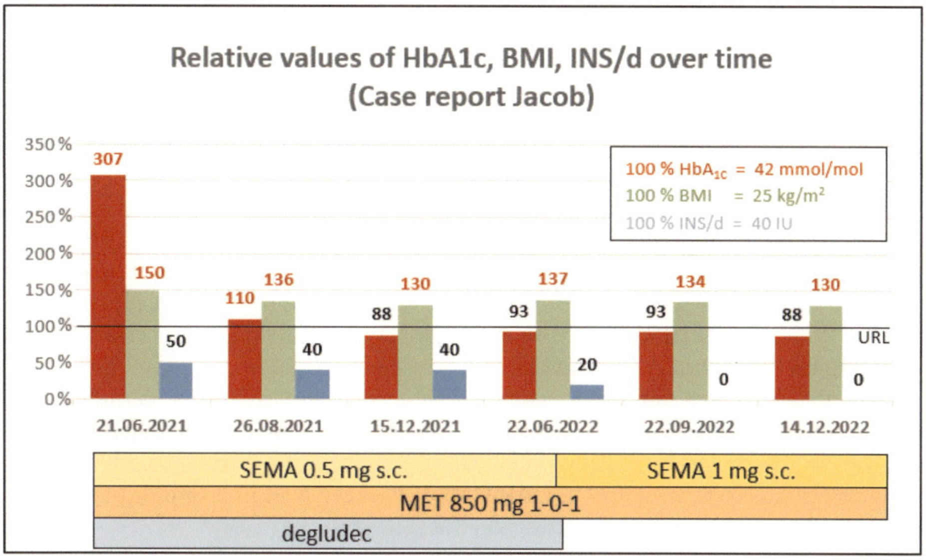

Figure 27.
The relative HbA_{1c} values demonstrate a noteworthy improvement in Jacob's response to treatment, decreasing from an initial value of 307–110% in relationship with the reference value. This indicates an effective treatment combination. Over 6 months, HbA_{1c} levels continued to decrease and remained below the highest reference value, shown in black. Insulin usage gradually declined and was discontinued in July 2022. Jacob's body mass initially decreased and remained relatively stable thereafter.

necessitating adjustments to his medication. The dose of insulin degludec was reduced, while the dose of SEMA was increased to 1 mg. This treatment adjustment resulted in further improvement in Jacob's condition.

By the end of July 2022, insulin degludec was completely discontinued, and Jacob continued his treatment with SEMA and MET alone. Despite the discontinuation of insulin, Jacob's HbA_{1c} remained stable at 39 mmol/mol, indicating sustained blood glucose control. Additionally, there was a slight decrease in body mass by 3 kg, demonstrating the ongoing success of the treatment approach in managing Jacob's body mass.

Looking ahead: To continue Jacob's treatment regimen to keep HbA_{1c} and INS/d under 100% of relative values. Reduction of his body mass is needed.

3. Discussion

Amy's case report highlights the important role of healthcare providers and families in managing the challenges imposed by both poorly regulated diabetes and advancing cognitive impairment.

Bejamin's case underscores the potential benefits of GLP-1 agonists in managing complex metabolic conditions. It provides valuable insights into developing personalized and effective treatment plans for individuals diagnosed with DM2 and Metabolic Syndrome, emphasizing the importance of body mass management in their overall health improvement.

Connor's case report highlights the significance of a comprehensive and tailored approach to managing T2D. Ongoing monitoring, frequent communication, and the timely implementation of interventions contributed to his improved glycemic control and overall well-being. This case underscores the importance of patient engagement and individualized care in optimizing the management of chronic conditions. The question is whether a person with T2D should have lower levels of HbA_{1c} at the expense of having a higher body mass or vice versa.

David's case report illuminates a pathophysiological approach to type 2 diabetes management, emphasizing the intricate interplay between external insulin utilization, glycemic control, and body mass modulation.

Managing diabetes in polymorbid patients like Emma requires a tailored and evolving treatment approach. Her successful glycemic optimization with the GLP-1 agonist and insulin therapy highlights the importance of exploring novel therapeutic options to address changing patient needs. Continuous monitoring and adjustments in treatment remain crucial to achieving and sustaining optimal glycemic control and mitigating the impact of comorbidities.

Fatima's case report underscores the intricate management approach in diabetes, emphasizing the synergistic use of insulin pump therapy, medication adjustments, and lifestyle modifications. Despite challenges, her glycemic control notably improved with a combination of oral SEMA, DAPA/MET, and the insulin pump, leading to a notable body mass decrease and reduced HbA_{1c} levels.

Henry's case report exemplifies the effectiveness of a comprehensive therapeutic approach utilizing a combination of MET, DAPA, and oral SEMA in HbA_{1c} and appetite control. Despite initial challenges in glycemic control, the incorporation of this medication resulted in improvements. The introduction of oral SEMA led to notable appetite reduction, body mass reduction, and decreased HbA_{1c} levels. This case emphasizes the potential of tailored multi-drug interventions in addressing complex metabolic conditions and underscores the importance of addressing lifestyle factors alongside pharmaceutical interventions for long-term success.

Gerry's case report highlights the intricate management of T2D and heart failure, emphasizing the significance of tailored medication adjustments and lifestyle modifications. The individualized approach employed to address Gerry's comorbid conditions led to improvements in glycemic control and cardiovascular health. Despite challenges in achieving optimal body mass and HbA_{1c} levels, his case underscores the complexity of managing multiple conditions and the need for adaptable treatment strategies.

Irene's case report complex medical history and combination therapy facilitated improvements in glycemic control and body mass reduction. The cautious adjustment of medication in response to her evolving needs, along with considerations for her cardiovascular health, played a pivotal role in achieving positive outcomes. Irene's case underscores the importance of tailoring treatment plans to address individual patient characteristics and comorbidities, with ongoing adjustments guided by both therapeutic efficacy and potential side effects.

Jacob's case exemplifies the potential benefits of a pathophysiology-oriented approach to treating type 2 diabetes mellitus. By combining SEMA and MET, Jacob achieved not only considerable body mass loss but also remarkable improvements in glycemic control. The tailored treatment regimen not only led to reduced reliance on external insulin but also demonstrated the dynamic relationship between body mass, glycemic control, and medication management.

4. Conclusion

Pathophysiology-oriented approach to treating type 2 diabetes, with early utilization of medication such as metformin and incretin-based therapies, offers a promising outcome of improvement of well-being. By targeting the underlying mechanisms driving insulin resistance and glucose dysregulation, this approach holds the potential to improve glycemic control and mitigate associated risks. Pairing pharmaceutical interventions with lifestyle modifications and education amplifies the efficiency of this strategy. As treatment plans continue to evolve, tailoring treatments to individual pathophysiological profiles could further refine type 2 diabetes management, leading to a more personalized and effective era of care.

Acknowledgements

Our deepest thanks go to the Department of Internal Medicine II – Gastroenterology and Geriatrics, University Hospital Olomouc, along with the Department of Physiology, Faculty of Medicine and Dentistry, Palacký University Olomouc, Czech Republic.

Abbreviations

ADA	American Diabetes Association
BM	Body mass
BMI	Body mass index
CGM	Continuous glucose monitoring
CSII	Continuous subcutaneous insulin infusion
INS/d	Insulin used per day
DAPA	Dapagliflozin
EASD	European Association for the Study of Diabetes
eGFR	Estimated glomerular filtration rate
Fiasp	Faster insulin aspart
GIP	Glucoso-dependent insulinotropic peptide
GLP-1 RA	Glucagon-like peptide receptor agonist
HbA_{1c}	Hemoglobin A_{1c}, glycated hemoglobin
HDL	High-density lipoprotein
IDegLira	Insulin degludec and liraglutide *fixed combination
INS/d	Insulin/day
LDL	Low-density lipoprotein
MDI	Multiple daily insulin
MET	Metformin
PG	Plasma glucose
SEMA	Semaglutide
SGLT2	Sodium-glucose cotransporter 2
SMPG	Self-monitoring of plasma glucose
T2D	Type 2 diabetes
TAG	Triacylglycerols
URL	Upper reference limit
IU	International unit of insulin

Author details

Noemi Nováková[1,2*], Martin Nezval[1,2] and Viktória Molnárová[1,2]

1 Department of Internal Medicine II – Gastroenterology and Geriatrics, University Hospital Olomouc, Czech Republic

2 Department of Physiology, Palacký University Olomouc Faculty of Medicine and Dentistry, Olomouc, Czech Republic

*Address all correspondence to: noemkak@gmail.com

References

[1] ElSayed NA, Aleppo G, Aroda VR, Bannuru RR, Brown FM, Bruemmer D, et al. On behalf of the American Diabetes Association, addendum. 2. Classification and diagnosis of diabetes: Standards of Care in Diabetes—2023. Diabetes Care. 2023;**46**(Suppl. 1):S19-S40. DOI: 10.2337/dc23-ad08

[2] Landgraf R, Aberle J, Birkenfeld AL, Gallwitz B, Kellerer M, Klein H, et al. Therapy of type 2 diabetes. Experimental Clinical Endocrinology Diabetes. 2019; **127**(S 011):S73-S92. DOI: 10.1055/a-1018-9106

[3] ElSayed NA, Aleppo G, Aroda VR, Bannuru RR, Brown FM, Bruemmer D, et al. Pharmacologic approaches to glycemic treatment: standards of care in diabetes—2023. Diabetes Care. 2023;**46** (Suppl 1):S140-S157. DOI: 10.2337/dc23-S009

[4] Kahn SE, Cooper ME, Del Prato S. Pathophysiology and treatment of type 2 diabetes: Perspectives on the past, present, and future. Lancet. 2014; **383**(9922):1068-1083. DOI: 10.1016/S0140-6736(13)62154-6

[5] ElSayed NA, Aleppo G, Aroda VR, Bannuru RR, Brown FM, Bruemmer D, et al. Glycemic targets: Standards of care in diabetes—2023. Diabetes Care. 2023; **46**(Suppl. 1):S97-S110. DOI: 10.2337/dc23-S006

[6] ElSayed NA, Aleppo G, Aroda VR, Bannuru RR, Brown FM, Bruemmer D, et al. Older adults: Standards of care in diabetes—2023. Diabetes Care. 2023; **46**(1):S216-S229. DOI: 10.2337/dc23-S013

[7] Davies MJ, Aroda VR, Collins BS, et al. Management of hyperglycemia in type 2 diabetes, 2022. A consensus report by the American Diabetes Association (ADA) and the European Association for the Study of diabetes (EASD). Diabetologia. 2022;**65**:1925-1966. DOI: 10.1007/s00125-022-05787-2

[8] Sanchez-Rangel E, Inzucchi SE. Metformin: Clinical use in type 2 diabetes. Diabetologia. 2017;**60**: 1586-1593. DOI: 10.1007/s00125-017-4336-x

[9] Artasensi A, Pedretti A, Vistoli G, Fumagalli L. Type 2 diabetes mellitus: A review of multi-target drugs. Molecules. 1987;**2020**:25. DOI: 10.3390/molecules25081987

[10] ElSayed NA, Aleppo G, Aroda VR, Bannuru RR, Brown FM, Bruemmer D, et al. Obesity and weight management for the prevention and treatment of type 2 diabetes: Standards of care in diabetes—2023. Diabetes Care. 2023;**46**(Suppl. 1): S128-S139. DOI: 10.2337/dc23-S008

[11] Chlup R, Kaňa R, Hanáčková L, Zálešáková H, Doubravová B. Pathophysiologic approach to type 2 diabetes management: One Centre experience 1980–2020 [Internet]. In: Type 2 Diabetes - from Pathophysiology to Cyber Systems. London, UK, London, UK: IntechOpen; 2021. DOI: 10.5772/intechopen.96237

[12] Inzucchi SE, Bergenstal RM, Buse JB, Diamant M, Ferrannini E, Nauck M, et al. Management of hyperglycemia in type 2 diabetes, 2015: A patient-centered approach: Update to a position statement of the American Diabetes Association and the European Association for the Study of diabetes. Diabetes Care. 2015; **38**(1):140-149. DOI: 10.2337/dc14-2441

[13] Chlup R, Kaňa R, Polcerová J, Zálešáková H, Ramík Z. Možnosti léčby

diabetu 2. Typu při oslabení kognitivních funkcí. “Syndrom trosečníka (cast away)”. (outlook of T2D treatment in patient’s cognitive deterioration – “cast away syndrome”). Kazuistiky v diabetologii (Diabetes Case Reports). Czech. 2019;**17**(2):35-40

[14] Chlup R, Runzis S, Castaneda J, Lee S, Nguyen X, Cohen O. Complex assessment of metabolic effectiveness of insulin pump therapy in patients with type 2 diabetes beyond HbA1c reduction. Diabetes Technology and Therapeutics. 2018;**20**(2):153-159

[15] Freckmann G, Buck S, Waldenmaier D, Kulzer B, Schnell O, Gelchsheimer U, et al. Insulin pump therapy for patients with type 2 diabetes mellitus: Evidence, current barriers, and new technologies. Journal of Diabetes Science and Technology. 2021;**15**(4): 901-915. DOI: 10.1177/1932296820928100

[16] Rodbard HW, Lingvay I, Reed J, et al. Semaglutide added to basal insulin in type 2 diabetes (SUSTAIN 5): A randomized, controlled trial. The Journal of Clinical Endocrinology and Metabolism. 2018;**103**(6):2291-2301

[17] Marso SP, Bain SC, Consoli A, Eliaschewitz FG, Jódar E, Leiter LA, et al. Semaglutide and cardiovascular outcomes in patients with type 2 diabetes. The New England Journal of Medicine. 2016;**375**(19):1834-1844. DOI: 10.1056/NEJMoa1607141

Chapter 15

Outcomes of Type 2 Diabetes Management: One Center Experience 2015–2023

Rudolf Chlup, Hana Zálešáková, Jiřina Gottwaldová, Michal Trefil, Jana Zapletalová, Richard Kaňa, Lada Hanáčková, Milena Bretšnajdrová, Přemysl Falt and Zdenka Polzerová

Abstract

The purpose of this chapter was (1) to identify the frequency of employing different kinds of medication (beta-stimulators, metformin, gliflozins, incretins and/or insulins, pioglitazone, statins, fibrates), (2) to assess global metabolic effectiveness of this medication in a walk-in diabetes center, and (3) to estimate frequency of HbA1c measurements in people admitted to hospital. Methods: In 200 people with T2D (age 24–95 y, 105 men) HbA1c, BM, BMI, blood pressure [BP], lipoproteins HDL, LDL, TAG, eGFR, proteinuria were assessed. Individual observation periods took in the range of 0.5–8.8 years. Student's t-test, Wilcoxon signed-rank test with Bonferroni correction and Spearman analysis were used to asses changes between the first and the last visit. $P < 0.05$ was considered as significant. In conclusion, reduction of HbA1c from start values of 52.6 (31.5–173.0) to 46.6 (31.5–116.6) mmol/mol along with reduction of BMI from 26.7 (16.0–45.3) to 25.4 (15.4–42.2) kg/m^2 ($P < 0.0001$) and correlation of delta HbA1c with delta BMI ($r = 0.209$, $p = 0.003$) confirmed global metabolic effectiveness of medication used in the walk-in diabetes center where the HbA1c was estimated 2–3 times per year in each subject whereas in hospital wards mostly once in up to 15% of admitted T2D patients.

Keywords: HbA1c, lipoproteins, estimated glomerular filtration rate, albuminuria, blood pressure, body mass, metformin, insulin, incretins, dapagliflozin, statins, quality of life, education, glucometers, continuous glucose monitoring, insulin pumps

1. Introduction

This chapter is focused on outcomes of routine management of people with type 2 diabetes (T2D) carried out at a diabetes center (Moravský Beroun, Institute of Specialized Treatment Paseka) in close cooperation with the Diabetes Center of the Teaching Hospital and Palacký University Olomouc.

The terminal objective of T2D treatment has been defined as "long active life without frustrating complications." Clinical and laboratory surrogate markers of metabolic balance and cardiovascular/renal protectivity have served to measure the immediate therapeutic effect.

From the beginning of the third millennium, the pathophysiological approach has offered optimistic perspectives [1]. Important papers [2–62] are cited throughout the entire chapter. Several studies focused on individual drug classes such as insulin preparations [5–12, 17], incretin preparations [13–16, 18–29] and gliflozins [30–34]. New technologies such as SMPG [4], CGM [7, 37, 38], insulin pens [8] and CSII [5, 6] became a part of daily routine. However, assessment of effectiveness of center-related therapeutic methods has not been routinely performed. Therefore, the purpose of this retrospective observational study was (1) to identify how frequently the recent medication with metformin, gliflozins, incretins, insulins and hypolipidemics was prescribed in a single walk-in diabetes center, (2) to assess global effectiveness of this medication on individuals with T2D attending this center and (3) to compare frequency of HbA1c measurements in this center and in people admitted to two independent departments of internal medicine and geriatrics in a teaching hospital.

2. Methods

2.1 Schedule of routine check-ups in the diabetes center

- Routine clinical check-ups including assessment of a recent 10-point PG profile, body mass (BM), BMI, heart rate and BP have been performed in 3-month intervals.

- Laboratory parameters (fasting S-Glucose, HbA1c, blood count, U-glucose, U-protein, serum concentration of uric acid, bilirubin, C-reactive protein, sodium, potassium, chlorides, calcium, magnesium, ALT, AST, GMT, ALP, alfa amylase, lipoproteins cholesterol, HDL, LDL, TAG, total protein, albumin, thyroid-stimulating hormone [TSH], triiodothyronine [T3], free thyroxine [fT4], creatinine, estimated glomerular filtration rate [eGFR] and urinalysis) have been estimated in 6-month intervals or more frequently. Laboratory analyzer COBAS Integra 400 and accredited methods were used [2, 3].

- Eye screening has been performed once a year. Other consultations (neurology, cardiology, gastroenterology, urology, gynecology, etc.) have been provided in specialized centers.

2.2 Characteristics of people with T2D attending the center in the course of the study (January 1, 2015: May 15, 2023)

All adults with T2D who, throughout the entire 9-year study period, have passed at least two routine visits involving estimation of HbA1c, BM and other surrogate markers were regularly followed with their routine check-ups and included in statistical evaluation.

	Absolute numbers (N)	Relative numbers	Age in the year 2023 [years]	
			Mean ± SD	Median, min, max
T2D (all)	200	100%	—	—
Men (all)	105	52.5%	—	—
Women (all)	95	47.5%	—	—
HbA1c estimations (all)	2662	100%	—	—
T2D followed continuously over the entire study period	66	33%	68.8 ± 10.6	70 32.4–91.5

Table 1.
T2Ds who (throughout the entire 9-year study period) have passed at least two routine visits comprising estimation of HbA1c and BM.

Year	2015	2016	2017	2018	2019	2020	2021	2022	2023
No of persons per year	135	163	161	163	151	139	138	132	97
Age mean of N total [years]	64.2	65.1	65.7	65.7	66.7	66.5	66.9	66.9	67.7
SD	10.9	11.2	11.2	11.4	11.3	11.4	11.6	11.5	11.0
Age Median of N total [years]	65.3	66.3	66.7	67.0	67.7	67.9	68.0	67.5	67.3
Min	24.4	25.4	26.4	27.4	28.4	29.4	30.4	31.4	32.4
Max	88.1	89.1	90.1	91.1	92.1	93.1	94.1	95.1	91.6
No of HbA1c per year	415	400	366	358	297	263	279	284	n/a
No of HbA1c per person/year	3.0	2.5	2.3	2.2	2.0	1.9	2.0	2.2	n/a

Mean ± SD, median (min, max). Number of HbA1c estimations per year.

Table 2.
Number (No) and age [years] of all individuals with T2D attending the diabetes center in respective year.

There was a total of 200 T2Ds, but only 66 (33%) of them were routinely followed until 2023, which was a variable period of time. In addition, in 2023, only 97 out of 132 people attended their last check-up before the terminal study date of May 15, 2023 (**Tables 1** and **2**).

2.3 Clinical and laboratory equipment and investigations

All T2Ds were trained in self-monitoring of plasma glucose (SMPG). Glucometers Calla (recently replaced by Galileo Glu/Ket), Wellion, Austria, employing generally glucose-oxidase strips were used (**Figure 1**). Glucometers Contour, Ascencia, employing glucose-dehydrogenase strips, were applied to people on the insulin pump paradigm (**Figure 2**) due to its wireless transfer of glucometer results to the insulin pump. Recently, a hybrid pump MiniMed 780 G, Medtronic, CA, USA, and glucometer Contour Plus One have been introduced.

Before each visit, each person was expected to provide a 10-point glycemic profile containing data on food and medication **Figure 3** [4]. People using hybrid insulin pumps with glucose sensors have their glycemic curves printed using software Carelink (**Figure 4**).

In each visit, BP, heart rate and BM were measured (**Figures 5** and **6**).

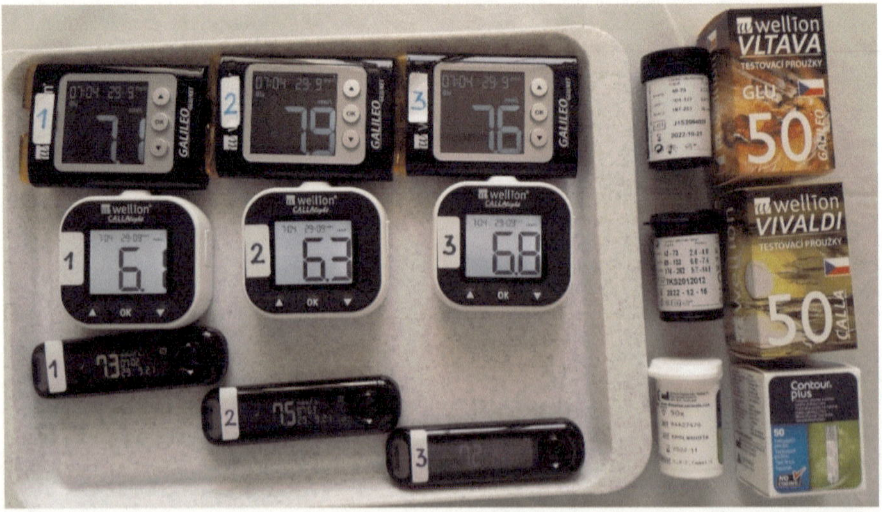

Figure 1.
Three glucometer strip systems: Galileo Glu/Ket (above), Calla (in the middle) and contour plus one (below). All nine glucometers are showing different values of plasma glucose concentration estimated in the same drop of blood collected from one finger-prick. Variability of the results appears to be lower when comparing the same-name glucometers.

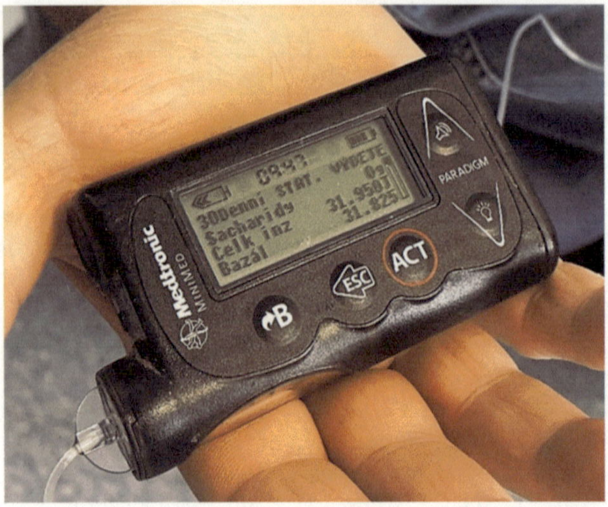

Figure 2.
Insulin pump paradigm 754 MiniMed, Medtronic, CA, USA, displaying: Mean INS/d (31.950 U in a span of 30 days) [5–7].

2.4 Design of the chapter

The data was obtained from electronic files of the walk-in diabetes center, protected with codes and ordered according to two scales, each scale aiming at specific targets:

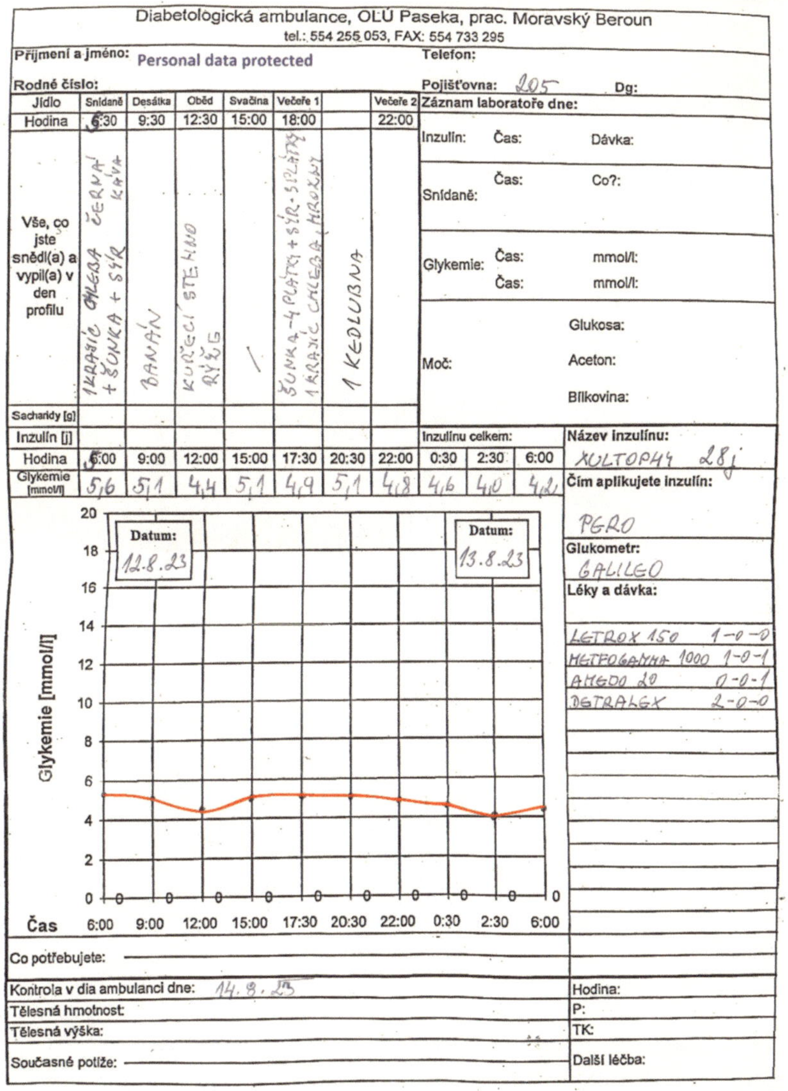

Figure 3.

Ten-point glycemic profile containing self-monitoring data including nutrition and medication. This document is provided by each person with T2D before each check-up.

1. *Study-period-related time scale* considering all individuals with T2D in each individual year. This scale has been employed to demonstrate the routine capacity of the diabetes center including frequency of individuals treated according to recommended pathophysiology-based principles with beta cell stimulators, metformin, dapagliflozin, DPP4 inhibitors, incretin preparations, insulins and hypolipidemics.

2. *The person-related visit scale considers* each individual from his/her first visit (V-START) to his/her last visit (V-END). Only visits where HbA1c was measured have been considered. In each individual, 1 to 4 HbA1c measurements per year (along with other surrogate markers) were performed. Mean values of HbA1c

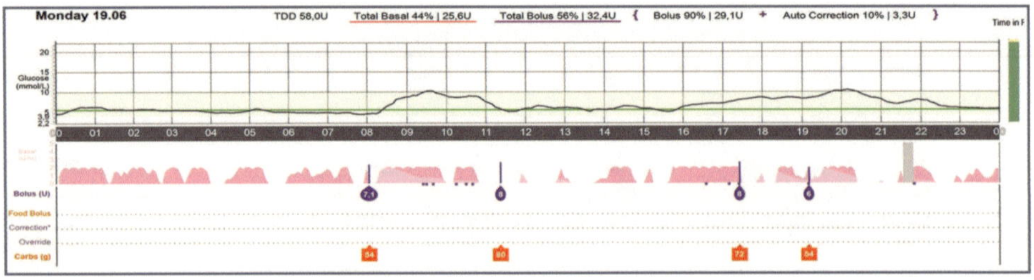

Figure 4.
The graph shows data collected with a hybrid pump MiniMed 780G within the span of 1 day. Glycemia-black line, target range (3.9–10.0 mmol/l) highlighted in green, INS basal in pink, INS bolus in blue, meals in brown. Accessible with name and password. Taken from www.carelink.minimed.eu.

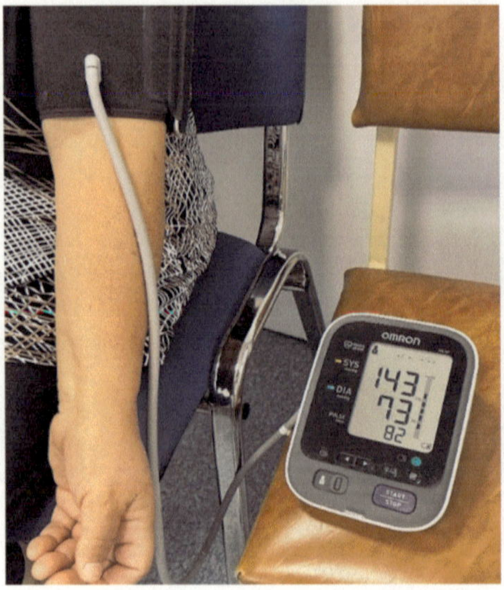

Figure 5.
Clinical investigation: Measuring blood pressure and heart rate using a digital tonometer.

calculated in each individual person for each individual year of his/her observational period was considered as a Visit, e.g.: V1 = mean of all HbA1c values estimated in the first year of one's observation; V2 = mean of HbA1c values estimated in the year following the V1 year, etc. Difference between HbA1c values at V-START and V-END was assessed, as well as differences of BMI and other relevant surrogate markers, to assess effectiveness of global diabetes management on individuals with T2D attending the center.

Next, the frequency of HbA1c estimations in patients admitted to internal (INT) and geriatric (GER) departments in the years 2015–2022 was recognized from the electronic database of the authors' institution.

2.5 Statistical analysis

Statistical analysis was performed using the IBM SPSS Statistics for Windows, version 23 (IBM Corp., Armonk, NY, USA). Standard descriptive statistics were used to summarize the data for continuous non-normal variables (checked by means of the

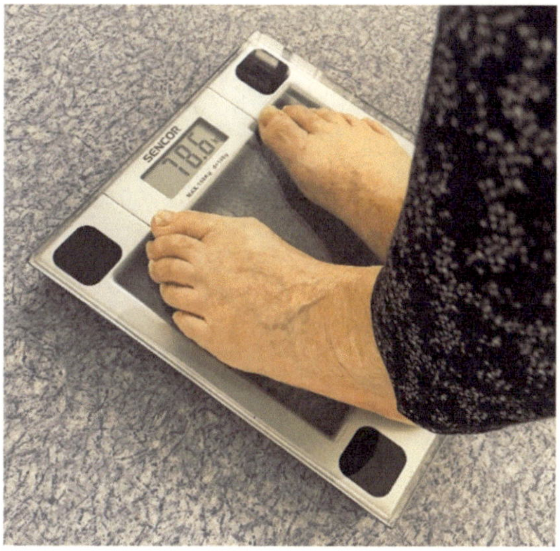

Figure 6.
Clinical investigation: Measuring body mass by means of a digital scale.

Shapiro–Wilk test). Wilcoxon signed-rank test with Bonferroni correction was used to assess the changes (Δ delta) of the parameters depicting the therapeutic effectiveness. Spearman correlation analysis was used to find an association between BMI and HbA1c. A significance level of $P < 0.05$ was considered meaningful.

3. Results

3.1 Frequency of various kinds of medication over the study years 2015–2023

The absolute/relative numbers of individuals with T2D treated with beta-stimulators, metformin, dapagliflozin, incretin preparations, insulins and hypolipidemics are presented according to the study period-related time scale (**Table 3**, **Figures 7** and **8**).

Year	**2015**	**2016**	**2017**	**2018**	**2019**	**2020**	**2021**	**2022**	**2023**
N of attending T2D/y	135	163	161	163	151	139	138	132	97
Beta-stimulator (glinide)	2	1	1	1	1	1	1	1	1
Beta-stimulator (S-urea)	0	0	0	0	0	0	1	1	1
Metformin[a]	119	111	105	102	92	106	109	82	54
Metformins' % of N	88%	68%	65%	63%	61%	76%	79%	62%	56%
Dapagliflozin	32	10	4	3	2	3	2	6	5
Dapagliflozin+Metformin	19	48	47	44	57	53	52	46	43
DAPAs'sum (n)	51	58	51	47	59	56	54	52	48
DAPAs' % of N	38%	36%	32%	29%	39%	40%	39%	62%	50%

Year	2015	2016	2017	2018	2019	2020	2021	2022	2023
iDPP4 (gliptin+ met)	32	27	19	22	14	6	6	5	4
Incretin Exenatide	5	6	4	3	3	0	0	0	0
Incretin Liraglutide	15	22	21	12	5	0	0	0	0
Incretin in IDegLira	0	2	11	26	27	28	26	25	19
Incretin Semaglutide sc.	0	0	0	0	14	17	28	33	22
Incretin Semaglutide tbl.	0	0	0	0	0	0	4	10	17
Incretins' sum (n)	20	30	36	41	49	45	58	68	58
Incretins' % of N	15%	18%	22%	25%	32%	32%	42%	52%	60%
Insulin Aspart lag	31	33	29	8	3	0	0	0	0
Insulin Aspart pen	33	42	38	14	9	8	5	2	2
Insulin Aspart lag+pen	64	75	67	32	12	8	5	2	2
Insulin Fiasp (lag+pen)	0	0	19	42	38	37	32	29	23
Short INSs' sum (n)	64	75	88	74	50	45	37	31	25
Short INSs' % of N	47%	46%	55%	45%	33%	32%	27%	23%	26%
Insulin Detemir	14	28	31	25	9	4	2	2	0
Insulin Degludec	0	0	0	0	18	22	22	18	14
Insulin IDegLira	0	2	11	26	27	28	26	25	19
Long INSs' sum (n)	14	30	42	51	54	54	50	45	33
Long INSs' % of N	10%	18%	26%	31%	36%	39%	36%	34%	34%
Pioglitazon	0	0	0	0	1	1	2	3	1
Atorvastatin	N/A	48	79	84	75	69	59	55	46
Rosuvastatin	0	30	34	25	27	28	28	23	22
Statins' sum (n)	N/A	78	113	109	102	97	87	78	68
Statins' % of N	N/A	48%	70%	67%	68%	70%	63%	59%	70%
Fibrates	0	0	5	7	11	12	15	14	11

Data were taken from the electronic database of the center. The percentage is related to the number (N) of all individuals who attended the diabetes center in the given year.
[a]Consider also the numbers of combined preparations DAPA+MET and gliptin +MET.

Table 3.
Absolute numbers (N) of all subjects attending the diabetes center and numbers of subjects treated with respective medication (highlighted by colors), in each year from January 1, 2015 to May 15, 2023.

3.2 The development of metabolic surrogate markers over person-related observation periods V1–V9

In a total of 200 adults who attended the diabetes center from 2015 to 2023, the following parameters (surrogate markers of therapeutic efficiency) were estimated and assessed:

- Glycated hemoglobin HbA1c (**Table 4, Figure 9**)
- BM (**Table 5, Figure 10**)

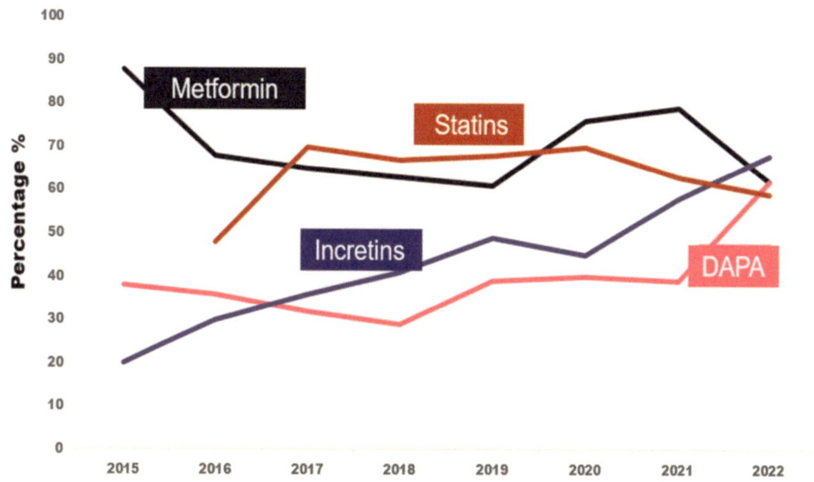

Figure 7.
Relative numbers (% related to N of subjects with T2D attending the diabetes center in the given year) of individuals, who were treated with metformin, dapagliflozin and incretin preparations are plotted according to the study-period-related time scale.

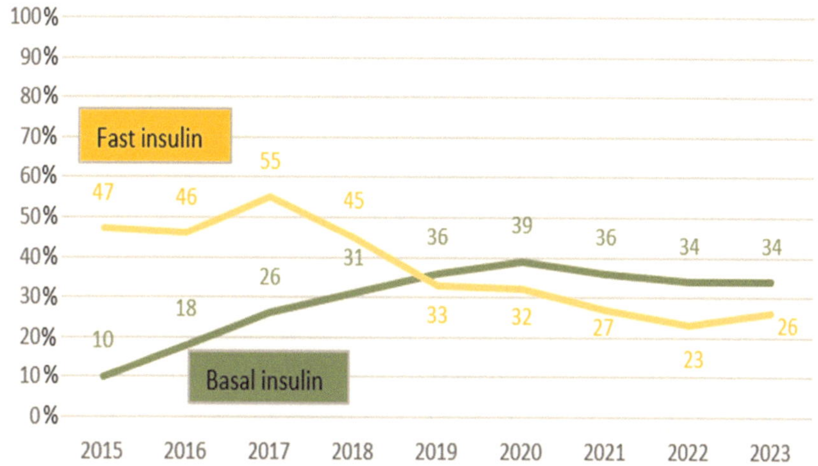

Figure 8.
Relative numbers (% related to N of subjects with T2D attending the diabetes center in the given year) of individuals who were treated with basal insulins and bolus (short-acting) insulins are plotted according to the study-period-related time scale.

- BMI (**Table 6**)
- Heart rate (beats per minute), blood pressure systolic, blood pressure diastolic (**Table 7**)
- Lipoproteins: high-density lipoprotein cholesterol (HDLC), low-density lipoprotein cholesterol (LDLC), TAG; TSH, C-reactive protein (CRP) (**Table 8**)
- Bilirubin, GMT, AST, ALP, uric acid (**Table 9**)
- Albumin, creatinine, urea, eGFR (**Table 10**)

- Blood count, hemoglobin concentration in blood, packed cell volume (**Table 11**)
- Proteinuria and glycosuria (absolute numbers (N) and percentage (%) of positive findings at respective visits (V1–V9) (**Table 12**).

Person-related Visit	HbA1c V1	HbA1c V2	HbA1c V3	HbA1c V4	HbA1c V5	HbA1c V6	HbA1c V7	HbA1c V8	HbA1c V9
N	200	199	176	160	142	127	110	100	66
Mean	56.5	50.9	50.9	51.6	50.0	50.5	51.9	51.5	53.8
SD	18.8	12.4	12.6	14.0	12.2	13.7	14.2	14.5	14.7
Minimum	31.5	30.2	33.2	31.5	33.1	29.3	36.3	36.4	36.3
25th percentile	43.0	42.0	42.1	42.2	41.3	41.5	42.0	41.4	43.7
Median	53	48**	49**	48**	46**	46*	48	47	49
75th percentile	65.8	57.3	55.5	55.9	54.9	54.7	57.3	56.9	59.6
Maximum	173.0	98.9	116.4	116.6	100.7	131.9	118.7	114.6	100.1

Mean ± SD, Median. Significant differences (compared to V1) are highlighted yellow.
P = 0.025.P < 0.001. See **Figure 7** for the upper reference limit (URL).*

Table 4.
The development of HbA1c [mmol/mol] from a person-related visit 1 (N = 200) to a person-related visit 9 (N = 66).

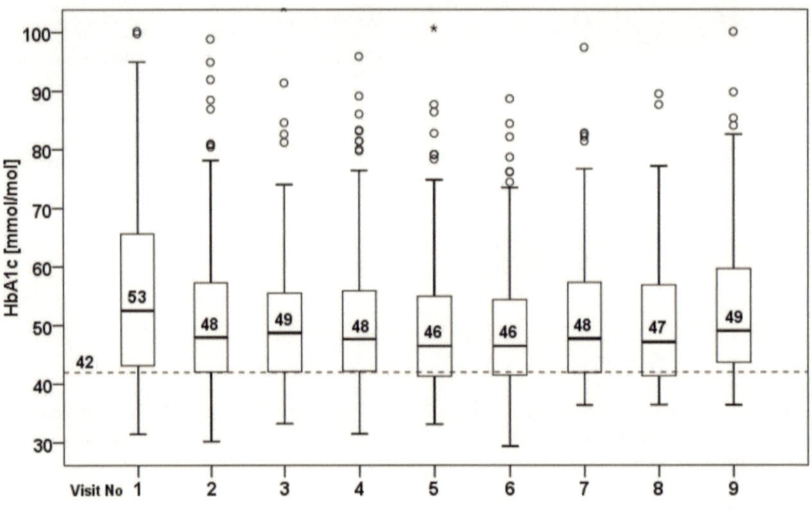

Figure 9.
*The development of HbA1c was recorded according to person-related visits (V1–V9) in T2D who attended the diabetes center from 2015 to 2023. Length of person-related observational periods varies from 1 to 9 years. Total number of people N = 200. Number (N) of people in individual visits is equal to the number of each individual person-related mean value of HbA1c in each year (**Table 4**). Upper reference limit (URL) = 42 mmol/mol.*

Person-related visit	BM V1	BM V2	BM V3	BM V4	BM V5	BM V6	BM V7	BM V8	BM V9
N	195	192	173	159	140	129	113	102	81
Mean	91.5	91.1	90	89.6	90.6	90	88.4	86.6	86.4

Person-related visit	BM V1	BM V2	BM V3	BM V4	BM V5	BM V6	BM V7	BM V8	BM V9
SD	19.9	19.3	19.1	19.2	19.1	19.4	18.8	19.2	18.5
Minimum	52	52	52	47	50	53	51	49	53
25th percentile	75	75	75	74	75	74	75	73	73
Median	91	91**	90**	90**	91**	91**	89**	87**	86**
75th percentile	104	104	104	103	102	101	98	97	96
Maximum	180	175	172	173	174	180	178	179	167

Mean ± SD, median (IQR). Significant differences (compared to V1) are highlighted in yellow.
$^*P < 0.05$.
$^{**}P < 0.001$.
The dates of visits are identical with the dates of visits estimating the HbA1c.

Table 5.
The development of BM [kg] over the person-related observation period, i.e., from visit 1 to visit 9.

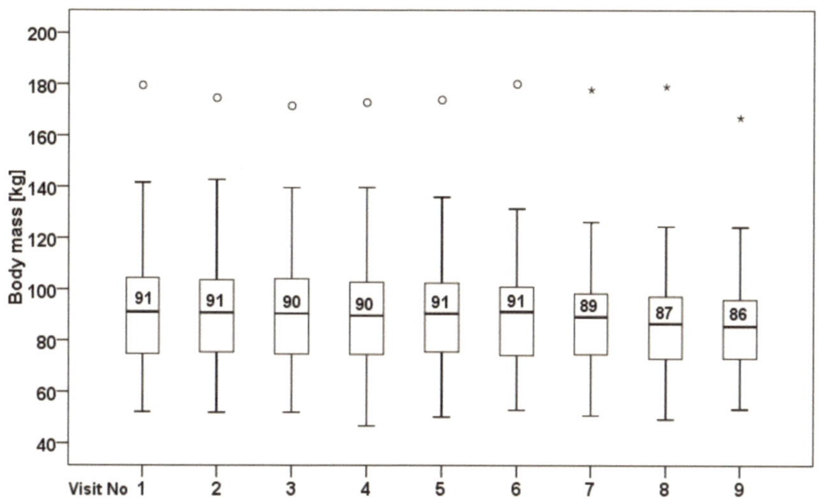

Figure 10.
*The development of BM [kg] in T2D individuals who attended the diabetes center from 2015 to 2023. Median (IQR). Number of people (= number of each individual person-related mean values of BM in each individual year) see **Table** 5. This number need not to be identical with the number of HbA1c estimations due to occasional lack of BM measurement, e.g., the body mass could not be measured in individuals if they were unable to operate the scale.*

Person-related visit	BMI V1	BMI V2	BMI V3	BMI V4	BMI V5	BMI V6	BMI V7	BMI V8	BMI V9
N	195	192	173	159	140	129	113	102	80
Mean	32.1	32.0	31.8	31.7	31.8	31.7	31.2	30.6	30.8
SD	6.0	5.8	5.6	5.6	5.5	5.4	5.4	5.4	5.4
Minimum	20.6	19.6	18.5	17.7	19.1	21.5	21.1	20.7	21.9
25th percentile	27.8	28.0	28.0	27.7	27.9	27.7	27.4	26.9	27.0
Median	32.0	31.8**	31.4**	31.1**	31.3**	31.3**	30.1**	29.8**	30.0**
75th percentile	35.7	35.4	35.5	35.6	35.3	35.0	34.0	33.6	33.4

Person-related visit	BMI V1	BMI V2	BMI V3	BMI V4	BMI V5	BMI V6	BMI V7	BMI V8	BMI V9
Maximum	55.3	55.8	54.5	54.5	53.1	50.1	48.5	47.8	48.5

Mean ± SD. Median (IQR). Significant differences (compared to V1) are highlighted in yellow.
***P < 0.001.*

Table 6.
The development of BMI [kg/m²] over person-related observation periods, i.e., from visit 1 to visit 9.

		Reference range	Visit 1	Visit 5	Visit 7	Visit 9
Heart rate [BPM]	Median		78	80	79	79
	Min	60	56	51	51	53
	Max	90	109	107	107	112
BP syst [mmHg]	Median		138	147**	144**	150**
	Min	(90)	100	91	105	109
	Max	130	193	188	195	202
BP diast [mmHg]	Median		80	85**	84**	85**
	Min	(40)	50	52	66	67
	Max	85	116	110	107	112

Median (min, max). Significant differences (compared to V1) are highlighted in yellow.
***P < 0.001.*

Table 7.
The development of heart rate (BPM – beats per minute) and blood pressure (BP) in person-related visit 1, visit 5, visit 7 and visit 9.

		Reference range	Visit 1	Visit 5	Visit 7	Visit 9
S-HDLC [mmol/l]	Median		1.20	1.13**	1.13**	1.17
	Min	1.00	0.56	0.42	0.46	0.56
	Max	2.10	2.86	2.85	2.04	1.93
S-LDLC [mmol/l]	Median		2.27	1.97	1.80**	1.76**
	Min	1.20	0.79	0.79	0.77	0.87
	Max	2.60	4.79	4.97	3.24	4.37
S-TAG [mmol/l]	Median		1.49	1.48	1.42	1.33
	Min	0.45	0.61	0.49	0.60	0.59
	Max	1.70	6.71	9.34	5.90	6.06
S-TSH	Median		2.50	2.67	2.53	2.67
	Min	0.27	0.01	0.17	0.01	0.01
	Max	4.20	35.3	64.1	19.0	9.6

		Reference range	Visit 1	Visit 5	Visit 7	Visit 9
S-CRP	Median		2.10	1.70	1.55	1.30
	Min	0.00	0.13	0.05	0.30	0.50
	Max	5.00	58.5	44.3	26.7	92.5

Median (min, max). Significant differences (compared to V1) are highlighted in yellow.
***P < 0.001. No difference in TAG, TSH and CRP.*

Table 8.
Data on lipoproteins, thyroid function and inflammation: high-density lipoprotein cholesterol (HDLC), low-density lipoprotein cholesterol (LDLC), triacylglycerols (TAG), thyroid-stimulating hormone (TSH) and C-reactive protein (CRP) in person-related visit 1, visit 5, visit 7 and visit 9.

		Reference range	Visit 1	Visit 5	Visit 7	Visit 9
S-Bil	Median		7.70	7.50	7.48	7.10
	Min	3.4	2.95	3.00	3.15	2.30
	Max	17.0	30.3	28.3	28.5	25.5
S-GMT	Median		0.500	0.378*	0.385*	0.370*
	Min	0.00	0.090	0.105	0.120	0.110
	Max	0.92	26.15	6.17	1.33	7.30
S-AST	Median		0.350	0.385*	0.380	0.353
	Min	0.00	0.180	0.200	0.225	0.210
	Max	0.58	1183	5.980	1.170	1.190
S-ALP	Median		1.23	1.24*	1.17	1.19
	Min	0.66	0.52	0.54	0.57	0.56
	Max	2.20	9.98	4.22	2.88	3.42
S-Uric acid	Median		346	343	332	332
	Min	180.0	167	151	123	152
	Max	420.0	700	648	562	647

Significant differences (compared to V1) are highlighted in yellow.
**P < 0.05. No difference in bilirubin and uric acid.*

Table 9.
Laboratory findings in hepatobiliary disorders: bilirubin (Bil), GMT, AST, ALP and uric acid.

		Reference range	Visit 1	Visit 5	Visit 7	Visit 9
S-albumin [g/l]	Median		45.9	45.0**	45.5	45.6
	Min	35.00	37.0	31.6	39.4	37.8
	Max	50.00	53.3	51.7	50.9	52.7
S-creatinine [umol/l]	Median		71	77**	79	—
	Min	62.0	38	38	37	—
	Max	115.0	714	486	152	—

		Reference range	Visit 1	Visit 5	Visit 7	Visit 9
S-urea [mmol/l]	Median		5.1	5.7**	5.8**	5.8**
	Min	2.90	2.5	2.5	2.3	3.1
	Max	7.50	16.7	21.0	15.9	16.1
eGFR [ml/s]	Median		1.59	1.40**	1.37**	1.38**
	Min	1.000	0.54	0.34	0.36	0.53
	Max	1.500	2.44	2.51	2.17	2.24

*Median (min, max). Occasional small deviations from N (**Table 4**) need to be considered. Significant differences (compared to V1) are highlighted in yellow.*
$^{**}P < 0.001$.

Table 10.
Parameters of renal function: Albumin, creatinine, urea, estimated glomerular filtration rate (eGFR) in person-related visit 1, visit 5, visit 7 and visit 9.

		Reference range	Visit 1	Visit 5	Visit 7	Visit 9
B-Hb [g/l]	Median		142	142	140*	143
	Min	135	94	98	96	78
	Max	175	181	178	179	180
B-Ery [n]	Median		4.78	4.92	4.62*	4.65
	Min	$4.0*10^{12}/l$	3.33	3.20	3.22	3.20
	Max	$5.8*10^{12}/l$	5.76	6.20	6.76	5.79
B-HTC	Median		0.419	0.426	0.415	0.423
	Min	0.400	0.302	0.296	0.276	0.269
	Max	0.500	0.527	0.545	0.598	0.524
B-Leu [n]	Median		8.10	8.40*	7.80	7.70
	Min	$4.0*10^{9}/l$	4.07	4.95	3.50	3.70
	Max	$10.0*10^{9}/l$	15.0	20.0	49.0	17.9
B-Thromb [n]	Median		238	236*	239*	246*
	Min	$150*10^{9}/l$	79	109	100	76
	Max	$400*10^{9}/l$	388	517	405	431

Significant differences (compared to V1) are highlighted in yellow.
$^{*}P < 0.05$. No difference in B-HTC.

Table 11.
Blood count, hemoglobin (B-Hb) and packed cell volume (B-HTC).

	V 1	V 2	V 3	V 4	V 5	V 6	V 7	V 8	V 9
Measurements of proteinuria (N)	186	186	166	154	136	122	108	95	70
Proteinuria positive (n)	21	17	15	11	10	7	6	9	5
Relative (% n out of N)	11.3	9.1	9.0	7.0	7.4	5.7	5.6	9.5	7.1

	V 1	V 2	V 3	V 4	V 5	V 6	V 7	V 8	V 9
Measurements of glycosuria (N)	177	186	168	153	135	122	109	94	73
Glucosuria positive (n)	52	75	68	62	63	58	52	49	36
Relative (% n out of N)	29.4	40.3	40.5	40.5	46.7	47.5	47.7	52.1	49.3

Table 12.
Qualitative urine examination on proteinuria and glucosuria at V1–V9.

The length of person-related observational periods varied. The date (year) of V-START might vary from person to person. Number of people (N) in consequent visits is decreasing as people entering the center later than in 2015 and/or leaving before the terminal visit on May 15, 2023, could attend only a lower number of visits.

3.3 Impact of pathophysiological approach applied over the study period

The study period lasted 9 years (from 2015 to 2023); however, only 66 of 200 attendees took part in all scheduled check-ups.

The person-related observational period started in all individuals (N = 200) at the first measurement (V-START), which might appear in any year, and various timeslapsed until the terminal measurement (V-END) (**Table 13**).

Comparison of the descriptive characteristics of principal surrogate markers, namely, HbA1c and BMI estimated at first and at the last person-related measurement and their delta (V-START) minus (V-END), was applied to assess the impact of the therapeutic approach (**Table 14**).

Spearman correlation analysis revealed a weak positive correlation ($r = 0.209$, $p = 0.003$) between delta (START–END) HbA1c and delta (START–END) BMI.

Figures 11 and **12** demonstrate the distribution of values of HbA1c and BMI at the first measurement (V-START) and at the last measurement (V-END) of the study.

Observational period	**Mean**	**SD**	**Median**	**Minimum**	**Maximum**
Time span [years] between V-START and V-END	5.5	2.4	6.8	0.5	8.8

Table 13.
Length of the person-related observational period in the entire group (N = 200).

Parameter	**Unit**	**Mean**	**SD**	**Median**	**Minimum**	**Maximum**	**p-value**
HbA1c-START	mmol/mol	57.5	20.1	52.6	31.5	173.0	0.0001
HbA1c-END	mmol/mol	51.4	15.0	46.6	31.5	116.6	
DELTA HbA1c	mmol/mol	6.09	20.12	3.27	−41.67	116.68	
BMI-START	kg/m^2	27.0	5.1	26.7	16.0	45.3	< 0.0001
BMI-END	kg/m^2	25.8	4.9	25.4	15.4	42.2	
DELTA BMI	kg/m^2	1.27	2.39	1.21	−5.06	10.37	

Table 14.
Descriptive characteristics of HbA1c and BMI at the START (V-START) and at the end (V-END) of subject-related observational periods and statistical analysis of changes START–END.

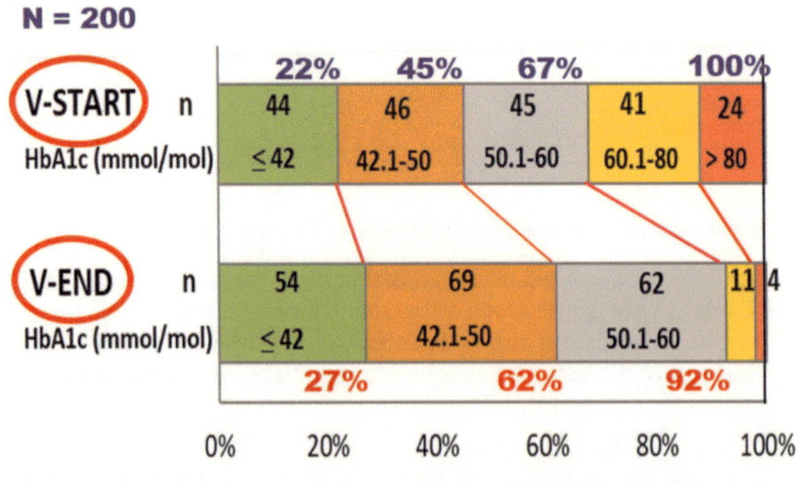

Figure 11.
Distribution of values of HbA1c at the first measurement (V-START) and at the last measurement (V-END) of each individual observation period. N = 200 (=100%).

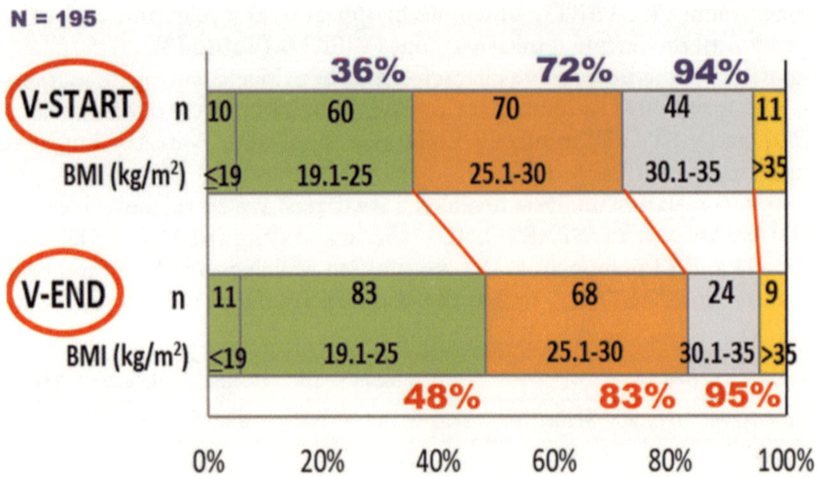

Figure 12.
Distribution of values of BMI at the first measurement (V-START) and at the last measurement (V-END) of each individual observation period. N = 195 (=100%).

3.4 Frequency of HbA1c measurements in people admitted to general hospital

To compare the outcomes of this trial with a routine "state of the art" of everydays' practice, the frequency of HbA1c estimations in people admitted to internal and geriatric departments of a large hospital in the Czech Republic was sought for (**Table 15**).

So, in individual years 2015–2022, HbA1c was measured in approximately 1.4%–6.3% of patients with T2D admitted to the Department of Medicine and in 3–44.6% of patients with T2D admitted to Department of Geriatrics.

	Parameter	2015	2016	2017	2018	2019	2020	2021	2022
INT	N all admitted patients/year	2980	2797	2852	3028	3358	3570	3444	3581
	N T2D on admission/registry	225	257	252	348	354	641	652	653
	Susp. N T2D (=30% of N all)	864	839	856	908	1007	1071	1033	1074
	N of HbA1c estimations/year	54	35	33	19	23	48	14	16
	% of HbA1c related to susp.N T2D	6.3%	4.2%	3.9%	2.1%	2.3%	4.5%	1.4%	1.6%
	% T2D related to N total	7.6	9.2	8.8	11.5	10.5	18.0	18.9	18.2
	% of HbA1c related to N total	1.8%	1.3%	1.2%	0.6%	0.7%	1.3%	0.4%	0.5%
	Mean Age of admitted T2D (years)	73.3	64.8	70.8	74.7	73.3	76.1	70.7	72.4
GER	N of all admitted patients/year	430	535	459	612	656	679	898	710
	N of T2D on admission/registry	70	118	85	158	137	198	236	176
	Susp. N T2D (=30% of N all	129	161	138	184	197	204	269	213
	N of HbA1c estimations/year	6	29	30	23	19	18	120	7
	% of HbA1c related to susp.N T2D	4.7%	18.0%	21.7%	13.0%	9.6%	8.8%	44.6%	3%
	% T2D related to N total	16.3	22.1	18.5	25.8	20.9	29.2	26.3	24.8
	% of HbA1c related to N total	1.4%	5.4%	6.5%	3.8%	2.9%	2.7%	13.4%	1.0%
	Mean age of admitted T2D (years)	75.5	72.0	77.8	77.7	82.5	78.0	74.7	77.7

Data from the electronic database of the authors' institution. N T2D on admission/registry in this table comprises only those people where T2D is registered in the database as the main (principle) condition of admission. The susp. (real) N T2D is assessed to be 30% of N all admitted patients/year to hospital due to various conditions/diagnoses.

Table 15.
Frequency of HbA1c estimations in all patients admitted to internal (INT) and geriatric (GER) departments in the years 2015–2022.

4. Discussion

This chapter focuses on three concerns: (1) to identify the frequency of application of recent drugs, namely, beta-stimulators, metformin, gliflozins, incretins and/or insulins, pioglitazone, statins and fibrates, in a diabetes center and (2) to assess global effectiveness of the T2D management based on medication, physical exercise, meal plan, education, self-monitoring, technical equipment, family background and personal cooperation within the healthcare system and (3) to estimate the frequency of HbA1c measurements in people admitted to hospital (which were used as "control group" attempting to identify potential involvement of non-diabetologists in routine diabetes care).

In the course of previous decades, glycemia and HbA1c were considered to be key markers of therapeutic effectiveness in T2D. Changes in body mass usually took place among marginal side effects of inappropriate diet and lifestyle [17]. On the other hand, changes of current amount of adipose and muscle tissues in the body are associated with availability of endogenous and/or injected insulin along with production of incretins in gut or their therapeutic administering and/or the sensitivity of respective receptors [18–28].

In addition, insulin stimulates appetite. Without insulin, symptoms of T1D including hyperglycemia and reduction of body mass appear. Without incretins, increased appetite leads to obesity and hyperglycemia. In addition, hyperglycemia is supported by escalated activity of SGLT2 in kidneys, resulting in increased reabsorption of glucose from primary urine.

So, euglycemia, optimal body mass and normal lipoproteinemia may be regulated using insulin and/or incretin preparations and/or gliflozins and other medication without delay [16–29].

Despite of frequent discussions dealing with the optimal/acceptable target values of respective metabolic parameters, our attempts aimed to

- good clinical condition without hypoglycemic risks and then
- usual reference range of parameters, i.e., fasting glycemia < 6.0 mmol/l, HbA1c < 42 mmol/mol, BMI < 25 kg/m_2, LDLC < 1.6 mmol/l, etc.
- maximal protection against cardiovascular and renal complications [6–8, 21–36, 51, 52]

The schedule of current clinical and laboratory check-ups, as stated at the beginning of this chapter, was always kept in mind.

The frequency of application of individual drugs (**Table 3**) allowed us to observe that:

- Metformin (including combinations with DAPA or iDPP4) has been widely used (in >95% of N) throughout the entire study.
- Dapagliflozin has been constantly administered to about 50 subjects, mostly in combination with metformin (even though the relative percentage of subjects on DAPA has increased from about 40 to 60% subjects, **Figure** 7).
- The percentage of people on incretins (exenatide, liraglutide and semaglutide) has continuously increased from 15% in 2015 to 60% in 2023 (**Figure** 7).
- The percentage of people on short-acting and faster-acting bolus-insulins decreased from about 50% before 2018 to 26% in 2023 (**Figure 8**). Based on results of impacted studies [9–12], insulin aspart was replaced by Fiasp. Even though in the “mini-trial” from 2019 [8] Fiasp did not lead to any significant improvement of metabolic parameters, 29 out of 31 subjects kept administrating Fiasp.
- The percentage of long-acting insulin users increased from 10% in 2015 to 34% in 2023 (**Figure 8**). We have replaced insulin detemir with insulin degludec in all of them.
- Administrating of beta cells stimulators and/or pioglitazone have always been close to zero.
- Statins have mostly been used in more than 60% of subjects, whereas the LDLC concentration dropped from 2.27 (0.79–4.79) mmol/l at visit 1 to 1.76 (0.87–4.37) mmol/l ($P < 0.001$) at visit 9 (**Table 8**).

The development of key metabolic surrogate markers, namely, HbA1c, BM and BMI may be recognized from **Tables 4-6, Figures** 7 and **8**. In general, their changes appear to be substantially impacted by optimized medication indicated in **Table 3**.

The assessed values of metabolic markers at individual visits are means mostly of two values in each individual year. A significant reduction of HbA1c at V2, V3, V4, V5 and V6 vs. V1 may be seen (**Table 4, Figure 9**). Similarly, a continuous decrease of BM between V1 and V9 was observed (**Table 5, Figure 10**).

In **Figure 11** (distribution of HbA1c values at the START vs. the END) and in **Figure 12** (distribution of BMI at the START vs. the END) is the effect of a complex T2D management clearly recognized: at the end of the study the number of T2D with HbA1c values <60 mmol/mol increased from 135 out of 200 (67%) people with T2D to 185/200 (92%) and only 15/200 (8%) remained higher than 60 mmol/mol. The final BMI < 25 kg/m^2 reached 93 out of 195 (48%) people with T2D in comparison to 70/195 (36%) individuals at the START visit.

Reduction of HbA1c median from start values of 52.6 (31.5–173.0) to 46.6 (31.5–116.6) mmol/mol (P = 0.0001) along with reduction of BMI median from 26.7 (16.0–45.3) to 25.4 (15.4–42.2) kg/m^2 (P < 0.0001, **Table 14**) demonstrated important benefits of a pathophysiology-based management of T2D which has been included into daily routine in the course of subject-related observational period lasting 6.8 (0.5–8.8) years (**Table 13**).

The current state of the art of precision medicine [16, 21–52] does not allow the select "the person related optimal medication" as early as the T2D had been recognized. To date, more therapeutic attempts appear to be necessary to find the most effective and acceptable combination of various drugs.

By reading **Table 3**, it is hard to identify which particular medication resulted in observed metabolic benefits. Two topics appear to be worth the particular assessment, namely, impact of fixed combination IDegLira and incretin receptor agonist semaglutide.

- The impact of combination of incretin with insulin (such as IDegLira) instead of CSII has already been presented [13, 20] and demonstrated the development of HbA1c and BMI over the first period on CSII and over the following period on IDegLira. In the CSII period, the HbA1c decreased in 3/8 T2D individuals and BMI in 4/8. Over the IDegLira period, the HbA1c decreased in 7/8 T2D people (**Figure 13**) and BMI in 7/8 (**Figure 14**). Medication with metformin (2000–3000 mg/day) and other drugs remained without substantial changes over the whole study period. Continuing observation of subject No 4 beyond the last study visit revealed progressive cognitive deterioration resulting in the omission of any medication. So, the increase of HbA1c (**Figure 13**) along with the decrease in BMI (**Figure 14**) may be explained by this condition (see Case report 1 in [20] for details). Finally, IDegLira was preferred in 7/8 T2Ds due to simplicity. Only one lady found the insulin pump more convenient due to the option of prandial boluses, enabling additional meals at any time.

So, management of T2D with a fixed combination of insulin degludec and liraglutide appears to be a promising pathophysiologic approach that is equally or even more effective than long-lasting CSII. A person-related approach needs to be considered.

- Therapeutic potential of a GLP1 receptor agonist semaglutide has already been demonstrated by Sustain and Pioneer studies [1]. In the period 2019–2023, we attempted to assess the impact of injectable and oral semaglutide on BMI, HbA1c and insulin needs in people with T2D [1, 14, 15, 20, 52, 53]. In 2023, a total of 48 T2D (28 men, 20 women), median age of 62.8 (45.0–87.4) years, diabetes duration median of 15.8 (0–27.8) years were assessed. Some of them were treated with injectable SEMA (n sc = 33) using doses up to 1.0 mg/week. The oral SEMA dosing (n oral = 15) started with 3 mg/day and was increased to 14 mg/day within 3 months. **Table 16** shows a significant reduction of HbA1c, BM and INS/d from the Start Visit A to the End Visit C. At Visit C, there were 2 out of 33 PWD2 who refused further treatment with injectable SEMA (due to maldigestion and increase of HbA1c) and 3/15 PWD2 who refused to continue with oral SEMA (due to maldigestion). Hence, 43/48 (90%) PWD2 appreciate their routine treatment with SEMA.

Hence, oral or injectable SEMA appears to be effective means of routine, long-lasting T2D management. Higher doses are worthy of consideration [15]. Our observation is consistent with other studies [1, 18–20] and with recommendations of respected bodies [16]. Preference of its oral or injectable form remains worth further research. Nevertheless, in 5 out of 48 (10%) T2D, maldigestion has not allowed to continue the semaglutide treatment in either form.

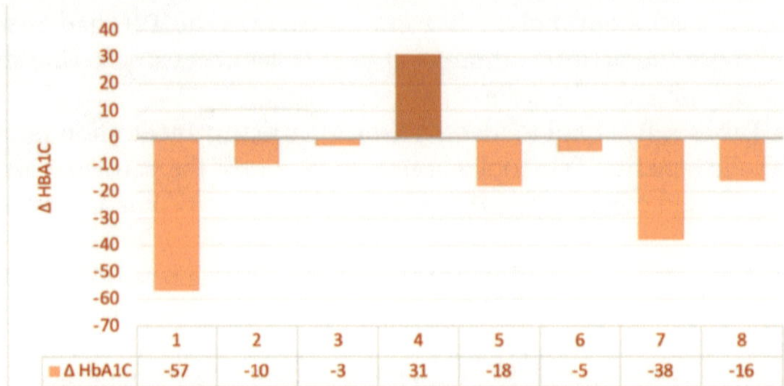

Figure 13.
Reduction of HbA1c [mmol/mol] following the switch from CSII to IDegLira in 7/8 individuals. The increase of HbA1c in subject No 4 became obvious beyond the end of this study: Cognitive deterioration resulting in unrecognized omitting of any medication [20].

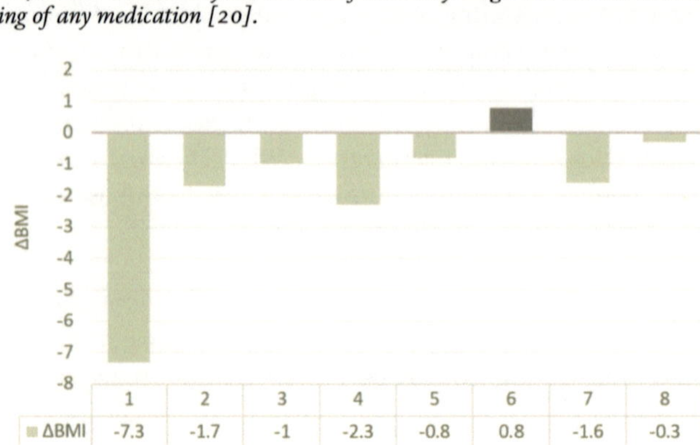

Figure 14.
Reduction of BMI [kg/m²] following the switch from CSII to IDegLira in 7/8 individuals.

Parameter	Visit A (Start)			Visit B (check-up)			Visit C (End)		
	Median	Min	Max	Median	Min	Max	Median	Min	Max
Days from Visit A	n/a	n/a	n/a	154	64	847	439	64	1414
HbA1c [mmol/mol]	60.1	39.9	129.2	51.9	36.0	86.4	48.0	36.7	108.9
Body mass [kg]	99.2	69.4	181.0	96.3	63.4	172.5	93.0	59.5	172.5
BMI [kg/m^2]	34.0	24.6	53.7	32.0	22.1	50.2	31.3	20.7	47.9
Insulin [U/day]	32.5	0.0	80.0	36.0	8.0	80.0	22.1	0.0	68.0
delta HbA1c (C-A)[a]							−6.5	−92.4	37.0
delta BM (C-A)[b]							−5.2	−23.1	4.5
delta BMI (C-A)[b]							−1.9	−10.3	1.7
delta insulin (C-A)[c]							−6.0	−43.9	13.0

Visit A – SEMA start, Visit B – SEMA increase, Visit C – SEMA last check-up. Significant reduction (compared to Visit A) I highlighted in yellow.
[a]P = 0.001;[b]P < 0.0001;[c]P = 0.019.

Table 16.
Changes (delta) of HbA1c, BM, BMI and INS/d.

Routine check-ups of clinical parameters (**Table 7**) revealed a significant increase of systolic and diastolic blood pressure at visit 5, visit 7 and visit 9. Hence, when taking into account the WHO Recommendations from 2023 [54], this finding has been a challenge, resulting in a timely implementation of regular blood pressure self-monitoring by means of a personal meter to make adequate antihypertensive therapy more flexible.

Additional clinical and biochemical parameters such as CRP, TSH (**Table 8**), bilirubin, GMT, alkaline phosphatase, AST, uric acid (**Table 9**), blood count (**Table 11**) have occasionally revealed relevant deviations (e.g., acute bronchitis, cholelithiasis, liver cirrhosis, hypothyroid disease, heart failure, anemia, etc.) which were solved in cooperation with general practitioners.

Renal function was measured using eGFR (**Table 10**). Despite a significant decrease of median eGFR from 1.59 ml/s at visit 1 to 1.38 ml/s at visit 9 the percentage of values in reference range increased. Qualitative urine examination showed the frequency of proteinuria up to 11,3% without any significant change between visit 1 and visit 9 (**Table 12**).

Adverse side effects such as activation of urinary infection when on DAPA, gastrointestinal discomfort at the beginning of incretin administration, and diarrhea when on metformin, appeared occasionally and mostly mild. Hypoglycemia appeared rarely. These complications were treated by adaptation of therapy as recommended. Nevertheless, maldigestion resulting in interruption of semaglutide therapy appeared in about 10% of T2D which need to be further studied.

HbA1c is a basic parameter assessing the effectiveness of diabetes management. In this trial, the real frequency of HbA1c measurements in a specialized diabetes walk-in center was 1.9–3.0 measurements per person per year (**Table 2**).

However, not all hospitals/departments are specialized in diabetes. That is why we attempted to compare some data from this specialized trial with 200 T2D with non-specialized diabetes care in routine practice of a hospital ward.

About 3000 people admitted (due to various diagnoses) yearly to internal and geriatric units of a teaching hospital were used as a control group (**Table 15**).

Frequency of HbA1c estimations in admitted patients served as potential marker of involvement of respective professional departments in diabetes care.

In hospital wards, the HbA1c was estimated in 0.4–13.4% of all patients admitted per year, such as about 2 HbA1c estimations in 100 patients per year. There was a slight difference between the two departments: HbA1c was measured in 1.4–6.3% of patients with T2D yearly admitted to the Department of Medicine and in 3 to 44.6% of patients with T2D yearly admitted to Department of Geriatrics. The high number of HbA1c investigations in 2021 is probably related to the COVID-19 epidemics when special attention was paid to early recognition of diabetes and its complications.

Considering the exciting history of medical research, unexpected complications may interfere with any fascinating perspective [55]. More questions, but enough answers remain [56]. However, human life span on insulin has already exceeded 50- and recently even 80 fruitful years [57, 58].

5. Summary and Conclusions

1. A total of 200 adults were treated in a single walk-in diabetes center. Their individual observation periods took in the range of 6.8 (0.5–8.8) years (median, min-max). At the end of the study, individually adapted antidiabetic and hypolipidemic medication contained metformin (in >95% out of 200 subjects) and/or gliflozins (in up to 60%) and/or incretins (in about 60%) and/or insulins (in about 50%) and/or statins (in up to 70%) and fibrates (in up to 15%).

2. The effectiveness of the global T2D management in the walk-in center was assessed by employing the differences of the HbA1c and BMI values between the first and last visit of subjects. Reduction of HbA1c from start values of 52.6 (31.5–173.0) mmol/mol to 46.6 (31.5–116.6) mmol/mol along with reduction of BMI from 26.7 (16.0–45.3) kg/m^2 to 25.4 (15.4–42.2) kg/m^2 demonstrated important benefits of complex management comprising variable lifestyle, medication, physical exercise, meal plan, education, self-monitoring, technical equipment, family background and personal cooperation within the healthcare system.

3. Frequency of HbA1c measurements in people admitted to the hospital was used as a blinded attempt to identify the potential involvement of non-diabetes departments in routine diabetes care. HbA1c was mostly investigated in less than 15% of yearly admitted patients with T2D whereas in specialized diabetes walk-in center 2.0–3.0 HbA1c measurements per person per year were performed.

So, the outcomes of the presented global approach focusing on implementation of recent medication in people with T2D are challenging. Last but not least, scheduled education, incretin/insulin pens, glucometers, CGM sensors and a flexible health care systém constitute the background of an effective management.

Parts of this review were presented at the Congress of the German Diabetes Association in Berlin, 2021 [13] and 2022 [15], at the Student Scientific Research Conference, Faculty of Medicine and Dentistry, Palacký University Olomouc, 2023 [52] and at the Annual Research Meeting of the Slovakian Diabetes Society, Topolčianky, 2024 [53].

Dedication

This chapter is dedicated to the memory of three professors [59, 60, 61, 62] born in different countries, working at different universities/institutes under oscillating friendly and unfriendly conditions whose lifelong empathy and open minds created fruitful perspectives for people with diabetes and motivated many health care professionals along with students for future diabetes care and research activities:

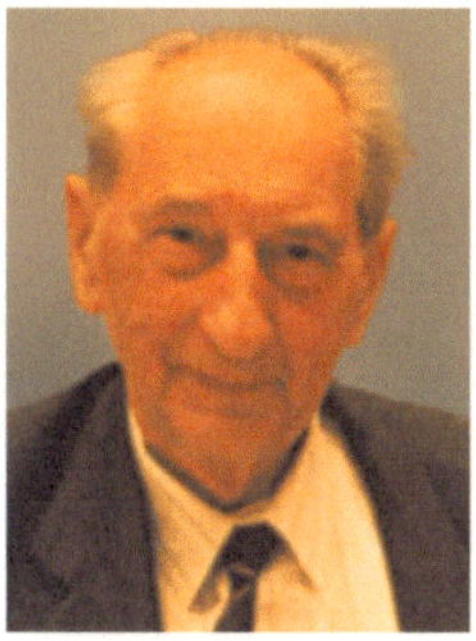

Rudolf Korec
Pavel Josef Safarik Uni Kosice
1921 - 2003

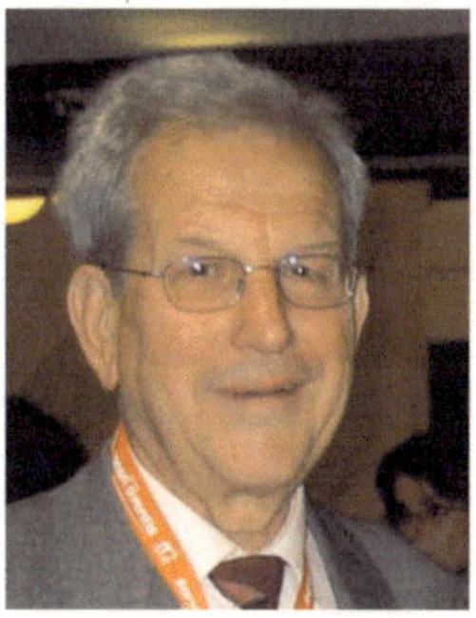

Waldemar Bruns
Institut Karlsburg, Sanatorium Saalfeld
1929 - 2024

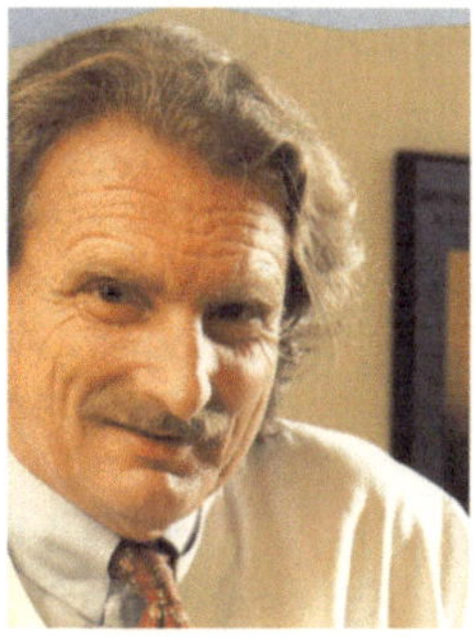

Michael Berger
Heinrich Heine Uni Düsseldorf
1944 - 2002

Acknowledgements

R.C. was in charge of the manuscript design and final text review; H.Z. was responsible for data collection, blood samples and data files; J.G. took care of biochemical investigations; M.T. was in charge of electronic data files and IT operations; J.Z. performed the statistical analysis and provided Figures and Tables; L.H. supervised the performance of therapeutic protocols including HbA1c and 10-point glycemic profiles, R.K., M.B., P.F. and Z.P. supervised the cooperation between walk-in diabetes center and hospital wards, and reviewed the manuscript. There is no conflict of interest.

Special thanks to Stanislava Dudová, Emilia Ďurajková, Lenka Kratochvílová, Michaela Nádvorniková, Jana Polcerová, Svatava Tancosová, Jana Ferancová, Pavel Kolčava, Eva Malá, Dana Masnikosová, Hana Peniaková, Jiří Podivínský, Jana Svobodová, Rastislav Šramko and their teams for outstanding neverending support.

Final acknowledgment belongs to specialists, nursing and other staffs, and students of Palacký University Olomouc (in particular to Zdeněk Ramík, Tzu Hsuan Cheng, Monika Slezáková, Romana Kotačková, Veronika Šálková, Tal Goldstein, Samuel Benyaminov, Biayni Minasyan, Dominika Šimková, Viktória Molnárová, Noemi Nováková, Martin Nezval, Jitka Bačíková), compliant people with diabetes, as well as to Insurance Companies and pharma industry in the Czech Republic.

Those who found this chapter worth of reading surely appreciate the support provided by Palacký University, Teaching Hospital Olomouc, Institute of Specialized Treatment Paseka and other important institutions.

Abbreviations

ADA	American Diabetes Association
B-HTC	packed cell volume

BP	blood pressure
BM	body mass
BMI	body mass index
CGM	continuous glucose monitoring
CSII	continuous subcutaneous insulin infusion
CRP	C-reactive protein
DAPA	dapagliflozin
EASD	European Association for the Study of Diabetes
eGFR	estimated glomerular filtration rate
Fiasp	faster insulin aspart (insulin aspart + vitamin B3)
fS-glucose	fasting serum glucose concentration
fT4	free thyroxin
GIP	glucose-dependent insulinotropic peptide
GLP1 RA	glucagon-like peptide receptor agonist
HbA_{1c}	hemoglobin A_{1c}, glycated hemoglobin
HDLC	high-density lipoprotein cholesterol
IDegLira	insulin degludec + liraglutide (fixed combination)
iDPP4	inhibitors of dipeptidyl peptidase 4
IQR	interquartile ratio
INS/d	insulin/day (amount of insulin per 24 h)
LDLC	low-density lipoprotein cholesterol
LIRA	liraglutide
MDI	multiple daily insulin injections
MET	metformin
PG	plasma glucose
SD	standard deviation
SEMA	semaglutide
SGLT2	sodium-glucose transporter 2
SMPG	self-monitoring of plasma glucose
T2D	type 2 diabetes
TAG	triacylglycerols
U-glucose	presence of glucose in urine
U-protein	presence of protein in urine
URL	upper reference limit

Author details

Rudolf Chlup[1,2,3*], Hana Zálešáková[3], Jiřina Gottwaldová[3], Michal Trefil[3], Jana Zapletalová[4], Richard Kaňa[3], Lada Hanáčková[3], Milena Bretšnajdrová[1], Přemysl Falt[1] and Zdenka Polzerová[3]

1 Department of Medicine II, Gastroenterology and Geriatrics, Teaching Hospital Olomouc, Czech Republic

2 Faculty of Medicine and Dentistry, Department of Physiology, Palacký University Olomouc, Czech Republic

3 Department of Diabetes Moravský Beroun, Institute of Specialized Treatments Paseka, Czech Republic

4 Faculty of Medicine and Dentistry, Department of Biophysics, Palacký University Olomouc, Czech Republic

*Address all correspondence to: rudolf.chlup@fnol.cz

References

[1] Chlup R, Kaňa R, Hanáčková L, Zálešáková H, Doubravová B. Pathophysiologic approach to type 2 diabetes management: One centre experience 1980–2020. Available from: https://www.researchgate.net/publication/349698872_Pathophysiologic_Approach_to_Type_2_Diabetes_Management_One_Centre_Experience_1980-2020

[2] Friedecký B, Kratochvíla J, Springer D, Prázný M, Pelikánová T, Zima T, et al. Diabetes mellitus – Laboratorní diagnostika a sledování stavu pacientů. Diabetes mellitus – Laboratory diagnostics and observation of patients' condition. Klinická biochemie a metabolismus. 2019;**27**(48): 32-47

[3] Hanas R, John G, On behalf of the International HbA1c Consensus Committee. 2010 consensus statement on the worldwide standardization of the hemoglobin A1C measurement. Diabetes Care. 2010;**33**:1903-1904

[4] Chlup R, Doubravová B, Bartek J, Zapletalová J, Krystyník O, Procházka V. Effective assessment of diabetes control using personal glucometers (Contourlink, Bayer, Germany; Calla, Wellion, Austria; Linus, Agamatrix, USA). Disease Markers. 2013;**35**(6): 895-905

[5] Aronson R, Reznik Y, Conget I, et al, for the OpT2mise Study Group. Sustained efficacy of insulin pump therapy compared with multiple injections in type 2 diabetes: 12-month data from the OpT2mise randomised trial. Diabetes, Obesity and Metabolism. 2016;**18**(5):500–507

[6] Chlup R, Runzis S, Castaneda J, Lee S, Nguyen X, Cohen O. Complex assessment of metabolic effectiveness of insulin pump therapy in patients with type 2 diabetes beyond HbA1c reduction. Diabetes Technology and Therapeutics. 2018;**20**(2):153-159

[7] Šoupal J, Petruželková L, Grunberger G, et al. Glycemic outcomes in adults with T1D are impacted more by continuous glucose monitoring than by insulin delivery method: 3 years of follow-up from the COMISAIR study. Diabetes Care. 2020;**43**:37-43

[8] Chlup R, Zapletalová J, Zálešáková H, Kochtová J, Kaňa R. Vliv léčby inzulinem Fiasp na glykemii, HbA1c a tělesnou hmotnost u osob s diabetem 1. A 2. Typu: Studie z reálné praxe. (Benefits of insulin Fiasp for persons with diabetes type 1 and diabetes type 2. Czech.). Diabetes a Obezita. 2019;**19**(38):90-97

[9] Heise T, Hövelmann U, Brøndsted L, et al. Faster-acting insulin aspart: Earlier onset of appearance and greater early pharmacokinetic and pharmacodynamic effects than insulin aspart. Diabetes, Obesity & Metabolism. 2015;**17**(7): 682-688. DOI: 10.1111/dom.12468

[10] Bowering K, Case C, Harvey J, et al. Faster aspart versus insulin aspart as part of a basal-bolus regimen in inadequately controlled type 2 diabetes: Onset 2 trial. Diabetes Care. 2017;**40**(7):951-957. DOI: 10.2337/dc16–1770

[11] Rodbard H, Tripathy D, Vidrio Velazquez M, et al. Adding fast–acting insulin aspart to basal insulin significantly improved glycaemic control in patients with type 2 diabetes: A randomised, 18-week, open-label, phase 3 trial (onset 3). Diabetes, Obesity & Metabolism. 2017;**19**(10):1389-1396. DOI: 10.1111/dom.12955

[12] Olšovský J. Klinické zkušenosti s inzulínem faster aspart – Fiasp. (Clinical experience with faster insulin aspart – FIASP Czech.). Kazuistiky v diabetologii (Case Reports in Diabetology). 2018; **16**(2):25-26

[13] Chlup R, Zálešáková H, Zapletalová J, Ramík Z, Goldstein T, Benyaminov D. Ersatz der langfristigen kontinuierlichen subkutanen Insulininfusion (CSII) bei Typ 2 Diabetikern durch insulin Degludec und Liraglutide (IDegLira) einmal täglich hat meistens eine verbesserte Stofwechsellage zur Folge. (Replacement of the CSII in persons with T2D by IDegLira once daily mostly results in improved metabolic control. German.). Diabetologie und Stoffwechsel. 2021; **16**(1):14. (Abstract)

[14] Chlup R, Zapletalová J, Cheng TH, Ramik Z, Slezáková M, Zálešáková H. Effects of incretins in people with type 2 diabetes on CSII. Diabetes. 2017;(Suppl. 1):A623 2387-PUB. (Abstract)

[15] Chlup R, Zálešáková H, Zapletalová J, Šálková V, Gottwaldová J. Semaglutide: Dosiserhöhung auf 1 mg/ Woche hat breitere metabolische Auswirkungen zur Folge. (Semaglutide: Increasing the dose to 1 mg/week results in improved balance. German.). Diabetologie und Stoffwechsel. 2022; **17**(1):26. (Abstract)

[16] Davies MJ, Aroda VR, Collins BS, et al. A consensus report by the American Diabetes Association (ADA) and the European Association for the Study of diabetes (EASD). Diabetologia. 2022;**2022**(65):1925-1966. DOI: 10.1007/s00125-022-05787-2

[17] Lasserson DS, Glasziou P, Perera R, Holman RR, Farmer AJ. Optimal insulin regimens in type 2 diabetees mellitus: Systematic review and meta-analyses. Diabetologica. 2009;**52**:1990-2000. DOI: 10.1007/s00125-009-1468-7

[18] Kumar, Jha P, Shukla H, Makwana A, Kakkad A. Pharmacotherapy of type 2 diabetes mellitus [Internet]. In: Type 2 Diabetes in 2024 – From Early Suspicion to Effective Management. London, UK: IntechOpen; 2023. DOI: 10.5772/intechopen.1002309

[19] Bahn KL. Management of Type 2 diabetes mellitus [Internet]. In: Type 2 Diabetes in 2024 – From Early Suspicion to Effective Management. London, UK: IntechOpen; 2023. DOI: 10.5772/intechopen.1002478

[20] Nováková N, Nezval M, Molnárová V. Pathophysiology-oriented treatment of type 2 diabetes: 10 Case reports [Internet]. In: Type 2 Diabetes in 2024 – From Early Suspicion to Effective Management. London, UK: IntechOpen; 2023. DOI: 10.5772/intechopen.1002857

[21] Nauck MA, Müller TD. Incretin hormones and type 2 diabetes. Diabetologia. 2023;**66**:1780–1795. DOI: 10.1007/s00125-023-05956-x

[22] Tschöp M, Nogueiras R, Ahrén B. Gut hormone-based pharmacology: Novel formulations and future possibilities for metabolic disease therapy. Diabetologia. 2023;**66**:1796–1808. DOI: 10.1007/s00125-023-05929-0

[23] Drucker DJ, Holst JJ. The expanding incretin universe: From basic biology to clinical translation. Diabetologia. Oct 2023;**66**(10):1765-1779. DOI: 10.1007/s00125-023-05906-7. Epub 2023 Mar 28. PMID: 36976349

[24] Mathieu C, Ahmadzai I. Incretins beyond type 2 diabetes. Diabetologia. Oct 2023;**66**(10):1809-1819. DOI:

10.1007/s00125-023-05980-x. Epub 2023 Aug 8. PMID: 37552238

[25] Solini A, Tricò D, Del Prato S. Incretins and cardiovascular disease: To the heart of type 2 diabetes? Diabetologia. Oct 2023;**66**(10):1820-1831. DOI: 10.1007/s00125-023-05973-w. Epub 2023 Aug 5. PMID: 37542009; PMCID: PMC10473999

[26] Goldney J, Sargeant JA, Davies MJ. Incretins and microvascular complications of diabetes: Neuropathy, nephropathy, retinopathy and microangiopathy. Diabetologia. Oct 2023;**66**(10):1832-1845. DOI: 10.1007/s00125-023-05988-3. Epub 2023 Aug 19. PMID: 37597048; PMCID: PMC10474214

[27] Andreasen CR, Andersen A, Vilsbøll T. The future of incretins in the treatment of obesity and non-alcoholic fatty liver disease. Diabetologia. Oct 2023;**66**(10):1846-1858. DOI: 10.1007/s00125-023-05966-9. Epub 2023 Jul 27. PMID: 37498367

[28] Karagiannis T, Bekiari E, Tsapas A. Socioeconomic aspects of incretin-based therapy. Diabetologia. 2023;**66**:1859–1868. DOI: 10.1007/s00125-023-05962-z

[29] Blüher M, Rosenstock J, Hoefler J, et al. Dose–response effects on HbA1c and bodyweight reduction of survodutide, a dual glucagon/GLP-1 receptor agonist, compared with placebo and open-label semaglutide in people with type 2 diabetes: A randomised clinical trial. Diabetologia. 2024;**67**:470–482. DOI: 10.1007/s00125-023-06053-9

[30] McMurray JJV, Solomon SD, Inzucchi SE, et al. Dapagliflozin in patients with heart failure and reduced ejection fraction. The New England Journal of Medicine. 2019;**381**(21):1995-2008. DOI: 10.1056/NEJMoa1911303

[31] Wiviott SD, Raz I, Bonaca MP, et al. Dapagliflozin and cardiovascular outcomes in type 2 diabetes. The New England Journal of Medicine. 2019;**380**: 347-357. DOI: 10.1056/NEJMoa1812389

[32] Heerspink HJL, Stefánsson BV, Correa-Rotter R, et al. Dapagliflozin in patients with chronic kidney disease. The New England Journal of Medicine. 2020;**383**:1436-1446. DOI: 10.1056/NEJMoa2024816

[33] Solomon SD, McMurray JJV, Claggett B, et al. Dapagliflozin in heart failure with mildly reduced or preserved ejection fraction. The New England Journal of Medicine. 2022;**387**(12): 1089-1098. DOI: 10.1056/NEJMoa2206286

[34] Vícha M, Skala T, Jelínek L, Pavlu L, Jarkovsky J, Dusek L, et al. Pharmacotherapy of diabetes mellitus in patients with heart failure – A nation-wide analysis of contemporary treatment. Biomedical Papers of the Medical Faculty of the University Palacký, Olomouc, Czechoslovakia. 2023;**167**(2):177-184

[35] Kohnert KD, Augstein P, Heinke P, Zander E, Peterson K, Freyse EJ, et al. Chronic hyperglycemia but not glucose variability determines HbA1c levels in well-controlled patients with type 2 diabetes. Diabetes Research and Clinical Practice. 2007;77:420-426

[36] El Sayed NA, Aleppo G, Aroda VR, Bannuru RR, Brown FM, Bruemmer D, et al. Glycemic targets: Standards of Care in Diabetes—2023. Diabetes Care. 2023; **46**(Supplement_1):S97-S110. DOI: 10.2337/dc23-S006

[37] Peterson K, Chlup R, Zapletalová J, Kohnert K, Kudlová P, Bartek J, et al. Influence of oral antidiabetic drugs on hyperglycemic response to foods in

persons with type 2 diabetes mellitus as assessed by continuous glucose monitoring system: A pilot study. Journal of Diabetes Science and Technology. 2010;**4**(4):983-992

[38] Poljaková I, Elšíková E, Chlup R, Kalabus S, Hasala O, Zapletalová J. Glucose sensing module – Is it time to integrate in into real-time perioperative monitoring? An observational pilot study with subcutaneous sensors. Biomedical Papers of the Medical Faculty of the University Palacký, Olomouc, Czechoslovakia. 2013;**157**(4):346-357

[39] Gajdova J, Karasek D, Goldmannova D, Krystynik O, Schovanek J, Vaverkova H, et al. Pulse wave analysis and diabetes mellitus. A systematic review. Biomedical Papers. 2017;**161**(3):223-233. DOI: 10.5507/bp.2017.028

[40] Kuss O, Opitz ME, Brandstetter LV, et al. How amenable is type 2 diabetes treatment for precision diabetology? A meta-regression of glycaemic control data from 174 randomised trials. Diabetologia. 2023;**2023**(66):1622-1632. DOI: 10.1007/s00125-023-05951-2

[41] Elfa Gustanar LA, Fajari NM. Screening and testing for prediabetes and type 2 diabetes in asymptomatic adults [Internet]. In: Type 2 Diabetes in 2024 – From Early Suspicion to Effective Management. London, UK: IntechOpen; 2023. DOI: 10.5772/intechopen.1002298

[42] Gudat U. Fuelling life and managing surplus: Revisiting type 2 diabetes [Internet]. In: Type 2 Diabetes in 2024 – From Early Suspicion to Effective Management. London, UK: IntechOpen; 2023. DOI: 10.5772/intechopen.1002613

[43] Kumwenda MJ. Dyslipoproteinaemia: Important concern in type 2 diabetes [Internet]. In: Type 2 Diabetes in 2024 – From Early Suspicion to Effective Management. London, UK: IntechOpen; 2023. DOI: 10.5772/intechopen.1002514

[44] Mitrea A, Mihaela Vladu I, Magdalena Rosu M, Clenciu D, Mota E, Mota M. Paradigm of insulin resistance, type 2 diabetes, obesity, fatty liver and atherosclerosis in metabolic syndrome [Internet]. In: Type 2 Diabetes in 2024 – From Early Suspicion to Effective Management. London, UK: IntechOpen; 2023. DOI: 10.5772/intechopen.1002510

[45] Zaid AM. Complementary and alternative medicine in type 2 diabetes [Internet]. In: Type 2 Diabetes in 2024 – From Early Suspicion to Effective Management. London, UK: IntechOpen; 2023. DOI: 10.5772/intechopen.1002422

[46] Grover-Páez F, Maya Gómez A, Hernández Suárez A, Martínez EA. From a glycocentric approach to prevention of multi-organ damage in type 2 diabetes [Internet]. In: Type 2 Diabetes in 2024 – From Early Suspicion to Effective Management. London, UK: IntechOpen; 2023. DOI: 10.5772/intechopen.1002363

[47] Gică N, Huluță I. Gestational diabetes mellitus [Internet]. In: Type 2 Diabetes in 2024 – From Early Suspicion to Effective Management. London, UK: IntechOpen; 2023. DOI: 10.5772/intechopen.1002793

[48] Weber P, Weberová D, Meluzinova H. Diabetes in old age - particularities and specifics [Internet]. In: Type 2 Diabetes in 2024 – From Early Suspicion to Effective Management. London, UK: IntechOpen; 2023. DOI: 10.5772/intechopen.1002479

[49] Waataja J, Ikramuddin S, Gal D, Billington C. Perspective chapter: Exploring the potential of Vagus nerve neuromodulation as a personalized and

enhanced therapeutic experience for type 2 diabetics [Internet]. In: Type 2 Diabetes in 2024 – From Early Suspicion to Effective Management. London, UK: IntechOpen; 2023. DOI: 10.5772/intechopen.1002713

[50] Dhanapalaratnam R, Issar T, Lee ATK, et al. Glucagon-like peptide-1 receptor agonists reverse nerve morphological abnormalities in diabetic peripheral neuropathy. Diabetologia. 2024;**67**:561–566. DOI: 10.1007/s00125-023-06072-6

[51] da Cruz RL, Araújo Cortines Laxe Renó A. The Angiosome concept and endovascular techniques for limb salvage [Internet]. In: Type 2 Diabetes in 2024 – From Early Suspicion to Effective Management. London, UK: IntechOpen; 2024. DOI: 10.5772/intechopen.1003988

[52] Molnárová V. Vliv semaglutidu na klinické a laboratorní ukazatele v léčbě diabetu 2. Typu. (Impact of semaglutide on clinical and laboratory parameters in treatment of T2D. Czech.). In: Supplementum of Students' Scientific Conference, Mai 2023 Faculty of Medicine and Dentistry. Czech Republic: Palacký University Olomouc; 2023. p. 98

[53] Chlup R, Zálešáková H, Nováková N, Molnárová V, Zapletalová J. Pathophysiologic approach in type 2 diabetes – Single center study 2015 – 2023. In: Slovakian Diabetes Society: Supplementum, 18th Annual Research Meeting 22nd March, 2024, Topolčianky, Slovakia. Publisher J+K, Nemšová, Slovakia; 2024. pp. 14-21 ISBN978-8089788-72-9

[54] World Health Organization. Global Report on Hypertension: The Race against a Silent Killer. Geneva: World Health Organization; 2023. Licence: CC BY-NC-SA 3.0 IGO, ISBN 978-92-4-008106-2 (electronic version), ISBN 978-92-4-008105-5 (print version)

[55] Jörgens V. Die Geschichte der Diabetes-forschung vom Opium zum Insulin. 1st ed. Mainz: Verlag Kirchheim +Co GmBH; 2022. p. 303

[56] Rothberg A, Lean M, Laferrère B. Remission of type 2 diabetes: Always more questions, but enough answers for action. Diabetologia. 2024;**67**(4):602-610. DOI: 10.1007/s00125-023-06069-1. Epub 2024 Jan 8. PMID: 38189935; PMCID: PMC10904507

[57] Fovenyi J. Eighty six years duration of type 1 diabetes mellitus. Journal of Clinical Diabetes. 2019;**3**:e104

[58] Fövényi J, Greschik I, Jermendy AL, Kocsis G. Clinical observations in patients with type 1 diabetes of over 50 years duration in one practice in Hungary. International Journal of Clinical Science and Medical Research. 2023;**3**(01):11-17. Available from: https://journalofmedical.org

[59] Korec R. Experimental and Spontaneous Diabetes Mellitus in the Rat and Mouse. Košice, ČSFR, Košice: Edition Center of University PJ Šafárik; 1991. pp. 1-246

[60] Bruns W, Fiedler H, Altman B, Lundershausen R, Menzel R, Worms F, et al. Insulintherapie Bei Typ 2 Diabetes Pathophysiologisch begründete Therapie Mit Insulin Unter Besonderer Berücksichtigung der Insulinresistenz Und Des Inkretineffektes. (Insulin Treatment in T2D Pathophysiology-Based Insulin Treatment with Particular Consideration of Insulin Resistance and Incretins. German.). 2nd ed. Bremen: UNIMED Verlag, AG; 2010

[61] Bruns W, GHW Preuße. Opus 99 ... und andere Fragmente aus der

Geschichte der deutsch-russischen Familie Bruns. Versuch einer literarischen Annäherung. [Opus 99 ... and other particles from the real past of a German-Russian family. Attempt of a prosaic construction. German.] 1st ed. Berlin: Trafo Verlagsgruppe Dr. Wolfgang Weist, trafo Literaturverlag Reihe Autobiographien Band; 2014. p. 47. ISBN 978-3-86465-034-5

[62] Berger M, Jörgens V, Mühlhauser I. Rationale for the use of insulin therapy alone as the pharmacological treatment of type 2 diabetes. Diabetes Care. 1999; **22**(Suppl. 3):C71-C75